AF335412

**EVELYN FRANK BURNS M.Ed., R.T.(R)**
Officer of Allied Health Programs
Houston Community College Systems
Houston, Texas

# Radiographic
# Imaging

. . . . . . . . . . .

## A Guide for Producing Quality Radiographs

**W.B. SAUNDERS COMPANY**
*A Division of Harcourt Brace & Company*
Philadelphia   London   Toronto   Montreal   Sydney   Tokyo

**W. B. SAUNDERS COMPANY**
*A Division of*
*Harcourt Brace & Company*

The Curtis Center
Independence Square West
Philadelphia, Pennsylvania 19106

**Library of Congress Cataloging-in-Publication Data**

Burns, Evelyn Frank.

Radiographic imaging: a guide for producing quality radiographs/
Evelyn Frank Burns.

p.    cm.

Includes index.

ISBN 0–7216–3246–7

1. Radiography, Medical—Image quality.    I. Title.
   [DNLM: 1. Quality Control.    2. Radiography—standards.
   3. Technology, Radiologic—standards.    WN 200 B967r]

RC78.B853 1992        616.07′572—dc20

DNLM/DLC                                    92–19465

Radiographic Imaging: A Guide for Producing Quality Radiographs                    ISBN 0–7216–3246–7



Last digit is the print number:    9    8    7    6    5    4    3

# Preface

The purpose of this book is to describe the principles for producing quality radiographs. Chapters 1 through 4 contain introductory material that is required for students to master the content of the chapters that follow. The introductory material in Chapters 1 through 4 is not intended to serve as a replacement for a good radiologic physics textbook.

Chapters 5 through 18 present a comprehensive discussion of the basic factors integral to the production and evaluation of radiographs.

This textbook is designed for use by beginning radiography students to cover the first year of study of factors that control the production of quality radiographs. It is also intended as a review guide for sophomore students as they prepare for the certification examination and as a reference for staff radiographers.

To support these concepts, students may use the *Laboratory Manual to Accompany Radiographic Imaging: A Guide for Producing Quality Radiographs* that has been written to accompany this textbook. The laboratory guide can be used to apply the theories learned in this textbook.

To enhance the student's ability to learn this material, each chapter begins with learning objectives and key words to be learned. Suggested questions for discussion are included as the material is presented. This is to keep students focused on the topic and identify the concepts to be learned. Using this approach, students can master the difficult concepts of contrast scale, contrast, density, definition, and visibility of detail and master the critique of radiographs.

# Acknowledgments

This book is a culmination of lecture notes and lesson plans developed during 20 years of teaching radiography students. I am very thankful to many radiologic technologists who have provided guidance and support for the preparation of this manuscript.

To my husband, Barry, I owe a great deal because he took on many additional duties in our home in order for me to have the time to complete this manuscript.

Individuals who spent many hours reading my notes and providing feedback as the manuscript was developed are Teresa Rice, Director of the Radiography Program at Houston Community College, Detna Kacher, faculty member at Houston Community College, and Lynn Arrington, Gulf Coast X-ray Co.

I thank Aubrey Bread, El Centro College in Dallas, Texas, Betty Palmer, Portland Community College, Portland, Oregon, and especially Charles Francis, Idaho State University, Pocatello, Idaho, for the many hours they spent reviewing this manuscript. Their critiques were extremely valuable. I am grateful for their willingness to support this project.

I thank my photographer, Mr. Glen Edwards, faculty member of the Houston Community College Photography Department, for his dedication and the numerous evening and weekend hours he spent preparing the photographs.

I thank the staff of Kelsey Seybold Clinic, P.A., in the Texas Medical Center for allowing me to take photographs in their radiology department. Special thanks to Ida Murray, Manager, Netta Kenner, Linda Womack, Bonnie Gardener, and Mr. Bob Millis from the nuclear medicine department.

I have been tremendously blessed by the support and encouragement of my Division Chairperson, Janet L. Schanutz, who is a former director of radiography programs. I also owe thanks to two very special personal friends: Stewart Bushong, Sc.D., and Milton Gray, M.D. They have always moved me to the next higher level of achievement.

To two personal friends, Robert (Bob) I. Phillips and Mary Lou Phillips, I give credit for giving me the confidence that I needed to begin to write this manuscript.

Preparing this manuscript has taught me two very important things: self-discipline and time management. A real supporter and counselor has been Lisa Biello, Editor-in-Chief for Health-Related Professions, W. B. Saunders Company. Her support, encouragement, and suggestions were always timely and on target.

During the last 20 years as an educator in a radiography program, I have received tremendous guidance from students. They are the best reviewers of educational materials. These wonderful people have guided me in developing ways to better understand contrast and density and the related theories. Their suggestions have been incorporated into this manuscript. To all of my former students, I thank you.

Finally, a very special group of people have provided me with spiritual and moral support—my Tuesday night home study group from St. John the Divine Episcopal Church in Houston. Their prayers and support have been the anchor to keep me on track, especially since I had to take a long break to have major surgery after I began writing this manuscript.

I encourage instructors to use the *Laboratory Manual to Accompany Radiographic Imaging* that has been written to supplement this book and that provides an opportunity for students to apply the concepts presented in this manuscript.

# Contents

**C H A P T E R   16**



**C H A P T E R   17**



**C H A P T E R   18**

# Overview of Radiographic Imaging Techniques

● ● ● ● ● ● ●

## CHAPTER OBJECTIVES

1. Describe radiographic imaging as an "art" and "science."
2. Explain the relationship between the terms *radiology, radiologic technologist,* and *radiologist.*
3. Describe the specialties included in the term *radiologic technology.*
4. Define or describe the following:

   radiology         radiograph
   radiologist       nuclear medicine technologist
   sonographer    radiation therapy technologist
   radiographer    radiologic technologist
   radiography

5. Describe the competencies and responsibilities a radiographer must possess to become a full member of the health care team.

## KEY WORDS AND TERMS

Radiography
"Art and science"
Radiology
Radiologist
Radiologic technologists
Radiographer
Radiograph
Nuclear medicine technologist

Radiation therapy technologist
Sonographer
Specialty
Specialist
American Registry of Radiologic Technologists
  (ARRT)
Competency

## RECOMMENDATIONS FOR GENERAL DISCUSSION QUESTIONS

1. Discuss the idea that radiography is both an art and a science.
2. Discuss the relationship between the radiographer and radiologist.
3. Name the specialty areas available to radiographers, and discuss accessibility to these areas.

## THE ART AND SCIENCE OF RADIOGRAPHY

Radiographic imaging can be described as an art and as a science. The term "art" refers to the production of something that is very well done. The American Heritage Dictionary* defines art as "a system of principles and methods employed in the performance of certain activities; a trade or craft that applies such a system of principles and methods." An artist is thought of as one who has special skills or one who practices an art or craft. The art of radiography implies there is need for specific skills in performance. As a science, radiography requires study and theoretical explanation of natural phenomena. Science implies knowledge, especially knowledge gained through experience.

RADIOGRAPHY REQUIRES SKILL IN PERFORMANCE. RADIOGRAPHY ALSO REQUIRES STUDY OF NATURAL PHENOMENA.

Radiography is an art and science acquired by study and practice in the use of x-rays to produce images. These images of the human body serve to assist physicians in the diagnosis of diseases and disorders. The art is in the use of x-ray equipment and accessories, such as film, cassettes, and protection devices, to produce images of the body. The art of radiography also includes the positioning of anatomic parts in such a way as to demonstrate specific features of the human anatomy. Inasmuch as radiography includes the use of x-rays, the "artist" (radiographer) must also be a "scientist." Science, in the practice of radiography, requires that a radiographer be able to understand the characteristics of x-radiation, how x-rays are produced, and how x-rays are used in producing images of the human body. With the skills of an artist and the knowledge of a scientist, radiographers produce radiographs providing maximum patient care and safety for the patient and technical personnel with the smallest amount of radiation dose to the patient.

## A REVIEW OF TERMINOLOGY

Entry into the profession of radiography introduces new terminology, such as the following: radiology, radiologist, radiologic technology, radiography, radiographer, and radiograph.

*Morris, William (ed): The American Heritage Dictionary of the English Language. Boston: Houghton Mifflin Co, 1976.

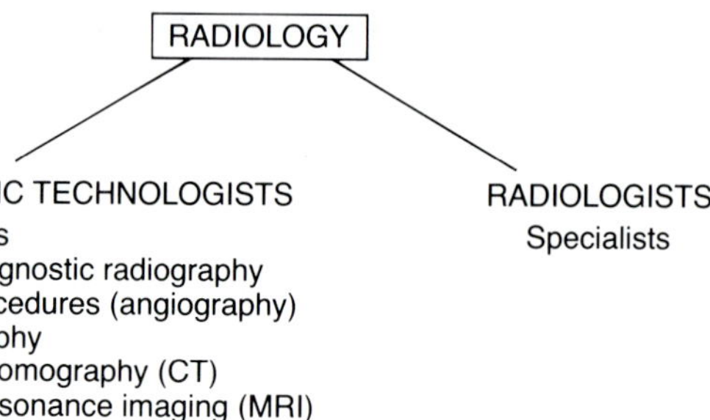


**FIGURE 1–1.** Professionals practicing within the specialty of radiology.

The full name of the medical specialty is *radiology*. Within the medical specialty of radiology, there are two groups of professionals: radiologists and radiologic technologists (Fig. 1–1).

*Radiologists* are medical doctors (M.D.'s) who are board certified to practice radiology. Many radiologists choose to specialize in such areas within radiology as neuroradiology, cardiovascular radiology, computed tomography, magnetic resonance imaging, nuclear medicine, radiation therapy, and sonography, some of which may require additional board certification.

RADIOLOGISTS ARE BOARD-CERTIFIED PHYSICIANS WHO PRACTICE RADIOLOGY.

*Radiologic technologists* are graduates of educational programs usually ranging in length from 2 to 4 years; they are certified to practice the profession by assisting physicians in the diagnosis of diseases (Fig. 1–2). Radiologic technologists are trained professionals who are skilled in the use of x-rays, radioactive materials, and/or ultrasonic sound waves to produce images of the human body for diagnosis and treatment of diseases.

RADIOLOGIC TECHNOLOGISTS ARE PROFESSIONALS WHO ARE SKILLED IN THE USE OF X-RAYS AND RADIATION FOR THE PRODUCTION OF IMAGES OF THE HUMAN BODY.

Radiologic technology has several specialties, which include radiography, nuclear medicine technology, radiation therapy technology, and diagnos-

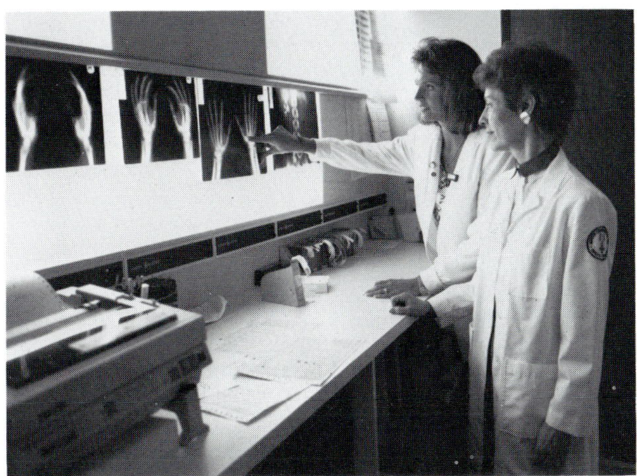

**FIGURE 1–2.** The radiologist and radiographer work very closely together. In this illustration, the radiographer is discussing the patient's medical history and the area of interest on the radiograph.

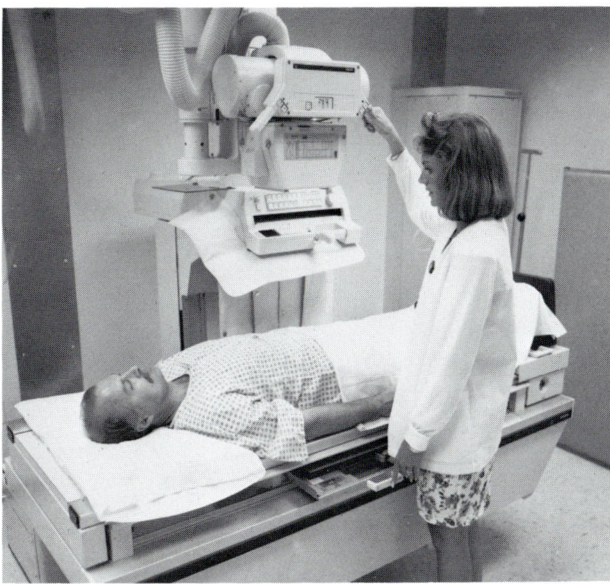

**FIGURE 1–3.** Radiographers must be able to work with patients to make them as comfortable as possible so as to produce high-quality radiographs that will allow adequate evaluation of the patient's condition.

tic sonography. *Radiographers* are trained professionals who are part of the health care team and are responsible for producing high-quality images using x-radiation (Fig. 1–3).

---

## RADIOGRAPHERS ARE PROFESSIONALS WHO ARE RESPONSIBLE FOR PRODUCING HIGH-QUALITY IMAGES USING X-RADIATION.

---

To become a radiographer, one must complete an educational program that requires a minimum of 2 years of training and supervised practice. Radiographers are certified by the successful completion of an examination given by the American Registry of Radiologic Technologists (ARRT). In the United States, radiographers must obtain a state license in order to be employed in more than 25 states. Radiographers work with patients to assist the radiologist in diagnosing diseases. Radiographers generally work under the direction of a radiologist.

The role of the radiographer is a key element in diagnosing disease. The radiographer's work must be of high quality, which comes as a result of a thorough understanding of how x-ray images are produced. The variety of roles available to a radiographer is great. The largest number of radiographers is needed for the general diagnostic area of imaging departments. Specialty areas available include cardiovascular angiography, mammography, computed tomography (CT), and magnetic resonance imaging (MRI).

*Nuclear medicine technologists* are technical personnel (often radiographers) trained in the use of radioactive drugs that are administered to patients for the purpose of evaluating and treating diseases (Fig. 1–4). Nuclear medicine technologists may obtain certification by ARRT or the Nuclear Medicine Technology Certification Board (NMTCB).

*Radiation therapy technologists* are also specially trained personnel (often radiographers) who assist physicians in the setup and dose calculation for patients who receive radiation for the treatment of cancer. Radiation therapists are certified by ARRT.

*Sonographers* are specially trained personnel who use high-frequency sound waves (ultrasonography) to produce images of the human body (Fig. 1–5). Certification is obtained through the Society of Diagnostic Medical Sonography.

Other common terms are "radiography" and "radiograph." *Radiography* is defined as the use of

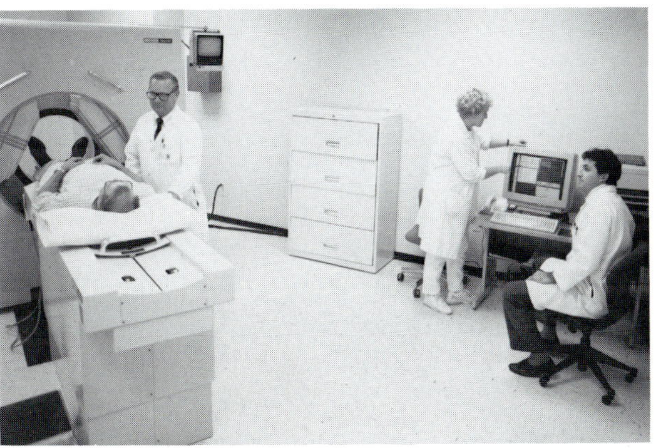

**FIGURE 1–4.** Nuclear medicine technologists working together as a team.

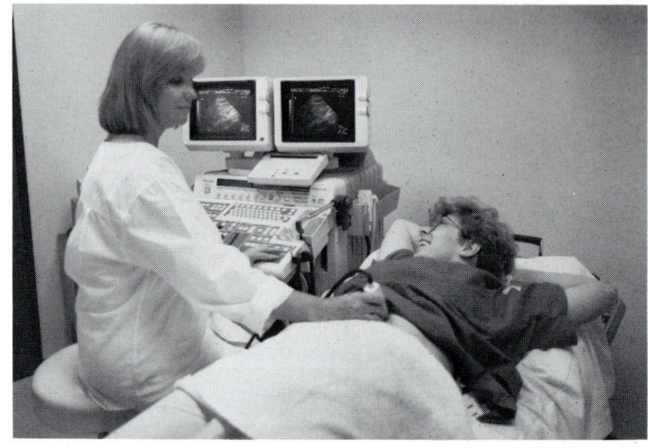

**FIGURE 1–5.** Sonographer performing an abdominal sonographic examination.

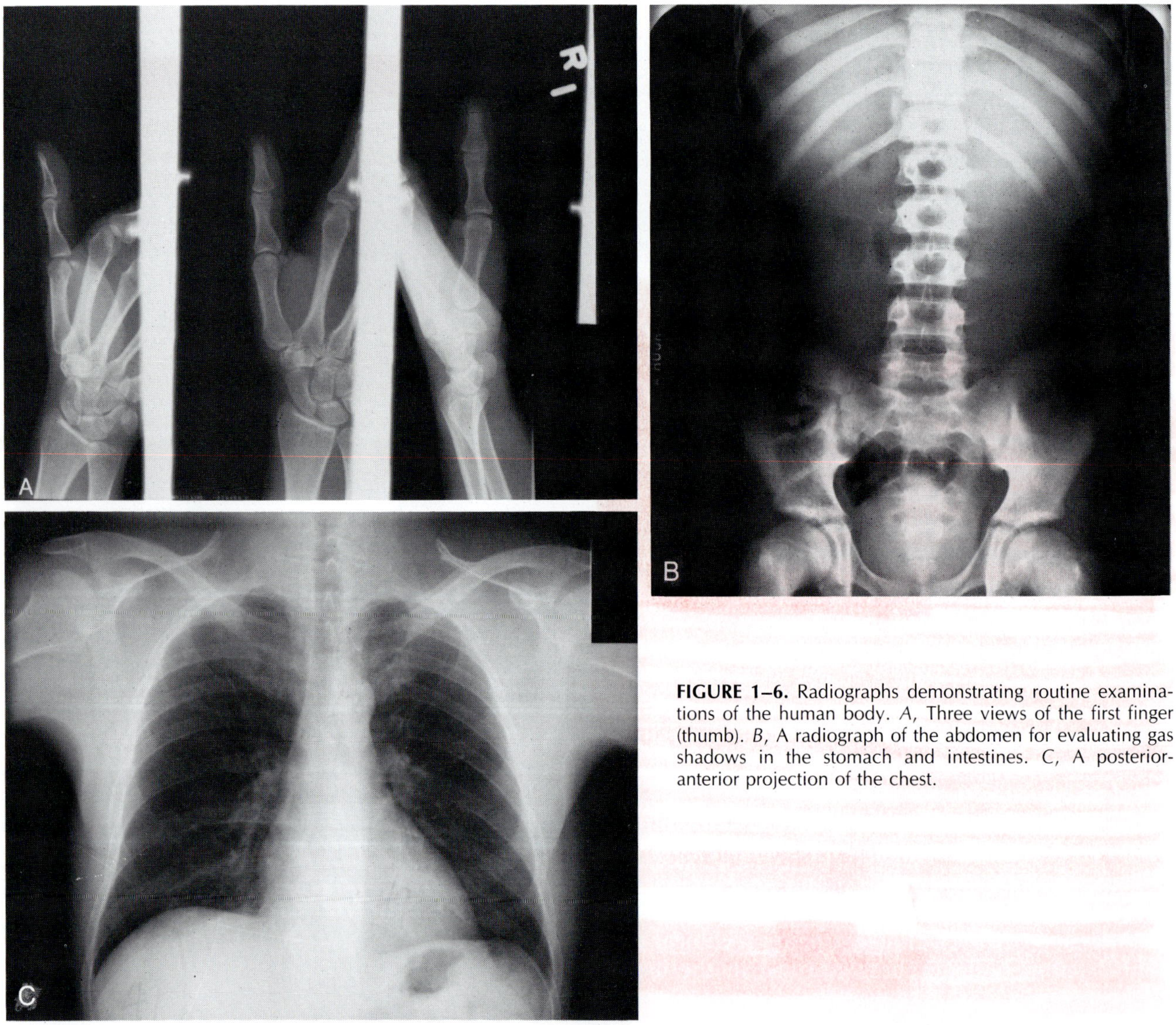

**FIGURE 1–6.** Radiographs demonstrating routine examinations of the human body. *A,* Three views of the first finger (thumb). *B,* A radiograph of the abdomen for evaluating gas shadows in the stomach and intestines. *C,* A posterior-anterior projection of the chest.

ionizing radiation to produce a recorded image on photosensitive material. The image produced using x-radiation is called a *radiograph*. A radiograph represents the image recorded on photosensitive material, which is usually called x-ray film. The production of high-quality radiographs and the evaluation of the finished product are the subject of this book.

---

RADIOGRAPHY IS THE USE OF IONIZING RADIATION TO PRODUCE A RECORDED IMAGE.

---

RADIOGRAPH IS THE IMAGE PRODUCED USING X-RADIATION.

---

## TECHNICAL COMPETENCIES

It is not within the scope of this text to identify all of the competencies of a radiographer. The text stresses those competencies needed for the making of a radiograph from the technical point of view.

Technical competencies include: operation of the control panel, selection of appropriate accessories, selection of correct factors to make exposures, use of the terminology in the evaluation of radiographs, measurement, and evaluation of results.

## CHARACTERISTICS OF A RADIOGRAPH

Figure 1–6A–C demonstrates three radiographs: hand, chest, and stomach. Review these three radiographs, which demonstrate examples of three different anatomic parts and required the use of different technical competencies to produce.

The responsibility of the radiographer must include a review of each radiograph for the following characteristics:

1. Exposure factors are adequate.
2. There has been adequate penetration of the part of interest.
3. Sufficient radiographic density and contrast are present.
4. Field size selection is appropriate.
5. Motion is eliminated during exposure.
6. The anatomic part is properly positioned.
7. Proper accessories have been selected.

The following chapters in this text expand each of these characteristics, with the exception of positioning of the anatomic part, which is not within the scope of this presentation of imaging techniques.

# The X-Ray Tube

## CHAPTER OBJECTIVES

1. Describe the design of the x-ray tube, including the glass envelope and housing.
2. Explain how the tube housing serves as a protective device.
3. Draw and label the glass envelope and the parts within the envelope.
4. Name the two electrodes found in the x-ray tube.
5. Explain the significance of the polarity of the anode and cathode.
6. Describe the design of the cathode filaments.
7. Explain the function of the large and small filaments.
8. Explain the purpose of the focusing cup.
9. Describe the process of thermionic emission.
10. Describe the structure and function of the anode.
11. Compare and contrast the rotating anode and the stationary anode.
12. Define and describe the line focus principle.
13. Differentiate between actual and effective focal spots.

## KEY WORDS AND TERMS

X-ray tube
Tube housing
Glass envelope
Electrode
Window
Cathode
Large filament
Small filament
Focusing cup
Tungsten
Thermionic emission
Electrons

Space charge
Anode
Rotating anode
Stationary anode
Stem
Rotor
Focal spot
Target area
Line-focus principle
Actual focal spot
Effective focal spot

## RECOMMENDATIONS FOR GENERAL DISCUSSION QUESTIONS

1. Name all of the parts of the x-ray tube, and explain how each part relates to the function of the tube.
2. Explain the origin of the "space charge."
3. Explain the difference between the actual focal spot and the effective focal spot, and discuss their importance in describing the line focus principle.

One of the primary responsibilities for a radiographer is to understand how x-rays are produced. A key factor in understanding this process is knowledge of the x-ray tube and its parts.

The x-ray tube and its housing are a vital component of the x-ray machine (Fig. 2–1).

## TUBE HOUSING

The x-ray tube is inside a heavy, lead-lined protective housing. When x-rays are produced by the x-ray tube, x-rays are emitted in all directions. The housing serves as a protective device, preventing x-rays from "leaking" to expose the patient and technical personnel unnecessarily.

WHEN X-RAYS ARE PRODUCED BY THE X-RAY TUBE, X-RAYS ARE EMITTED IN ALL DIRECTIONS.

There are several openings in the tube housing for electrical cable connections and the port or window, through which useful x-rays pass to expose the patient and produce radiographs (Fig. 2–2).

The housing also serves as a support for the x-ray tube and protects it from rough handling or other possible damage. Although the housing has been designed for protection from electrical hazards, it is imperative that technical personnel and the

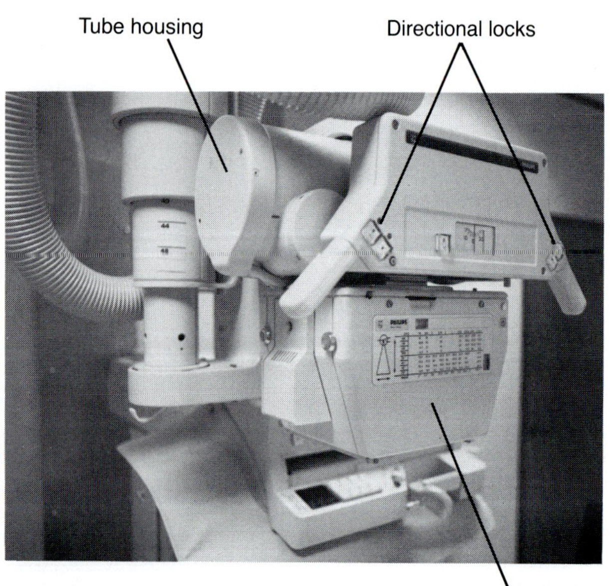


FIGURE 2–1. X-ray tube housing with collimator and directional locks attached.

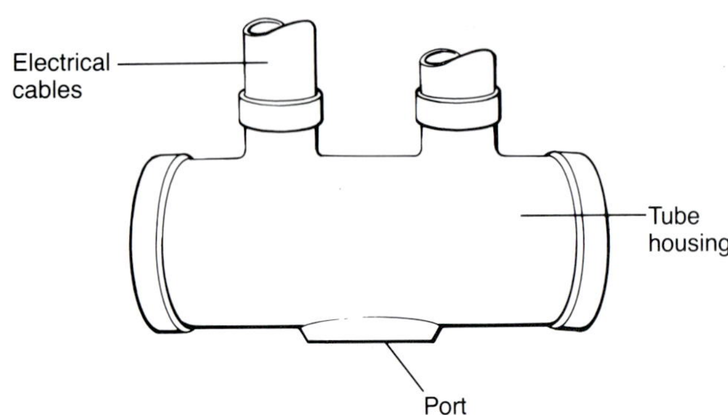


FIGURE 2–2. Lead-lined tube housing for the x-ray tube.

patient keep hands and fingers away from the housing during exposures.

THE TUBE HOUSING SERVES AS SUPPORT FOR THE X-RAY TUBE AND PROTECTS FROM ELECTRICAL HAZARDS.

## THE GLASS ENVELOPE

The x-ray tube is located inside the tube housing. The tube consists of two electrodes inside a glass envelope. The glass envelope is usually made of heat-resistant, chemical-resistant glass (Pyrex) to withstand the enormous amounts of heat produced during x-ray production. The x-ray tube is a special vacuum tube so that small quantities of gas, which might be found in a non-vacuum tube, will not interfere with the production of x-rays.

THE X-RAY TUBE IS LOCATED INSIDE THE TUBE HOUSING, ENCLOSED IN A GLASS ENVELOPE.

The window of the glass envelope is a small area in the Pyrex glass that is usually made thinner so that x-ray photons pass through the window with minimum absorption of the photons.

## THE X-RAY TUBE

The x-ray tube is sometimes referred to as a diode tube, meaning it has two electrodes (Fig. 2–3).

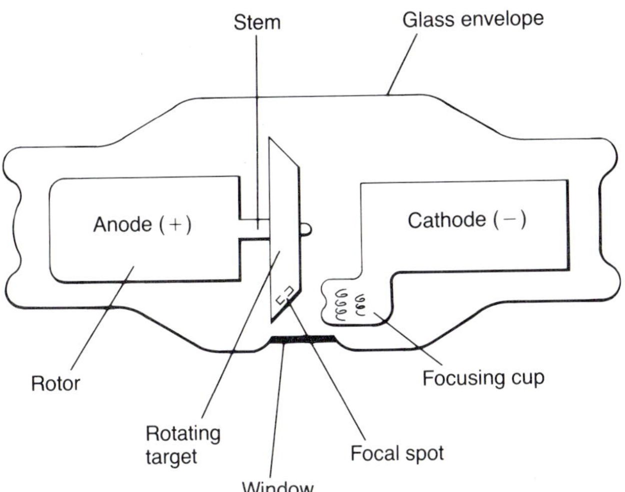



**FIGURE 2–3.** Glass enclosed x-ray tube located inside the tube housing.

The two electrodes found in the x-ray tube are the cathode and anode, which are designed to produce x-rays.

## The Cathode

The cathode is the negatively charged electrode; it consists of these major parts: the large filament, the small filament, and the filament cup, or focusing cup (Fig. 2–4).

### THE CATHODE IS THE NEGATIVELY CHARGED ELECTRODE.

The filament serves a vital function for the source of electrons in the production of x-rays. The filaments are small coils of tungsten wire about 1 to 2 cm in length. The longer coil of tungsten is the large filament, and the shorter coil is the small filament. Tungsten is the metal of choice because it is able to withstand the tremendous amounts of heat that are present at the time x-rays are produced and because it provides a good source of electrons, through the process known as thermionic emission.

### THE CATHODE FILAMENT IS THE SOURCE OF ELECTRONS FOR THE PRODUCTION OF X-RAYS.

Thermionic emission occurs when a current is applied to the filament, the coil of wire becomes very hot, and negatively charged electrons break away from the wire to form a "cloud." This cloud of electrons is called a "space charge" and becomes the source of electrons for producing x-rays (Fig. 2–5).

### THERMIONIC EMISSION OCCURS WHEN THE NEGATIVELY CHARGED ELECTRONS BREAK AWAY FROM THE HOT FILAMENT TO FORM A SPACE CHARGE.

The filament cup, or focusing cup, encases the two filaments. The cup serves to focus the space charge to a target area on the anode at the time of exposure. The cup is negatively charged, thus repelling the electrons. This causes the electrons to remain in a small cloud, as opposed to being more spread out. This results in the electrons being focused to a smaller area on the target.

Most diagnostic x-ray tubes have two cathode filaments: small and large focus (see Fig. 2–4). Each filament is encased in the filament cup and functions

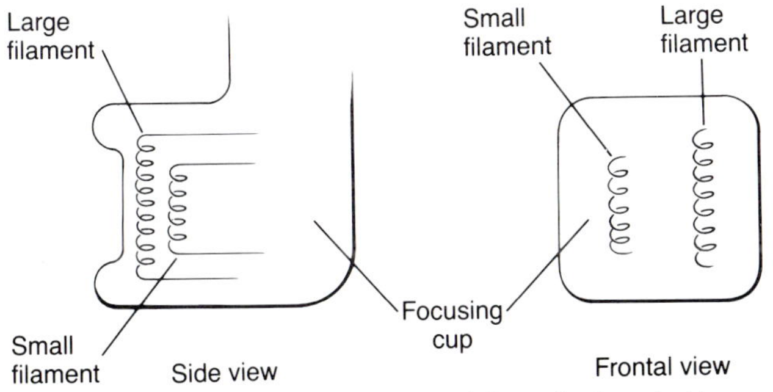

**FIGURE 2–4.** The focusing cup is part of the cathode. It holds two coils of tungsten wire. The longer coil serves as the large filament, and the short coil is the small filament.

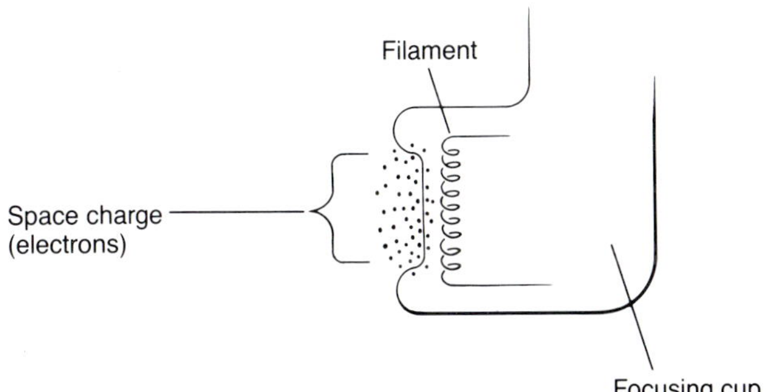



**FIGURE 2–5.** The filament shown with a space charge. The electrons in the space charge are a result of thermionic emission. The coil of wire is heated, and when it is very hot, electrons "boil off."

separately from the other. The smaller filament or small focus results in electrons being focused to a smaller target area on the anode, whereas the larger filament or larger focus directs the electrons to a larger target area on the anode.

## The Anode

The anode is the positive electrode in the x-ray tube. In diagnostic radiology, there are two types of anodes found in x-ray tubes: rotating and stationary. Most x-ray tubes, however, are of the rotating anode type.

---

THE ANODE IS THE POSITIVELY CHARGED ELECTRODE.

---

The rotating anode consists of three components: the rotating target, stem, and rotor (Fig. 2–6).

The rotor is a shaft-like structure made primarily of copper. It serves as the rotation device that turns the stem and target area. The stem, also usually made of copper, attaches the rotating target area to the rotor. Copper is the metal of choice because it is an excellent conductor and it facilitates the conduction of heat away from the target area.

The rotating target is a circular, disk-like structure with a slanted or beveled edge. It serves as the target for receiving electrons as they move from the cathode to the anode. The target area is made of tungsten to withstand the stress of heat when struck by the space charge.

---

THE ROTATING ANODE TARGET RECEIVES THE ELECTRONS AS THEY MOVE FROM THE CATHODE TO THE ANODE.

---

The part of the target that receives the electrons is angled, making the disk look as though it has a beveled edge. Angles on the edge of the rotating target may vary from 8 to 20°.

The target area of a rotating anode turns during the exposure. Most rotating anodes turn at approximately 3000 revolutions per minute (RPM), with higher speed rotating anodes turning at 10,000 RPM.

Rotation of the anode during the exposure results in the heat generated at that time being distributed over a larger area than would be true if the anode did not turn. During the exposure, the electrons in the space charge strike the target at a specific area

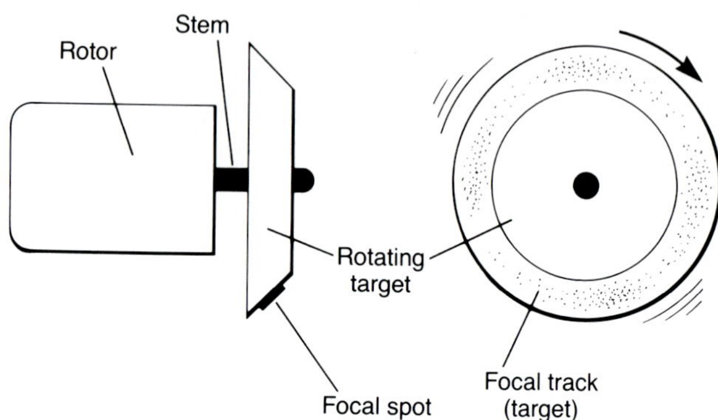


**FIGURE 2–6.** The anode with a rotating target.

or focal spot. The rotating target produces a focal track that runs the circumference of the rotating target disk. The focal spot is only the part (or area) on the focal track that is actually hit by the electrons during the exposure. The rotating target helps to dissipate heat. The copper stem and rotor serve as conductors to help conduct heat away from the rotating target.

### Line-Focus Principle

The design of an anode target area, which is angled, is known as the line-focus principle. As demonstrated in Figure 2–7, the angle on the anode target area makes the actual physical target area appear smaller. As the electrons strike the area of

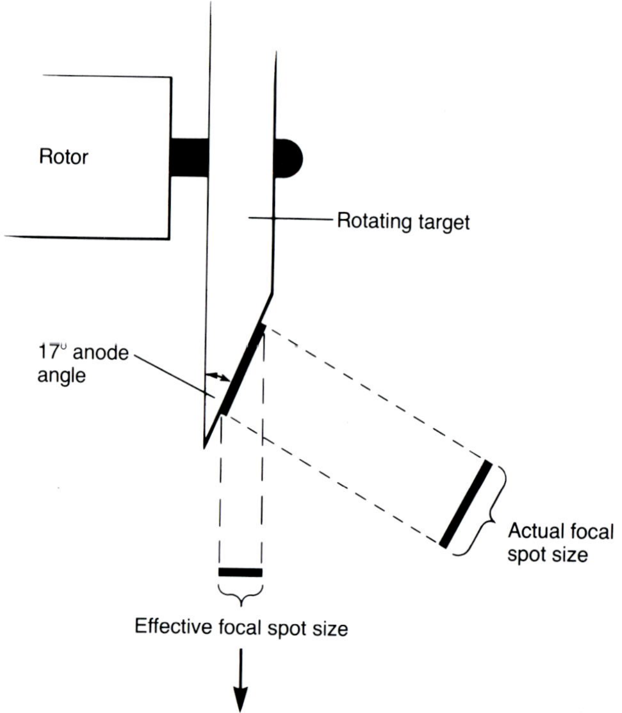


**FIGURE 2–7.** The line focus principle results in an effective focal spot size that is smaller than the actual focal spot size.

the target, x-rays are produced and projected toward the body part to be imaged. This results in a smaller "effective focal spot." The effective focal spot is evaluated as only that area directly below the target and over the window, or that area which is projected toward the patient.

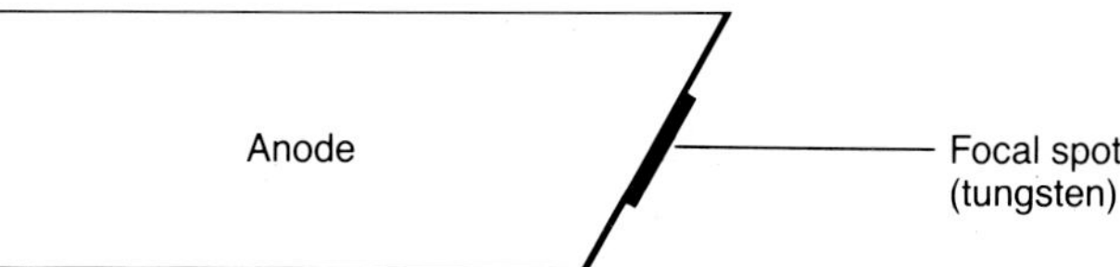



**FIGURE 2–8.** A stationary anode is a long shaft made with a tungsten target embedded in the slanted surface.

## THE LINE-FOCUS PRINCIPLE RESULTS IN A SMALLER EFFECTIVE FOCAL SPOT SIZE.

The line-focus principle results in the actual area of the target where electrons hit being larger than the effective target area projected toward the patient. The significance of this principle will become more evident in subsequent chapters relating to image formation. The line-focus principle also allows for an increase in the heat loading capacity at the focal spot as a result of the increased physical size, but at the same time, it allows for a relatively small effective or projected focal spot size.

## Stationary Anode

Stationary anode tubes are designed in a similar fashion to rotating anodes but without rotation capacity (Fig. 2–8).

Stationary anodes resemble a long shaft made of copper with a tungsten target area embedded on a slanted surface. The slanted surface establishes the line-focus principle, allowing for a larger area to be hit by electrons. This allows for a smaller effective focal spot to be projected toward the patient. These types of x-ray tubes are usually found in dental units and some mobile radiographic units as a result of the reduced output of these x-ray machines.

# Producing X-Rays

## CHAPTER OBJECTIVES

1. Describe the function of the following components on x-ray generator control panels:

   On/off switch      Rotor switch
   Exposure timer      Exposure switch
   Milliampere selector      Accessory controls
   mA/mAs meter      Kilovoltage meter
   Kilovoltage selector

2. Name and describe three types of exposure timers.
3. Discuss the advantages for using electronic timers with x-ray equipment.
4. Describe at least two methods used to evaluate x-ray generator timers.
5. Describe thermionic emission.
6. Describe the origin and function of the "space charge."
7. Explain tube current (mAs).
8. For given values of mA and time, calculate mAs.
9. Discuss kilovoltage and the "force" needed to produce x-rays.
10. Explain the importance of the kilovoltage meter.
11. Differentiate between the rotor and exposure controls.
12. Describe the purpose for accessory controls, and give examples.
13. Differentiate between phototimer and ionization chamber as used to terminate x-ray exposures.
14. Describe the sequential use of the components on the control panel to produce x-rays.
15. Describe advantages for using a daily "warm-up" procedure for the x-ray tube.

## KEY WORDS AND TERMS

Control panel
Kilovoltage (kV)
Milliampere (mA)
Milliampereseconds (mAs)
Exposure time (S)
On/off switch
mAs meter
kV meter
Rotor switch
Exposure switch
Accessory controls
Warm-up procedure
Preheat anode

Mechanical timer
Synchronous timer
Electronic timer
Back-up timer
Ionization chamber
Phototimer
Automated exposure time
Tube current
"Kilo"
"Space charge"
Thermionic emission
Calibrated oscilloscope
Spinning top test

# RECOMMENDATIONS FOR GENERAL DISCUSSION QUESTIONS

1. Discuss the role of the radiographer at the control panel in preparing for making x-ray exposures.
2. Explain how each component on the control panel contributes to the production of x-rays.
3. Describe how the spinning top test supports the concept of "pulsating x-radiation."
4. Explain the relationship of the rotor control switch to the exposure switch and describe the sequence for operating these controls.
5. Discuss the concept of mAs and how it is different from kilovoltage.
6. Compare and contrast phototimer and ionization chamber as devices used to terminate x-ray exposures.
7. Discuss the sequence of events for producing x-rays, and prepare a procedure guide that outlines these events.

As described in Chapter 1, two of the primary responsibilities for a radiographer are the operation of the control panel for producing x-rays and the selection of exposure factors. The knowledge and understanding of equipment operation is very important in producing high-quality radiographs and at the same time protecting the patient from injury or exposure to unnecessary radiation.

Because there are many manufacturers of radiographic equipment, different characteristics are produced in the equipment. However, almost all x-ray generators have certain controls in common—the controls used by the radiographer to make selections on the control panel. Many newer x-ray generator controls have sophisticated computerized panel displays requiring greater knowledge and understanding in the operation of the equipment. Radiographers must be able to make proper selections for kilovoltage, milliamperes, length of exposure time, and focal spot size.

> TO PRODUCE A RADIOGRAPH, RADIOGRAPHERS SELECT KILOVOLTAGE, MILLIAMPERES, TIMES, AND FOCAL SPOT SIZE.

The control panel is a part of radiographic equipment that becomes very familiar to radiographers (Fig. 3–1).

The controls are the on/off switch, exposure timer, milliampere selector, mA/mAs meter, kilovoltage selector, kV meter, rotor switch, exposure switch, accessory controls for use of the Potter-Bucky diaphragm, and, with some units, automated exposure controls (Fig. 3–2).

## THE ON/OFF SWITCH

The main purpose of the on/off switch is to connect the electrical power to the radiographic generator control device. This switch allows the generator unit to be ready for x-ray production. The on/off switch is usually part of the control console, as shown in Figure 3–2, and the radiographer must be familiar with its location.

> THE ON/OFF SWITCH CONNECTS THE ELECTRICAL POWER TO THE X-RAY GENERATOR.

On arrival in the morning, the radiographic generator should be turned "on" to warm up. This is done with the on/off switch. In addition, the radiographer must be familiar with the location of the main power box. In an emergency, the main power switch would be turned "off," along with the on/off switch.

## EXPOSURE TIMER

The exposure timer is located on the control panel console and serves as a means to determine the

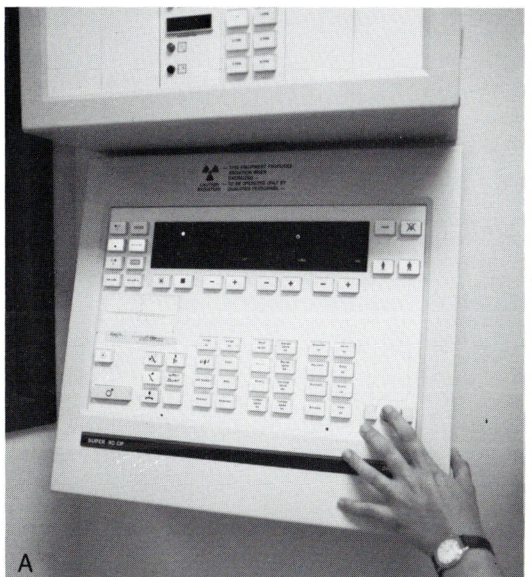
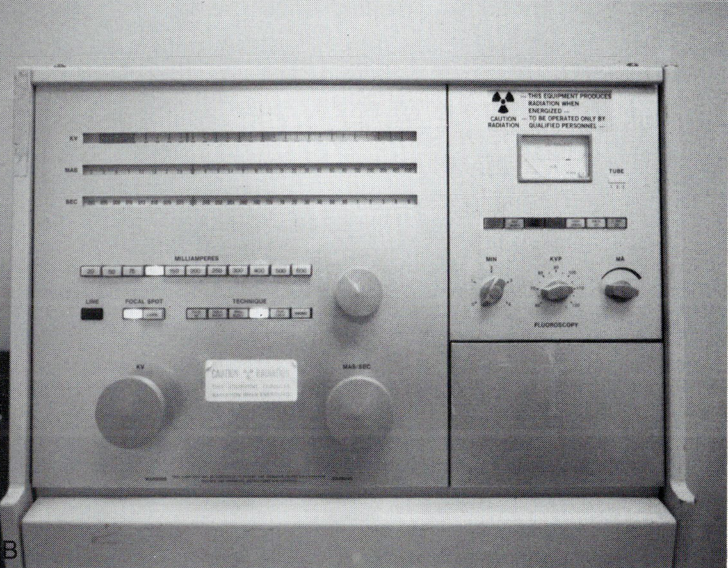

**FIGURE 3–1.** Control panels for the x-ray generator. *A,* A control panel with a variety of controls and options. The radiographer's hand is next to the rotor and exposure switch. *B,* A basic control panel for radiographic procedures, including fluoroscopy.

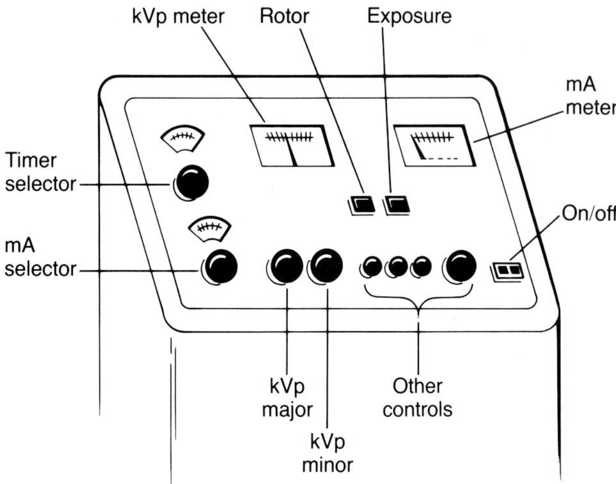

**FIGURE 3–2.** Illustration of a basic control panel console. The radiographer routinely uses these controls: kilovoltage peak (kVp), mA, timer, rotor, exposure switch.

length of time x-rays will be produced. A variety of timers may be found in radiographic equipment. Exposure timers are described as mechanical, synchronous, or electronic types.

> **EXPOSURE TIMERS DETERMINE THE LENGTH OF TIME THE X-RAYS WILL BE PRODUCED.**

Mechanical timers are simple types that work in a manner similar to a spring-set dial. The knob on the timer is turned to a specific mark, which winds a spring. When the exposure occurs, the spring unwinds in the time period set on the dial. Mechanical timers are limited to their shortest setting of 1/10 second. Shorter times are more advantageous for radiographic imaging of the body because of possible motion of the body part to be examined.

Synchronous timers are motor-driven devices that take advantage of the 60-Hertz alternating current used in the United States. Synchronous timers use exposure settings that are intervals related to 1/60 second (examples are 1/30 sec, 1/20 sec, and 1/10 sec.). The shortest time available is 1/120 second. Synchronous and mechanical timers are not considered to be as accurate as the electronic timer.

The electronic timer is the most common type found in radiographic equipment today. The electronic timer is more sophisticated, designed with complex circuitry, and considered to be the most accurate of exposure timers. The advantages of the electronic timer are exposure times of less than 1/120 second, reliability, and being less prone to malfunctions.

## Evaluation of Timers

The length of time that x-rays are produced is an important factor in controlling the amount of radiation to which the patient is exposed. It is very important for exposure timers to function properly. Evaluation of timers must be done periodically to guarantee accuracy.

Radiographers can perform a simple evaluation of exposure timers on single-phase, full-wave rectified radiographic units. The evaluation or test can be done using a device called the *spinning top* (Fig. 3–3).

The spinning top consists of two metal parts. The top part is a round disk approximately 3 inches in diameter. Near the edge of the top part is a small hole. The top part rests on a smaller circular pedestal and rotates freely.

To perform the test, place the spinning top on the upper surface of an x-ray cassette that contains unexposed x-ray film. Select exposure factors, beginning with 1/60, 1/30, or 1/10 second. The spinning top is set spinning by a flip of the fingers and the exposure is made while the top spins. The image produces dashes (or dots), and the number of dashes produced relates to the exposure time selected. The timer is considered to be operating within normal limits if two dashes are produced with 1/60 second,

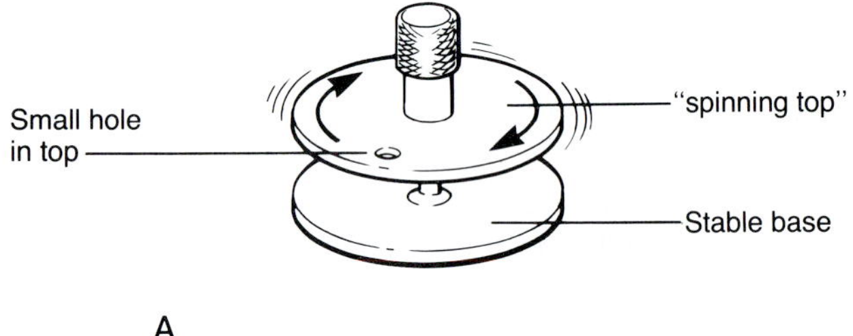


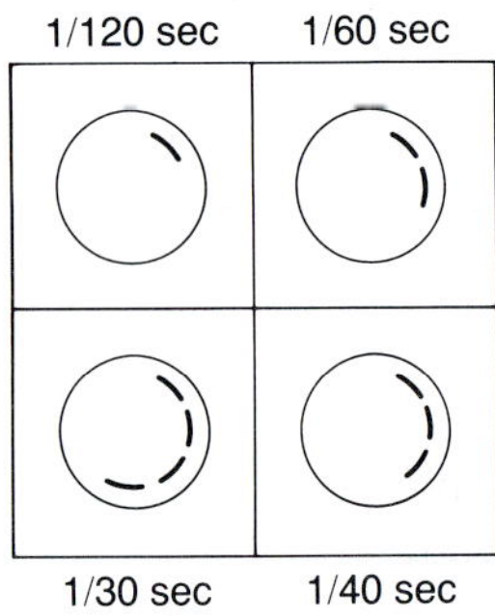


**FIGURE 3–3.** *A*, A spinning top to be used for testing exposure timers. *B*, Four exposures are illustrated. There is one dot for every 1/120-second exposure: 1/120 second produces one dot; 1/60 second produces two dots; 1/40 second produces three dots; 1/30 second produces four dots.

four dashes with 1/30 second, and 12 dashes with 1/10 second. With a single-phase, full-wave rectified x-ray unit, there will be one dot for every 1/120 second of exposure. To calculate, multiply the time of the exposure (in seconds) by 120 to determine the number of dots that should be present for a properly functioning machine.

Because other types of radiographic equipment such as three-phase and capacitor discharge units do not produce the same pulsed radiation, the spinning top would not be the instrument of choice to evaluate the exposure timer.

To test a three-phase x-ray generator, one uses a calibrated oscilloscope. The oscilloscope is connected in the circuit to the primary voltage going into the step-up transformer for measurement of actual time for the exposure. The actual time is compared with the selected time to evaluate the accuracy of the timer.

Single-phase and three-phase x-ray generator timers can be evaluated using a pulse-counter device. The counter is placed in the primary x-ray beam. The pulses are counted and recorded for evaluation.

## MILLIAMPERE SELECTOR

The milliampere selector controls the amount of electrical current flowing through the cathode filament. As current flows through the cathode filament, heat is produced, causing thermionic emission (see Fig. 2–5). Thermionic emission produces a "space charge" as a result of electrons breaking away from the hot cathode filament. During the exposure, the electrons in the space charge move from the cathode to the anode, constituting the tube current. (See Fig. 3–2 for an illustration of a milliampere selector.)

THE mA SELECTOR CONTROLS THE AMOUNT OF ELECTRICAL CURRENT FLOWING THROUGH THE CATHODE FILAMENT.

Radiographic units have a variety of mA selections, ranging anywhere from 25 to 2000 mA. In many general radiographic units, the selection of mA determines the focal spot size. In Figure 3–7, the "L" refers to selections using the large focal spot and "S" refers to selections using the small focal spot. Figure 3–2 demonstrates that 50 mA will use the small focal spot, thus causing current to flow through the small filament; 500 mA will use the

large focal spot, and current will flow through the large filament.

## MILLIAMPERE/MILLIAMPERESECOND METER

The milliampere (mA) or milliamperesecond (mAs) meter is also located on the control console. This meter will provide information for the radiographer by indicating the total amount of electrical current passing across the x-ray tube (from cathode to anode) at the time of the exposure (Fig. 3–4).

THE mAs METER INDICATES THE TOTAL AMOUNT OF ELECTRICAL CURRENT PASSING ACROSS THE X-RAY TUBE DURING THE EXPOSURE.

The total amount of tube current (mAs) passing across the tube is the product of the milliamperes and the exposure time.

Milliamperes × Time (seconds) = Milliampereseconds (mAs)
EXAMPLE: 50 mA × 1/10 sec = 5 mAs

Radiographers should make it a habit to look at this meter during the exposure in addition to keeping watch over the patient. The mA/mAs meter is located in the high-voltage section of the x-ray circuit and may indicate exposure problems relating to improper equipment calibration.

## KILOVOLTAGE SELECTOR

The kilovoltage (kV) selector permits increases or decreases in the voltage across the x-ray tube at the

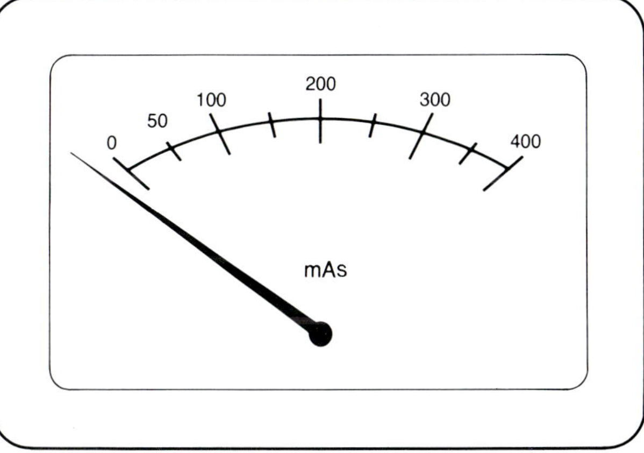


**FIGURE 3–4.** Milliamperesecond (mAs) meter. At the time of exposure, the meter dial moves to the right, indicating the mAs for the exposure.

time of the exposure. "Kilo" means one thousand and a kV setting of 80 means that 80 thousand volts will be produced to "push" the electrons across the x-ray tube at the time of the exposure. Selections made with the kV selector determine the specific tap on the autotransformer that is part of the x-ray circuit. The selection of kV determines the energy of the x-rays produced during the exposure. Figure 3–5 illustrates kV selector devices.

## KILOVOLTAGE CONTROLS THE AMOUNT OF VOLTAGE ACROSS THE TUBE DURING THE EXPOSURE.

Kilovoltage selections are made with two control selectors—labeled kV major and kV minor. The kV major selector permits changes of approximately 10 kilovolts with each turn, and the kV minor selector allows for changes of approximately 1 to 2 kilovolts per turn. The combination of these two kilovoltage control selectors permits easy selections for specific kilovoltage settings.

## KILOVOLTAGE METER

The kV meter is actually a prereading volt meter. The meter indicates the voltage selection. The position on the meter provides information for the

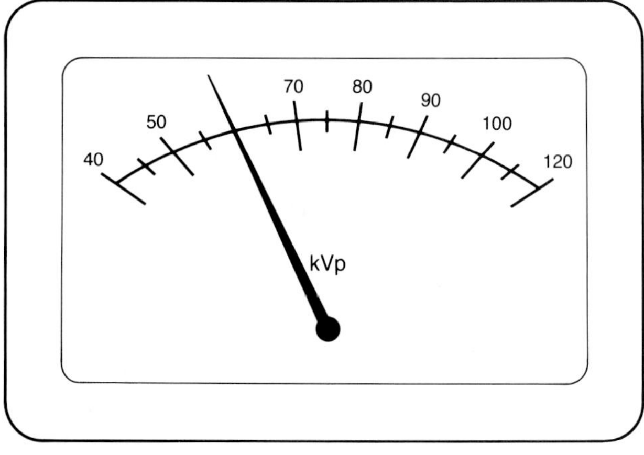
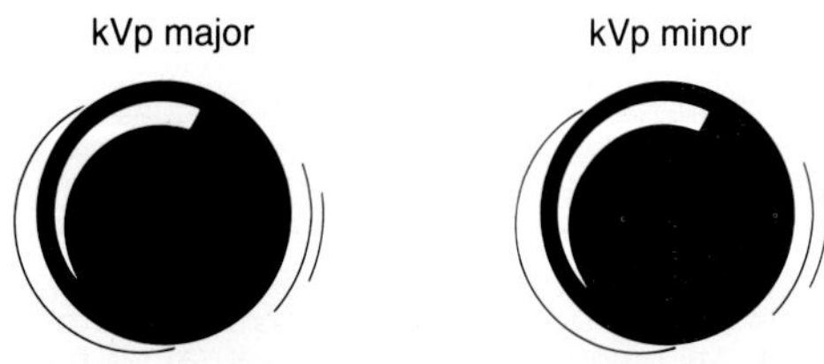

**FIGURE 3–5.** kVp selectors. The kVp major knob will move the dial about 10 points; the kVp minor knob will move the dial 1 to 2 points.

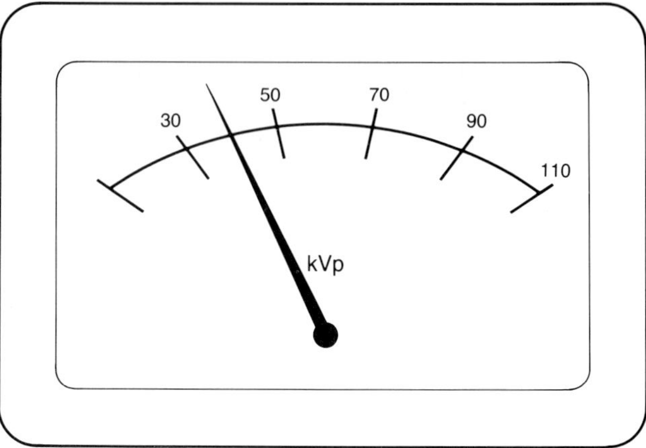

**FIGURE 3–6.** The kilovoltage meter gives a prereading for the amount of voltage across the x-ray tube during the exposure.

radiographer by indicating the amount of potential difference or voltage that will move across the x-ray tube at the time of exposure. "Prereading" means the meter gives a reading (at the time of selection) for the amount of voltage expected to pass across the x-ray tube as the exposure is made (Fig. 3–6).

## THE KILOVOLTAGE METER PROVIDES A READING OF THE PRESELECTED VOLTAGE.

## ROTOR AND EXPOSURE SWITCH

The rotor control switch may be a separate control or may be incorporated as part of the exposure switch. Operation of the rotor switch causes the anode to rotate, turning to its maximum speed before the exposure is made. Maximum rotation of the anode is accomplished in about 1 second. In addition, the activation of the rotor switch permits the full current to flow through the cathode filament (full current is determined by the mA selection made earlier), causing the filament to become very hot. If it were possible to look in the x-ray tube at this point, the filament would produce a bright red glow due to the amount of heat present as a result of the current flow.

## THE ROTOR CONTROL INITIATES THE ROTATION OF THE ANODE IN PREPARATION FOR THE EXPOSURE.

The rotor switch must remain engaged during the exposure. When the maximum RPM of the anode is reached, the exposure switch is activated.

The activation of the exposure switch results in the production of x-rays. X-rays are produced for a time period selected by the exposure timer. It is extremely important that the rotor and exposure switches be utilized only as needed for making an exposure. In order to permit a longer life for the x-ray tube, radiographers should not activate either switch unnecessarily or for long periods of time (Fig. 3–7).

## ACCESSORY CONTROLS

Accessory controls may include Potter-Bucky diaphragm utilization, vertical or horizontal devices, and line voltage adjustor. Before using these control switches, radiographers must obtain the appropriate instructions relating to how and when each switch is to be utilized.

## AUTOMATED EXPOSURE TIMERS

Automated exposure timers are designed to assist the radiographer in producing high-quality radiographs with adequate amounts of radiation exposing the film. This type of timer generally requires no direct operation by the radiographer.

Automated exposure timers are generally described as a phototimer or ionization chamber, based on the design. Both timers are designed to terminate the exposure automatically when the desired amount of exposure reaches the film.

---

AUTOMATED TIMERS ARE DESIGNED TO TERMINATE THE X-RAY EXPOSURE AUTOMATICALLY.

---

Phototimers are located behind the cassette holder. The phototiming device includes a highly sensitive photomultiplier tube. Facing the photomultiplier tube is a fluoroscopic screen that gives off light when exposed to x-radiation. The exposure will be terminated when the proper amount of fluorescent light from the screen reaches the photomultiplier tube. The phototimer is calibrated to a preset amount of exposure based on the type of procedure that is to be performed (Fig. 3–8B).

Another automated exposure device is an ionization chamber. The ionization chamber is radiolucent and therefore placed between the cassette holder

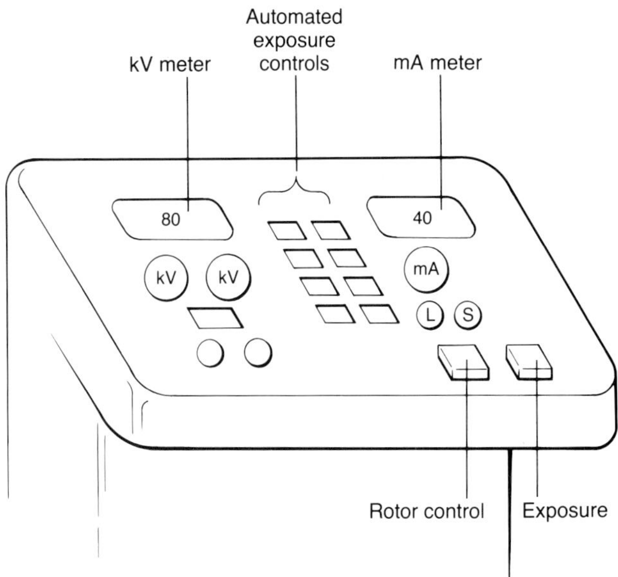


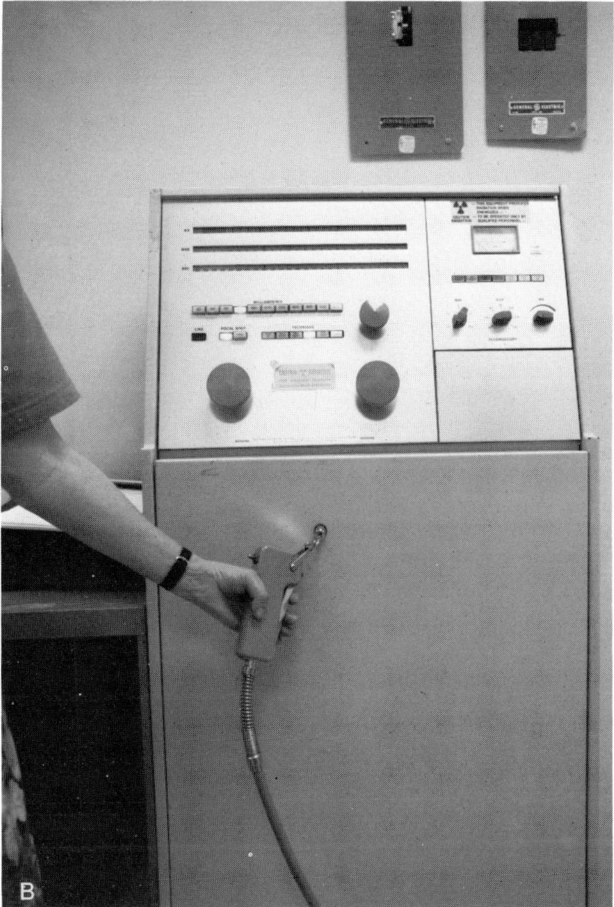


**FIGURE 3–7.** *A*, The rotor control is engaged to rotate the anode. When the maximum revolutions per minute (RPM) of the anode is reached, the exposure switch is activated. *B*, Radiographic control panel showing the rotor and exposure switch. The radiographer is holding the rotor/exposure control switch.

and the patient (Fig. 3–8A). The ionization chamber is more complex in design than the phototimer device but functions in a similar manner. As the

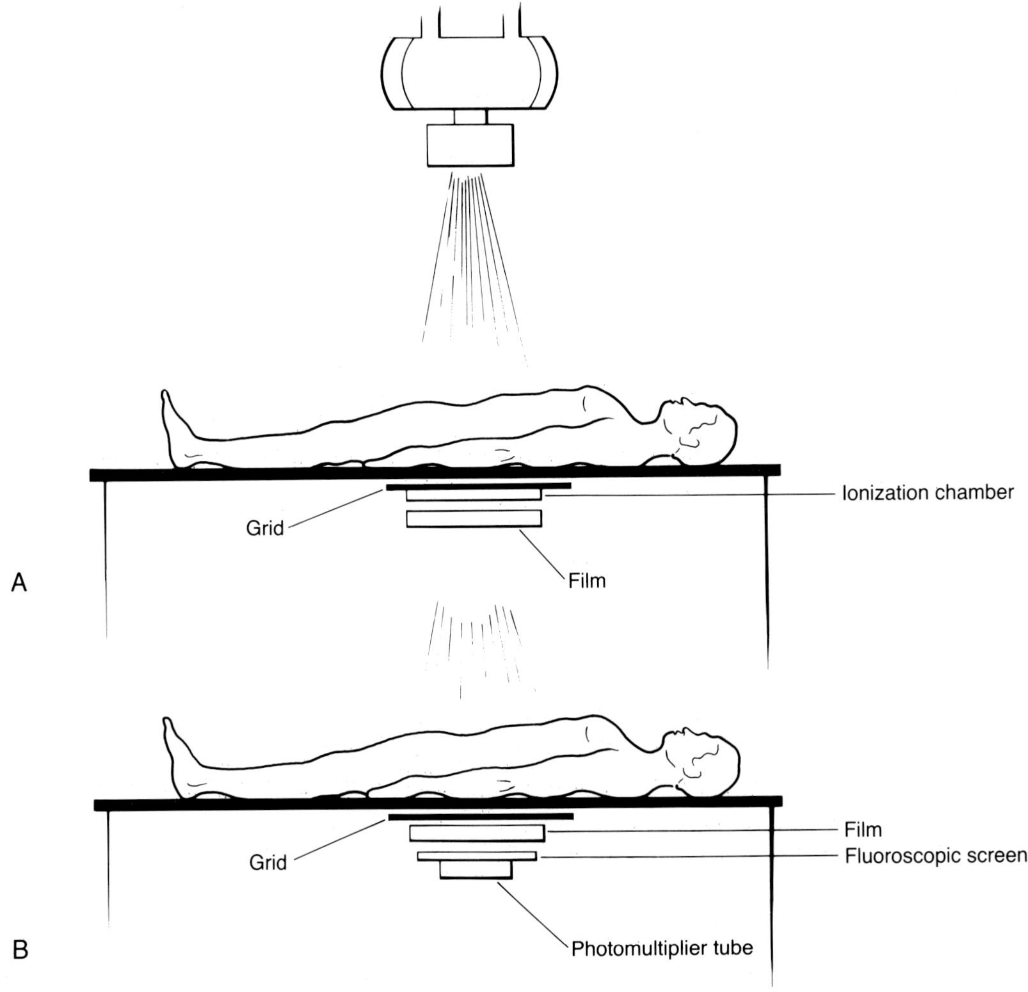

**FIGURE 3–8.** Automated exposure timer devices. *A*, The ionization chamber is located between the patient and film, underneath the grid. *B*, The phototiming device is located under the grid and the film. Both devices are designed to terminate the exposure when the proper amount of exposure to the film has been reached.

ionization chamber is exposed to x-radiation, it becomes charged or ionized. Once a preset charge is attained, the ionization chamber will initiate the termination of the exposure.

When exposures are made using automated exposure devices, the radiographer must usually select a back-up time using the manual exposure timer switch. A back-up timer selection serves as protection for the patient and the x-ray tube. For example, the back-up timer is set at 1 second, and if the automated exposure timer fails or is improperly set by the radiographer, the back-up timer will terminate the exposure after 1 second.

## SELECTION OF EXPOSURE FACTORS

In order to produce a high-quality radiograph, the radiographer must select proper factors on the control panel console. These factors include kilovoltage, milliamperes, exposure time, and table-top or Potter-Bucky diaphragm methods. Selection of factors is based on the type of procedure and the anatomic part to be radiographed (Fig. 3–9). Examples of exposure factors would be:

1. Hand—100 mA, 1/30 sec, 55 kV, table-top method
2. Abdomen—200 mA, 1/4 sec, 75 kV, Bucky method

## PRODUCTION OF X-RAYS

Before an exposure can be made, the radiographer has several duties to perform. The patient must be ready and placed in the proper position on the table. In addition, the equipment must be in place and appropriate factors selected on the control panel console.

The production of x-rays occurs as a result of a sequence of events. When ready, the radiographer begins the process by activating the rotor switch.

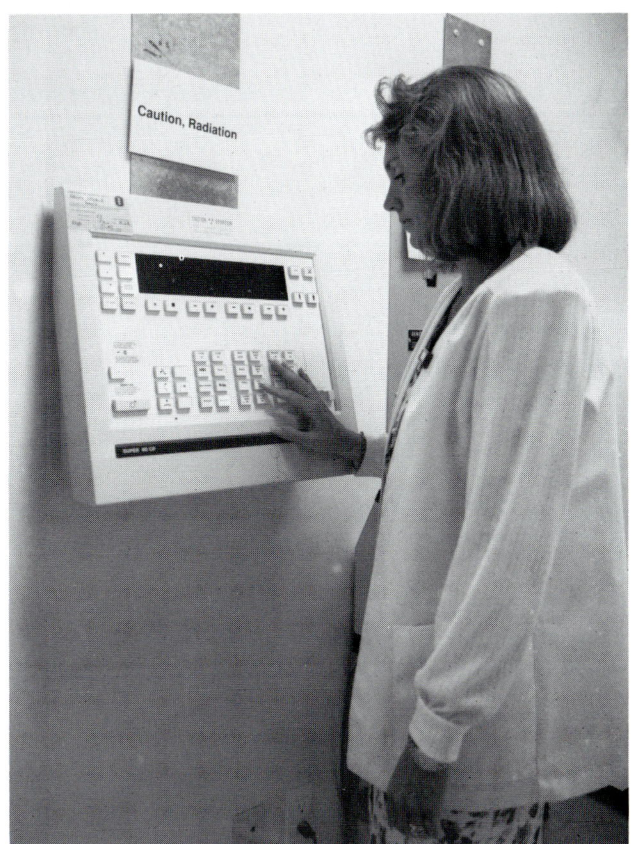

**FIGURE 3–9.** Radiographer selecting exposure factors in preparation for making the exposure.

The rotor switch allows the tube to be ready for producing x-rays. The anode apparatus begins rotating at the proper RPM and the cathode filament becomes very hot, resulting in thermionic emission. Thermionic emission creates the space charge as a result of the electrons that have broken away or "boiled off" from the *hot* tungsten filament.

With the filament hot, the space charge ready, and the anode rotating at peak revolutions per minute (RPM), the next step is to activate the exposure switch. As the exposure switch is activated, the current (electrons) will flow from the negative cathode to the positive anode target. The current flows as a result of the application of voltage or potential difference between the negative and positive electrodes. The electrons move with very high speed as a result of the thousands of volts (kilovoltage) applied to the electrodes during the exposure (Fig. 3–10).

CURRENT (ELECTRONS) FLOWS ACROSS THE TUBE AS A RESULT OF THE APPLICATION OF kV. AS THE ELECTRONS STRIKE THE TARGET, X-RAYS ARE PRODUCED.

As the electrons strike the anode target (focal spot), they hit with great force, resulting in several types of interactions with the target material. The dominant result is heat production. Another product is the production of x-rays. The conversion of electron kinetic energy to x-rays is only about 1% or less. The main result is heat.

When the exposure is terminated, x-rays are no longer present in the room or in the patient. Inasmuch as x-rays travel at the speed of light, when the switch is off or the exposure is terminated, x-rays are no longer present.

X-rays are produced traveling in all directions. The lead housing surrounding the x-ray tube will absorb most of the x-radiation. The useful rays are those x-rays that pass through the tube window and housing port to strike the patient and help produce a radiograph. The useful x-rays that leave the tube housing are called the primary x-ray beam, as illustrated in Figure 3–10.

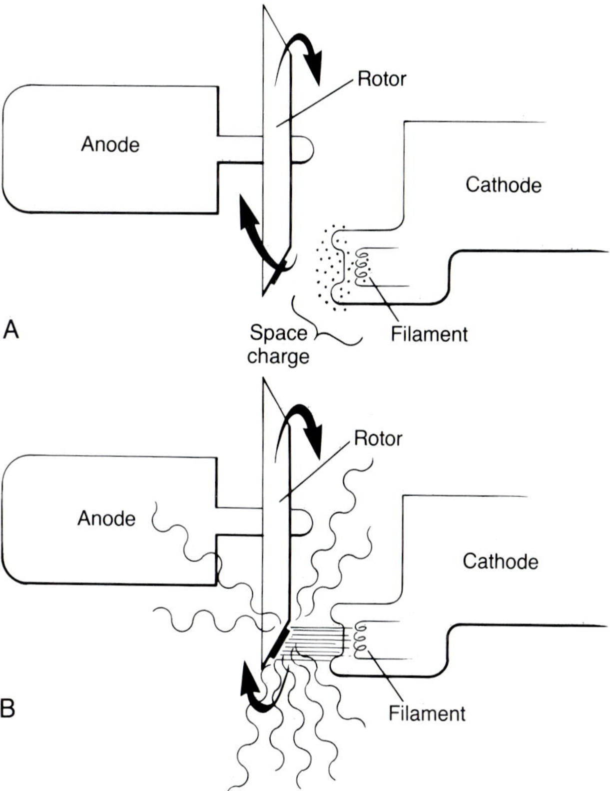


**FIGURE 3–10.** The production of x-rays. *A,* The anode is rotating at 3000 revolutions per minute (RPM); the cathode filament is hot, producing a space charge ready to produce x-rays. *B,* The exposure is taking place. The electrons in the space charge travel from the cathode to the anode and strike the target; x-rays are produced traveling in all directions.

## PROPER CARE OF RADIOGRAPHIC EQUIPMENT

The life of the x-ray tube will be directly related to the actions of the radiographer. X-ray equipment, especially the x-ray tube, is very expensive. The radiographer is accountable for using the equipment properly in order to prevent damage.

Before use, the x-ray tube should be preheated. The anode target area of the x-ray tube should be preheated routinely each morning before the x-ray tube is used. To accomplish this, exposures are made using a low milliampere setting (50 or 100 mA), a large focal spot, low to moderate kilovoltage (65 to 70 kV), and a long exposure time of 2 to 3 seconds. Three or four exposures are made, with several seconds between each exposure. If the tube is not used for several hours during the day and allowed to cool to about room temperature, the warm-up procedure should be used before regular exposures are made.

---

THE X-RAY TUBE SHOULD BE PREHEATED EACH MORNING BY FOLLOWING A ROUTINE WARM-UP PROCEDURE.

---

Another precaution mentioned earlier in this chapter relates to the rotor switch. Use only as needed; once adequate anode rotation is reached, the exposure should be made. Continual rotation of the anode with the presence of the "hot" filament will shorten the life of the anode and cathode filament.

It is important for radiographers to understand that their actions relating to the operation of the radiographic equipment will directly affect the life span of the x-ray tube.

# Characteristics of X-Radiation

●　●　●　●　●　●　●

## CHAPTER OBJECTIVES

1. Explain how the characteristics of x-rays contribute to assist physicians in the diagnosis of disease.
2. Discuss how x-rays are similar to light.
3. Describe three basic rules for radiographers to use for protection.
4. List six characteristics of x-rays.

## KEY WORDS AND TERMS

| | |
|---|---|
| Wilhelm Konrad Roentgen | Shielding |
| Wave-like motion | Photon |
| Speed of x-rays | Luminescence |
| Time | Protection |
| Distance | |

## RECOMMENDATIONS FOR GENERAL DISCUSSION QUESTIONS

1. Discuss the importance of x-rays in the diagnosis of disease.
2. Discuss each characteristic of x-rays and identify the advantages and disadvantages of each.
3. Discuss the importance and application of the three basic rules for radiation protection.

X-rays were discovered by Wilhelm Konrad Roentgen on November 8, 1895. The events leading to this phenomenal discovery took place in Dr. Roentgen's physics laboratory located at the University of Wurzburg, Germany. Very soon after his discovery, the medical world began to recognize how x-rays provided a new tool for the diagnosis of disorders, especially breaks in the skeleton. What is even more unusual—many of the characteristics described by Dr. Roentgen in his original work are the basics of x-ray physics students study today.

The use of x-rays became a vital tool in assisting physicians to diagnose diseases or disorders. X-rays are used to treat tumors. Research and tests have shown how x-rays cause biologic changes in tissue. This is an advantage in radiation therapy technology, where high energy x-ray photons are used to decrease the size of a tumor.

---

## THE USE OF X-RAYS IS VITAL IN ASSISTING PHYSICIANS WITH THE DIAGNOSIS OF DISEASES AND DISORDERS.

---

X-rays are a form of electromagnetic radiation, a spectrum of energies that includes visible light. X-rays have characteristics similar to visible light except that they travel with significantly shorter wavelength and with greater energy. X-ray photons travel in wave-like motion through air or matter with sufficient energy to penetrate the human body, including the dense bones of the skeleton. This characteristic is the true reason for the usefulness of x-rays in diagnosis of disease and abnormalities of the human body. X-rays travel at the speed of light and behave with some of the same characteristics as light; when the "switch" is turned off, the x-rays are no longer present.

---

## X-RAYS ARE A FORM OF ELECTROMAGNETIC RADIATION, A SPECTRUM OF ENERGIES INCLUDING VISIBLE LIGHT.

---

Because x-radiation can ionize tissue, causing biologic changes, the operators of radiographic equipment must follow appropriate guidelines in the use of the equipment to prevent unnecessary exposure. This is extremely important to protect the patient and other radiology personnel from the dangers associated with ionizing radiation.

Radiographers must observe the rules of time, distance, and shielding. Protection for the operator from ionizing radiation can be achieved by using the shortest possible exposure time, maintaining the longest distance possible from the source of x-rays, and always standing behind a shield containing the prescribed amount of lead or lead equivalent. Most radiographic departments are physically designed to accommodate these basic rules. Radiographers can, therefore, expect to be protected from exposure to ionizing radiation by adhering to these rules.

---

## RADIOGRAPHERS MUST OBSERVE THE RULES FOR TIME, DISTANCE, AND SHIELDING.

---

X-rays are often called "photons," which describe a "bundle of energy." The photons are known to be electrically neutral. This means that photons possess no electrical charge—they are neither positive nor negative. As x-rays travel through air, the air is ionized, causing the production of an electrical charge, thus making the photons detectable by specially designed detection devices called ionization chambers, which measure the ions produced.

X-rays photons are invisible to the human eye. Their presence can only be detected by the changes they produce in tissue or in the air. X-ray photons travel at the speed of light, or $3 \times 10^8$ m/sec.

Other characteristics of x-ray photons are important in understanding the use of x-rays for radiographic imaging of the body. Consider the following characteristics:

1. X-ray photons cannot be focused by a lens, as with photography.
2. X-ray photons travel in straight lines and diverge from the point of origin.
3. X-ray photons cannot be deflected by mirrors or other devices.
4. When x-ray photons strike certain substances, visible light is emitted. This is called luminescence.
5. X-ray photons will cause changes to occur in the sensitive emulsion of photographic film.
6. When x-radiation interacts with matter, secondary radiation and scatter radiation are produced.

Radiographic imaging can be accomplished only if the radiographer fully understands the nature and characteristics of x-rays. X-rays cause things to happen. When x-rays strike the substances found inside film holders (intensifying screen phosphors), the light produced plays an important role in exposing the sensitive film emulsion. The visible light enhances or intensifies the action of the x-rays.

When x-rays interact with matter, scatter radiation and secondary radiation are produced. When this happens, the object exposed to x-radiation becomes the source, producing scatter and secondary rays. The radiographer and other personnel must protect themselves from this radiation by the utilization of lead barriers such as leaded glass or lead-lined walls and doors. The control of secondary and scatter radiation will be the subject of subsequent chapters.

WHEN X-RAYS INTERACT WITH MATTER, SCATTER RADIATION IS PRODUCED; THE OBJECT BECOMES THE SOURCE BY PRODUCING SCATTER RADIATION.

## CHAPTER 5

# Imaging System: X-Ray Film, Film Holders, and Intensifying Screens

## CHAPTER OBJECTIVES

1. Name the basic components of x-ray film.
2. Describe the characteristics of the film base.
3. Describe the characteristics of the film emulsion.
4. Describe the significance of the silver halide crystal.
5. Define film speed or sensitivity.
6. Define film latitude.
7. Discuss the inherent film characteristics of speed, latitude, and contrast.
8. Differentiate between screen and direct exposure film.
9. Explain the parallax effect.
10. Differentiate between single- and double-emulsion x-ray film.
11. Define latent image.
12. Describe the process that creates the latent image.
13. List the guidelines for handling and storage of x-ray film.
14. Describe the construction and function of film holders (cassettes).
15. Explain why intensifying screens are important in imaging of the human body.
16. Define fluorescence and phosphorescence.
17. List the four basic components of intensifying screens.
18. Describe the purpose of base, reflective layer, phosphor layer, and protective coating.
19. Explain how rare earth screens differ from calcium tungstate.
20. Compare the conversion efficiency of calcium tungstate and rare earth screens.
21. Describe the advantages for using rare earth screens in radiographic imaging.
22. Identify the kilovoltage range that will produce the maximum efficiency with calcium tungstate and rare earth screens.
23. Define relative speed value.
24. Compare the advantages and disadvantages for speed values assigned to different types of screens.
25. Describe the test for evaluating film-screen contact.
26. Describe the care required for intensifying screens.
27. Explain "quantum mottle."
28. Explain the concept of light diffusion with screen phosphors.

# KEY WORDS AND TERMS

X-ray film
Intensifying screens
Film holder
Cassette
Film emulsion
Silver halide crystals
Film base
Polyester base
Sensitivity speck
Supercoat
Film speed
Imaging system
Film sensitivity
Film latitude
Film contrast
Screen film
Direct exposure film
Single-emulsion film
Blue-sensitive film

Green-sensitive film
Orthochromatic film
Parallax effect
Latent image
Backscatter
Screen base
Reflective layer
Phosphor layer
Screen protective coating
Screen unsharpness
Fluorescence
Phosphorescence
Calcium tungstate
Barium lead sulfate
Zinc sulfide
Rare earth phosphor
Yttrium
Conversion efficiency
Relative speed value

# RECOMMENDATIONS FOR GENERAL DISCUSSION QUESTIONS

1. Discuss the importance for using intensifying screens in radiography.
2. Describe how speed and conversion efficiency of screen phosphors become an important consideration in the selection of an imaging system.
3. Using examples of film screen combinations, compare speed, image resolution, contrast, and latitude.
4. Discuss the advantages and disadvantages for a medium-sized radiology department to change from calcium tungstate system to a 400-speed rare earth system.
5. Describe light diffusion with the use of intensifying screens and how it is influenced by thickness of the phosphor layer.

In an earlier chapter, x-ray photons were described as having the ability to affect the sensitive emulsion of photographic film. X-ray film is sensitive to a limited portion of the visible light spectrum, whereas photographic film responds to all colors of the visible light portion of the electromagnetic spectrum.

X-ray film is used in the recording of body images. When the very sensitive emulsion of x-ray film is exposed to light and x-radiation, chemical changes occur. After the x-ray film has been exposed and processed using chemicals that make the image visible, the film can be stored and kept as a permanent record (Fig. 5–1).

Because there are many manufacturers of x-ray film, numerous choices in film types are available. The type of x-ray film selected depends on many factors, such as body part, speed, film quality, etc.

## X-RAY FILM COMPOSITION

The type of x-ray film most commonly used is described as a product having a flexible and thin transparent base coated on both sides with sensitive emulsion. An adhesive layer is coated on the base before adding the emulsion to provide maximum contact with the important emulsion layer. A supercoat or protective coating is then used to protect the sensitive emulsion surface. The outer protective coating is essential for protection of the film surface at the time of use in a film holder (Fig. 5–2).

X-RAY FILM IS MADE OF A FLEXIBLE THIN TRANSPARENT BASE COATED ON BOTH SIDES WITH A SENSITIVE EMULSION.

### Base

The base is the foundation or support that allows the film to maintain shape and prevents unnecessary bending, which could cause artifacts. The base is usually thicker than the support structure used in the production of photographic film.

THE FILM BASE IS THE SUPPORT TO HOLD SHAPE, PREVENT BENDING, AND PROVIDE SUPPORT FOR THE EMULSION.

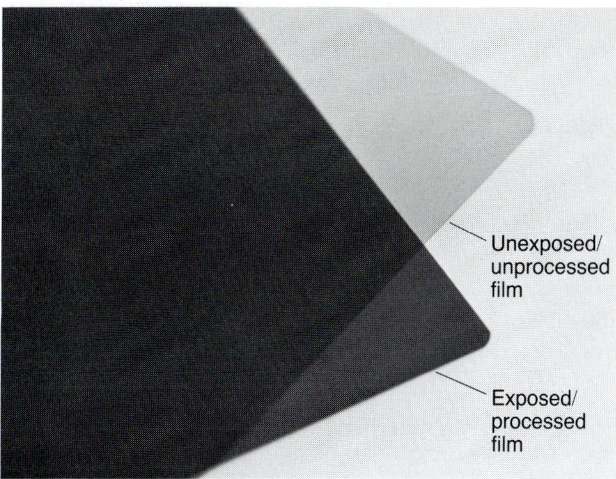

**FIGURE 5–1.** Photograph showing exposed and unexposed x-ray film. The darker film has been exposed and processed. The lighter film has not been exposed or processed, and the emulsion is present on both sides, producing opaqueness.

Certain characteristics are required for a good film base. The materials must be transparent or clear so as not to detract from the image. The base should also be flexible and sturdy to prevent damage in processing or handling of the film. The base contains a slight blue tint to provide a finished product that is pleasing to the eye.

The base is generally made of a strong polyester foundation. Polyester provides flexibility, transparency, and other characteristics listed above that are needed for an excellent film base. When the base is ready for finishing, an adhesive layer is coated on each side prior to the addition of the highly sensitive and complex emulsion.

### Emulsion

The emulsion is coated on both sides of the base and becomes the most important component of x-ray film. The emulsion is the ingredient that results in the sensitivity of x-ray film to light and x-ray photons.

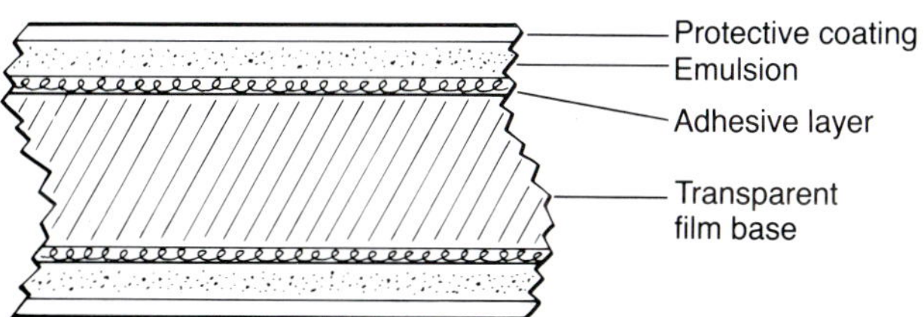

**FIGURE 5–2.** Cross-section of x-ray film. The transparent film base is coated on both sides with an adhesive layer, the sensitive emulsion and the outer protective coating.

THE FILM EMULSION IS THE LAYER WITH THE SENSITIVITY TO LIGHT AND X-RAYS.

X-ray film emulsion contains silver halide crystals suspended in a layer of gelatin. Gelatin is the ideal substance for suspending the halide crystals because it gives permanence to the emulsion. When placed in a solution, the gelatin will soften and swell so that processing chemicals can penetrate the emulsion. This becomes extremely important in processing the image so that it becomes visible and permanent. The gelatin does not dissolve in solution and will reharden after the invisible image becomes visible during the processing cycle.

Suspended in the gelatin is the active ingredient, silver halide crystals. The silver halide crystals are sand-like granules distributed throughout the emulsion. The crystals are tiny microscopic structures made primarily of silver bromide and silver iodide. The chemical mixture involved in the production of these tiny crystals does not produce a perfect structure. The imperfections found in the crystal structure are called "sensitivity specks" (Fig. 5–3).

THE SILVER HALIDE CRYSTALS ARE TINY GRANULAR STRUCTURES FOUND IN THE EMULSION; THE IMPERFECTIONS IN THEIR STRUCTURE ARE CALLED SENSITIVITY SPECKS.

The manufacturing procedure employed in producing the emulsion will determine how sensitive or how fast the x-ray film will respond to light and/or x-rays. The concentration of the halide crystals and the character of the sensitivity specks become basic elements in classifying film speed. After it is mixed, the film emulsion is coated on both sides as the next layer on top of the adhesive coating.

The final layer in film preparation is the "supercoat"—the protective layer that prevents abrasions, scratches, and other types of damage to the emulsion surface.

## CHARACTERISTICS OF X-RAY FILM

X-ray film possesses several characteristics important in the evaluation of the finished product. These characteristics are important because they represent the tools used to compare one film type with another. Film characteristics are identified as speed, latitude, and contrast.

X-RAY FILM CHARACTERISTICS ARE SPEED, LATITUDE, AND CONTRAST.

### Speed

The inherent characteristic of speed defines the sensitivity of the emulsion and its ability to respond to light or x-rays. In Figure 5–4, film A and film B are exposed under identical conditions using exposure factors 5 mAs, 60 kVp and the same screen type. Film A is a moderate or average speed film while film B is more sensitive and considered to be a fast film. The result shows film A to have adequate exposure for visualization of the image and film B to be overexposed (too dark, or too black).

SPEED IS THE FILM'S ABILITY TO RESPOND TO LIGHT OR X-RAYS.

Film speed is given an arbitrary value, with the average or medium being 100. Fast films may have a value of 200, 300, etc., with a slow value being 50 or less. Before the 1970s and 1980s, the old way to match x-ray film with an appropriate intensifying screen was to match speed values. A film with a 100 speed value would have been matched with a screen that had a speed value of 100. If the speed values were mixed, each product (film or screen) maintained its original speed value.

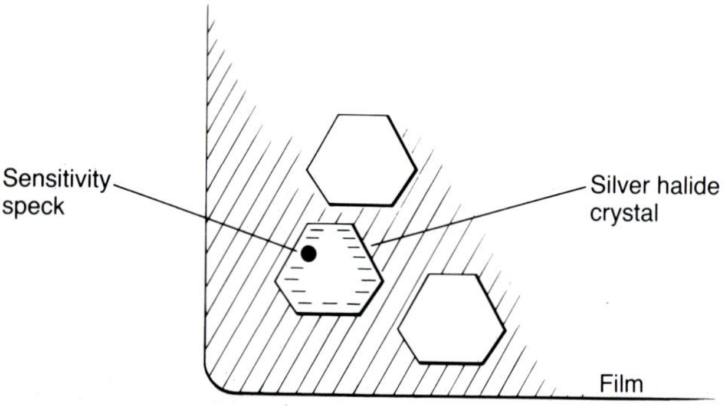


**FIGURE 5–3.** The sensitivity speck is an imperfection found in the halide crystal structure.

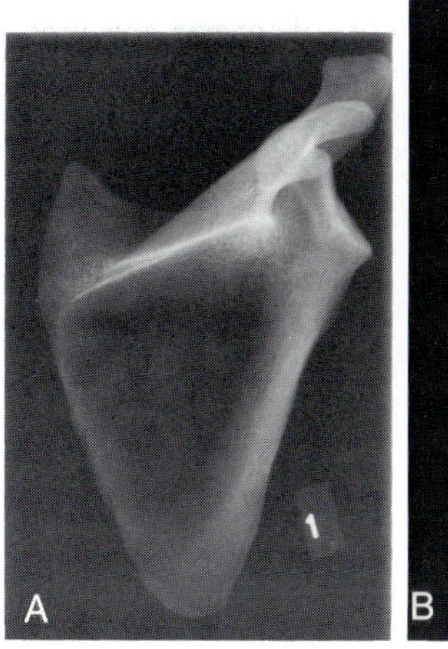
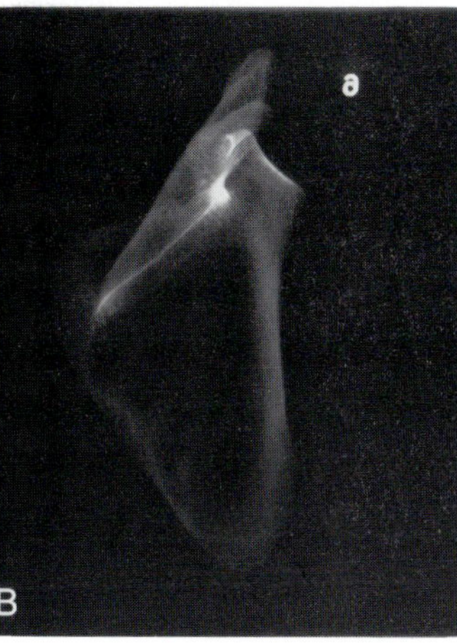



**FIGURE 5–4.** X-ray film that has greater sensitivity will have increased blackening on the film. *A* and *B,* Film A and Film B were exposed using the same exposure factors. Film A was produced using an average or medium speed film. Film B has increased blackening on the film as a result of increased sensitivity of the emulsion. Film B would be considered a faster film than Film A.

The most modern method to evaluate speed is with a "system" value, which includes the combined value of a particular film and screen type needed. Together the system may be described as a 100 or 300 system.

IMAGING SYSTEM IS THE COMBINATION OF A PARTICULAR FILM AND SCREEN TYPE.

## Latitude

Film latitude is the inherent characteristics in the film emulsion that allow a moderate or acceptable range of densities (different degrees of blackening) to be recorded. Exposure latitude and film latitude are similar by definition, but exposure latitude primarily refers to the ability of the exposure factors selected to record an image with the appropriate range of densities on the film.

FILM LATITUDE IS THE FILM'S ABILITY TO RECORD AN ACCEPTABLE RANGE OF DENSITIES.

## Contrast

The inherent characteristic of film contrast describes the ability of the emulsion to record minute differences in densities across the film. Contrast is the difference in blackening present and is necessary to visualize small details on the film.

FILM CONTRAST IS THE INHERENT ABILITY TO RECORD MINUTE DIFFERENCES IN DENSITY ACROSS THE FILM.

## TYPES OF X-RAY FILM

There are probably as many types of x-ray film as there are manufacturers. For simplicity, the types of film available for diagnostic radiology are categorized as screen film, direct exposure, single emulsion, duplication, subtraction, mammography, and dental. Screen-type film is generally the choice for diagnostic radiology. The other types are used mostly with special radiographic procedures.

For many years x-ray film was produced to be sensitive to blue-violet light, and we referred to it as blue-sensitive film. Panchromatic is the term used to describe film that is used in photography because it is sensitive to all colors in the visible light spectrum. Orthochromatic describes the type of film used in radiology, which is known as green-sensitive. It is sensitive to almost all colors in the spectrum except red. In diagnostic radiology, radiographers use primarily blue-sensitive and orthochromatic film.

Each film type has inherent characteristics relating to contrast, speed, and latitude. Although smaller silver halide crystals in the emulsion produce greater contrast, the speed is generally slower. The larger the halide crystals, the lower the contrast but the faster the speed. Frequently, these characteristics can be offset by the type of screen selected to combine with the film.

### Screen-type Film

Screen film requires fluorescent light (from the intensifying screens) in addition to x-rays to provide optimal efficiency. This means that it should be used with intensifying screens, which are found inside film holders.

SCREEN FILM IS MADE TO USE WITH INTENSIFYING SCREENS, BECAUSE OF THE FILM'S SENSITIVITY TO LIGHT.

Screen-type film has emulsion coated on both sides, which makes it more efficient. A negative

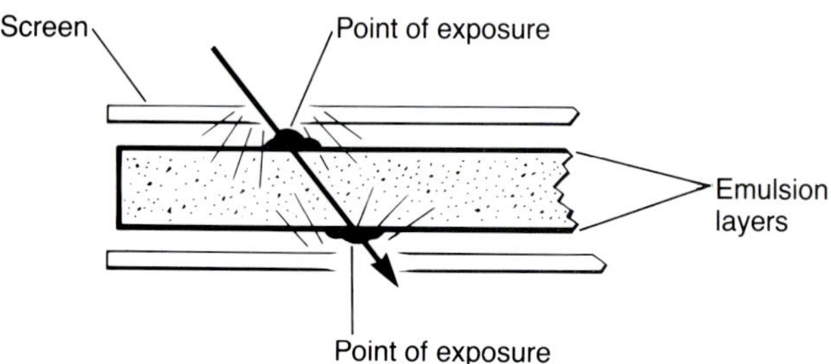


**FIGURE 5–5.** The parallax effect occurs when a light or x-ray photon strikes the film emulsion at an angle on one side, passes through the film, and exposes the emulsion at a point that does not correspond to the point where it originally exposed the emulsion. The parallax effect will result in a reduction in film quality.

aspect of the double emulsion is the "parallax" effect. In the parallax effect, light enters from an angle affecting a particular spot on the emulsion and travels through to the other side striking a spot not exactly corresponding to the opposite layer. The parallax effect results in decreased resolution on the image (Fig. 5–5).

### Direct Exposure Film

Direct exposure film is designed specifically for use without intensifying screens. This type of film is made for use with the direct exposure of x-ray photons. Direct exposure film has thicker emulsion, with an increased amount of silver halide crystals.

---

DIRECT EXPOSURE FILM IS DESIGNED FOR USE WITHOUT THE NEED FOR INTENSIFYING SCREENS.

---

Because direct exposure film is also less sensitive to light, the fluorescent light from the intensifying screens would be less effective. An increase in exposure factors is required with the use of this type of film compared with the use of screen film and intensifying screens. It is recommended for use with low-risk or low-exposure examinations of thin body parts.

### Single-Emulsion Film

Single-emulsion film has emulsion coated on one side of the base only. This factor alone would prevent the parallax effect. In producing single-emulsion film, manufacturers may add light-absorbing dyes to the emulsion. The absorbing dyes prevent

photons, particularly light, from striking adjacent silver halide crystals. Some manufacturers use an antihalation backing. This prevents the "bouncing around" of light photons as the screens fluoresce, thus improving the sharpness of the image.

Although single-emulsion film provides a radiograph with improved definition, it requires increased exposure to attain sufficient density on the film.

Subtraction and duplication films are also single-emulsion film types. *Subtraction* film is a single-emulsion film designed to produce a copy that is the exact opposite of the original radiograph. *Duplication* film is a type of single-emulsion film that responds differently to light photons. A decrease in density will occur if the film is exposed to light or the exposure is increased to lighten the film. Duplication film can be used to produce an exact copy of a radiograph.

## THE LATENT IMAGE

How is the image produced? The production of the latent image (also called the photographic effect) is the invisible change that takes place in the film emulsion when it is exposed to x-ray photons and fluorescent light from intensifying screens.

---

THE LATENT IMAGE IS PRODUCED BY THE INVISIBLE CHANGES THAT TAKE PLACE WHEN THE FILM EMULSION IS EXPOSED BY X-RAYS AND LIGHT.

---

Just prior to the time of exposure, the silver halide crystal has a negative surface charge (Fig. 5–6). As the emulsion is exposed by x-rays and light from the intensifying screens, the halide crystals absorb energy from light and x-ray photons. This absorption of energy and subsequent interactions in the crystals cause the negative electrons to move to the sensitivity speck. Silver ions, which have a positive charge, are then attracted to the area of the sensitivity speck because of the increased negative charge from the electrons. As this interaction occurs, atoms of metallic silver are formed. The number of silver ions that are attracted to the sensitivity speck and that form metallic silver depends on the amount of exposure received by the halide crystals. This process occurs across the entire surface of the emulsion, producing the "latent" or invisible image (Fig. 5–7).

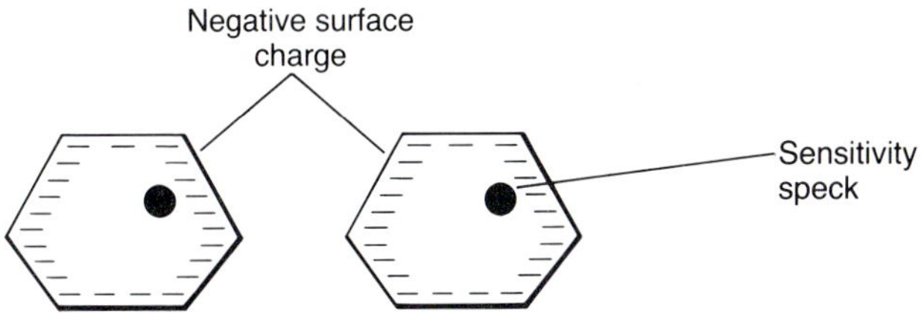



**FIGURE 5–6.** Prior to exposure, the silver halide crystals have a negative surface charge.

> **THE AMOUNT OF METALLIC SILVER DEPOSITS IN THE EMULSION DEPENDS ON THE AMOUNT OF EXPOSURE TO THE HALIDE CRYSTALS.**

During processing, the chemicals in the solutions are able to move through the softened gelatin to reach the atoms of metallic silver. This causes the metallic silver to blacken, which results in darkened areas on the finished film. The degree of blackening then depends on the amount of exposure the silver halide crystals received.

When the body is radiographed, x-rays must pass through parts of different thickness. The area of the x-ray film located underneath the thick parts will receive less radiation, causing less exposure to the halide crystals and producing light areas on the finished radiograph (Fig. 5–8).

## CARE OF X-RAY FILM

Radiographers must exercise caution in the use and storage of x-ray film. Rules related to the general handling of x-ray film should be as follows:

Handling:

1. Hands must be clean and dry.
2. Use no lotions or creams on hands.
3. Film should not be bent, buckled, or pinched.
4. Film should not be laid on cabinet or benches.
5. Film should not be dropped or slid across a surface.
6. Film should be opened in a darkened room using recommended safelight system.

Storage:

1. Store film in a cool and dry place approximately 50°F and with 5% humidity.
2. Store away from radiation areas or use protective barriers.
3. Note manufacturers' expiration dates.
4. Store upright and not in stacks.

## FILM HOLDERS

X-ray film is the primary recording medium used in radiography. In order for the radiographer to use x-ray film, a light-tight carrier must be available. Film holders used in radiography are called cassettes (Fig. 5–9). Cassettes are sturdy containers that protect the x-ray film from exposure to room light.

> **CASSETTES ARE FILM HOLDERS USED TO TRANSPORT FILM FOR USE WITHOUT EXPOSING THE FILM TO ROOM LIGHT.**

Cassettes have a metal frame with a thermosetting plastic (Bakelite) or magnesium front. The

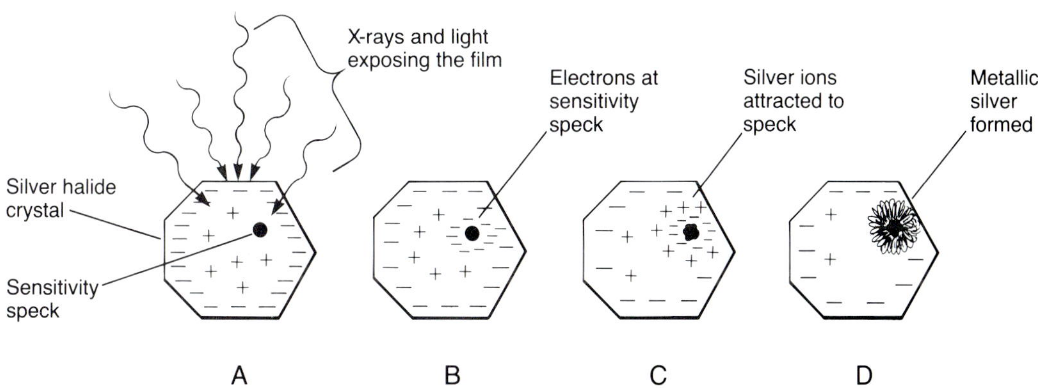



**FIGURE 5–7.** *A,* The halide crystal is exposed by x-rays and light from the intensifying screens. *B,* As energy is absorbed, negative electrons move to the sensitivity speck. *C,* The positive silver ions are then attracted to the area of the speck. *D,* The amount of silver attracted to the sensitivity speck depends on the amount of exposure received by the halide crystal. Development of the metallic silver will produce a black or darkened area on the film.

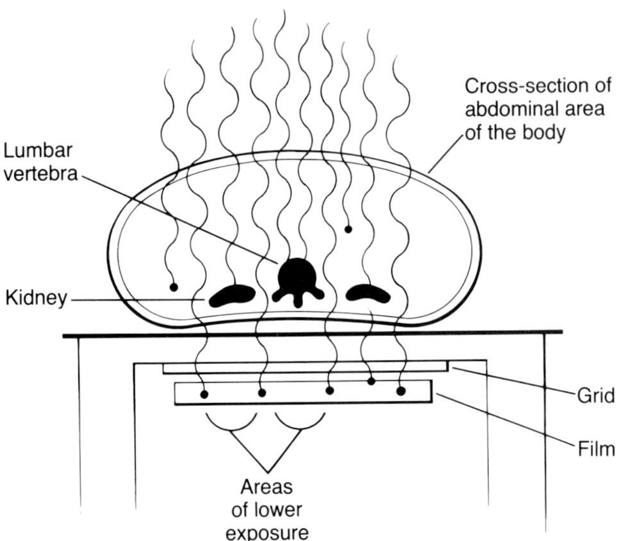


**FIGURE 5–8.** The abdominal area of the body contains organs and other structures of different thicknesses. The area of the x-ray film located under thick or dense structures, such as the vertebrae or kidneys, will receive less radiation as a result of the absorption or weakening of the photons. The halide crystals directly under these areas will receive less exposure.

light-tight seal is completed by snap or latch hinges (Fig. 5–9). Black felt was used in older style cassettes to provide a more effective seal.

Most cassettes have a lead backside to prevent backscatter x-radiation from reaching the film. Phototiming and automated exposure cassettes are often made with less leaded material and a thinner backside to allow x-rays to easily penetrate the anatomic part and reach the x-ray detector of the automated exposure control.

## INTENSIFYING SCREENS

The most important component is found inside the cassette and is called the "intensifying screen"

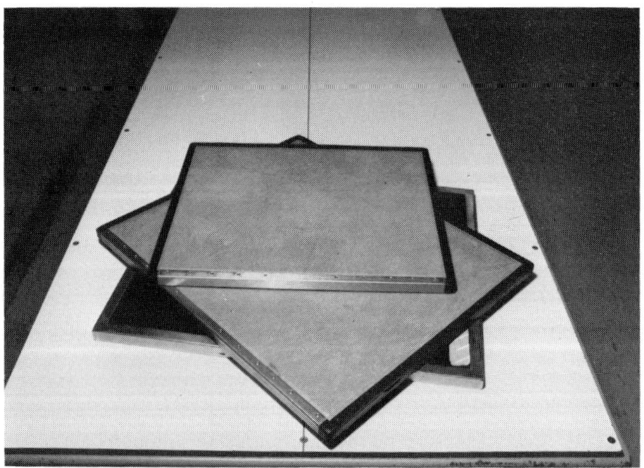

**FIGURE 5–9.** Film holders are called cassettes. Film holders are used to prevent light exposure to the sensitive x-ray film. Cassettes are available in a variety of sizes and exposure characteristics.

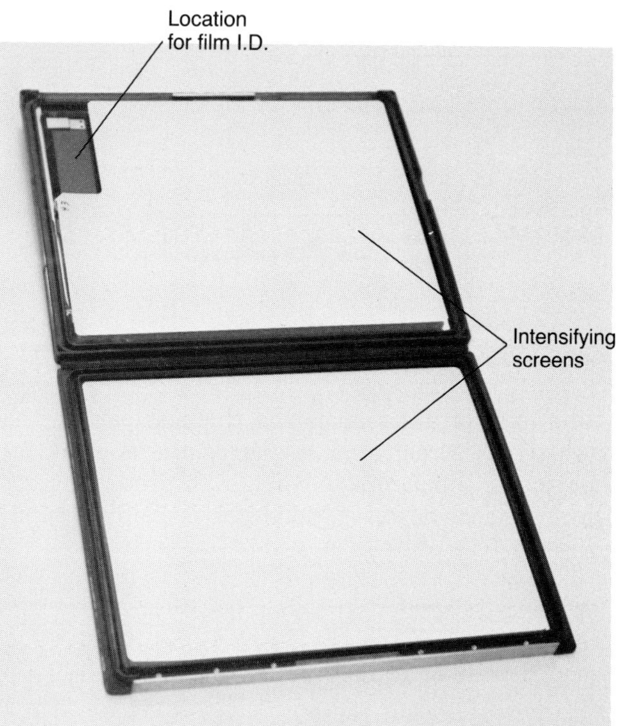


**FIGURE 5–10.** An open cassette. Inside the film holder are the intensifying screens. The rectangular open space on the upper screen is the space for film identification (patient's name, date, etc.).

(Fig. 5–10). Intensifying screens are extremely useful because they intensify the action of x-rays used in producing the image. Screens have been used in radiography since early in the 1900s and are as important as x-ray film in radiographic imaging systems.

### INTENSIFYING SCREENS INTENSIFY THE ACTION OF X-RAYS.

Intensifying screens are cardboard- or plastic-base structures that are usually found as pairs inside the cassette. The screens contain phosphors that cause luminescence or light to be given off from the screens at the time of x-ray exposure. Usually, more of the x-ray photons will interact with the screen phosphors than directly with emulsion of the x-ray film.

As described earlier in this chapter, because x-ray film is sensitive to x-rays and light, the light or "fluorescence" given off from the screens helps to produce the image on the film. It is important for radiographers to understand the characteristics of the phosphors found within these screens.

Intensifying screens have four basic components: base, reflective layer, phosphor layer, and protective coating (Fig. 5–11).

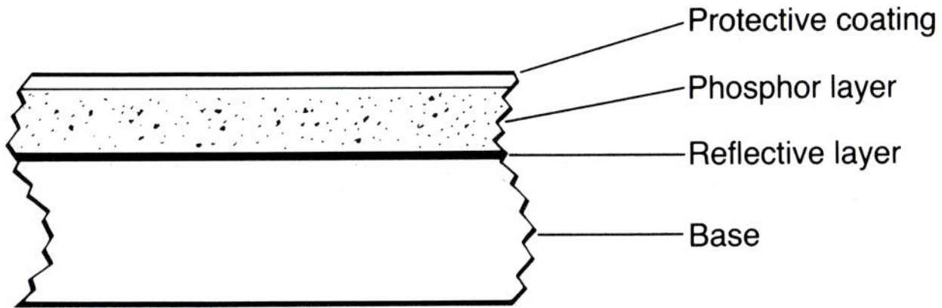

**FIGURE 5–11.** Cross-section of intensifying screen showing the four basic components: base, reflective layer, phosphor layer, and outer protective coating.

## Screen Base

The base of a screen is the thickest part of the intensifying screen and serves as the support for the other components. A very high grade of cardboard is used; however, polyester is gaining popularity because of its flexibility and durability.

---

THE BASE OF THE INTENSIFYING SCREEN PROVIDES SUPPORT FOR THE PHOSPHOR LAYER.

---

## Reflective Layer

The reflective layer is a very thin layer of a white shiny substance, usually titanium dioxide. The purpose of the reflective layer is to redirect light toward the film and improve the efficiency of the screen (Fig. 5–12).

---

THE REFLECTIVE LAYER SERVES TO REDIRECT LIGHT TOWARD THE FILM.

---

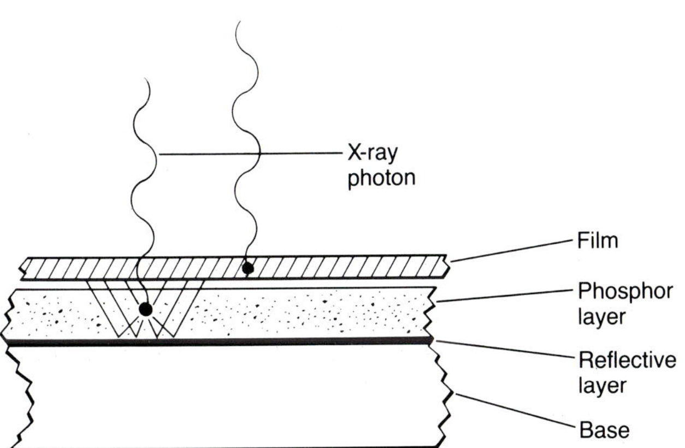

**FIGURE 5–12.** The reflective layer redirects light to the film, thus improving the efficiency of the screen. The disadvantage is the crossover of light photons as they are redirected toward the film. The crossover causes a loss of image sharpness.

As light is reflected or redirected toward the film, there is crossover of the photons, which causes a loss in sharpness of the image or "unsharpness." Screens may have a crossover effect of 30% or more. Manufacturers are also producing high-detail screens without the use of reflective backing because of the loss in image sharpness. Absorbing dyes have been used effectively in reducing this crossover effect.

## Phosphor Layer

The active layer within the screen is the phosphor layer. The phosphor layer is the most important component because the phosphors are able to convert the energy from the x-ray photons to visible light photons. In other words, fewer x-ray photons are needed to produce many light photons (Fig. 5–13).

---

THE MOST IMPORTANT LAYER IS THE PHOSPHOR LAYER; THE PHOSPHORS ARE ABLE TO CONVERT X-RAY ENERGY TO VISIBLE LIGHT.

---

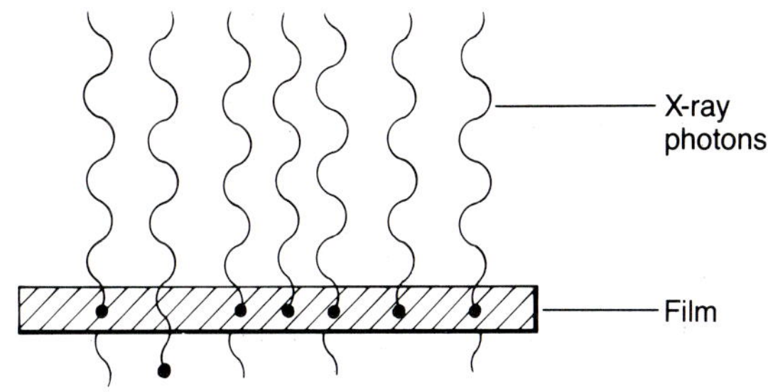

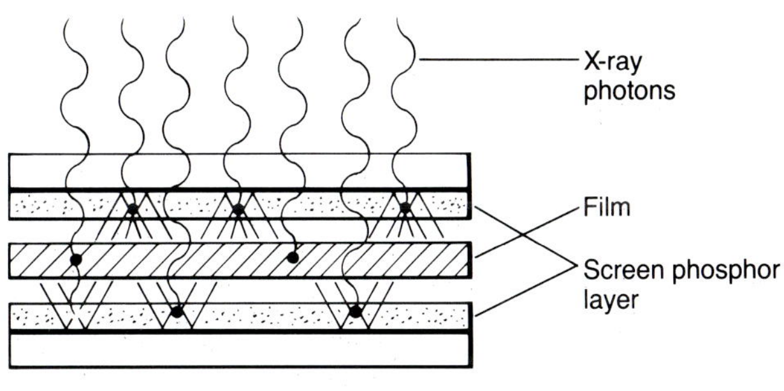

**FIGURE 5–13.** Exposure to the film with and without intensifying screens. *A,* Exposure to the film without screens; only x-rays will expose the film. *B,* Exposure to the film with the use of screens. X-rays and light from the screens expose the film. The phosphors are able to convert x-ray energy to light.

Phosphors used in the manufacture of screens have one characteristic in common—they are capable of luminescence, which means "the ability to give off visible light." The glow of light from the screens is called *fluorescence.* Fluorescence is the emission of visible light as a result of absorption of radiation. The fluorescence will continue as long as the stimulation from radiation is present.

---

LUMINESCENCE IS THE ABILITY TO GIVE OFF LIGHT. FLUORESCENCE IS THE EMISSION OF LIGHT AS A RESULT OF EXPOSURE TO RADIATION.

---

Radiographers can view the fluorescent phenomenon by placing an opened cassette on an x-ray table. The screens should be facing up toward the x-ray tube. Move the x-ray tube over the screens, darken the room, and make an exposure. The light given off by the screen is visible.

An important characteristic of the phosphor used in screens is minimal afterglow. Afterglow or "phosphorescence" is the glow of light after the exposure has stopped. Afterglow is undesirable because increased darkening on the film will result after the exposure has ended.

---

PHOSPHORESCENCE OR AFTERGLOW OCCURS WHEN SCREENS EMIT LIGHT AFTER THE EXPOSURE HAS BEEN TERMINATED.

---

The most common phosphor types used in producing intensifying screens are calcium tungstate and rare earth. Before the 1980s, the phosphor of choice was calcium tungstate. Calcium tungstate responded well to exposure from x-radiation, and manufacturers were able to vary the composition to produce different screen speeds, recognized as slow, medium or par, and high-speed or fast screens. Barium lead sulfate was another phosphor used to produce high-speed screens. Zinc sulfide was the phosphor of choice for the production of screens used with fluoroscopic devices because it responded well to radiation of low intensity.

---

CALCIUM TUNGSTATE AND RARE EARTH PHOSPHORS ARE THE MOST COMMON PHOSPHORS USED IN SCREENS.

Although calcium tungstate phosphors served radiographers well, the major disadvantage was related to speed. As speed was increased, the sharpness of the image decreased. Faster screens were available, but the result left more to be desired in terms of image sharpness.

## Protective Coating

The protective coating is a cellulose layer that serves to protect the phosphor layer and reduce static build-up from movement of the film across the screen. In addition, the protective coating reduces the possibility of damage to the phosphor layer during normal use and cleaning.

---

THE PROTECTIVE COATING SERVES TO PROTECT THE PHOSPHOR LAYER.

---

## Rare Earth Screens

Since the early 1980s, the phosphor of choice has changed to rare earth elements, which include gadolinium and lanthanum. Yttrium is another element used in newer screens because it has characteristics very similar to rare earth phosphors. The term "rare" does not mean that their occurrence in the earth is rare but instead, that the elements are quite difficult to refine.

The rare earth phosphors convert x-ray photon energy to light more efficiently. The result is greater energy conversion with less x-ray energy. Because the conversion is so efficient, the crossover effect does not increase, which results in improved sharpness of the image. When rare earth screens are compared with calcium tungstate screens having the same speed factor, the high-speed calcium tungstate screen will produce a significant increase in the crossover effect and a decrease in sharpness of the image.

---

RARE EARTH PHOSPHORS ARE MORE EFFICIENT IN CONVERTING X-RAY ENERGY TO LIGHT.

---

Rare earth phosphors need less x-ray energy to provide the same energy conversion as calcium tungstate but without sacrificing sharpness of the

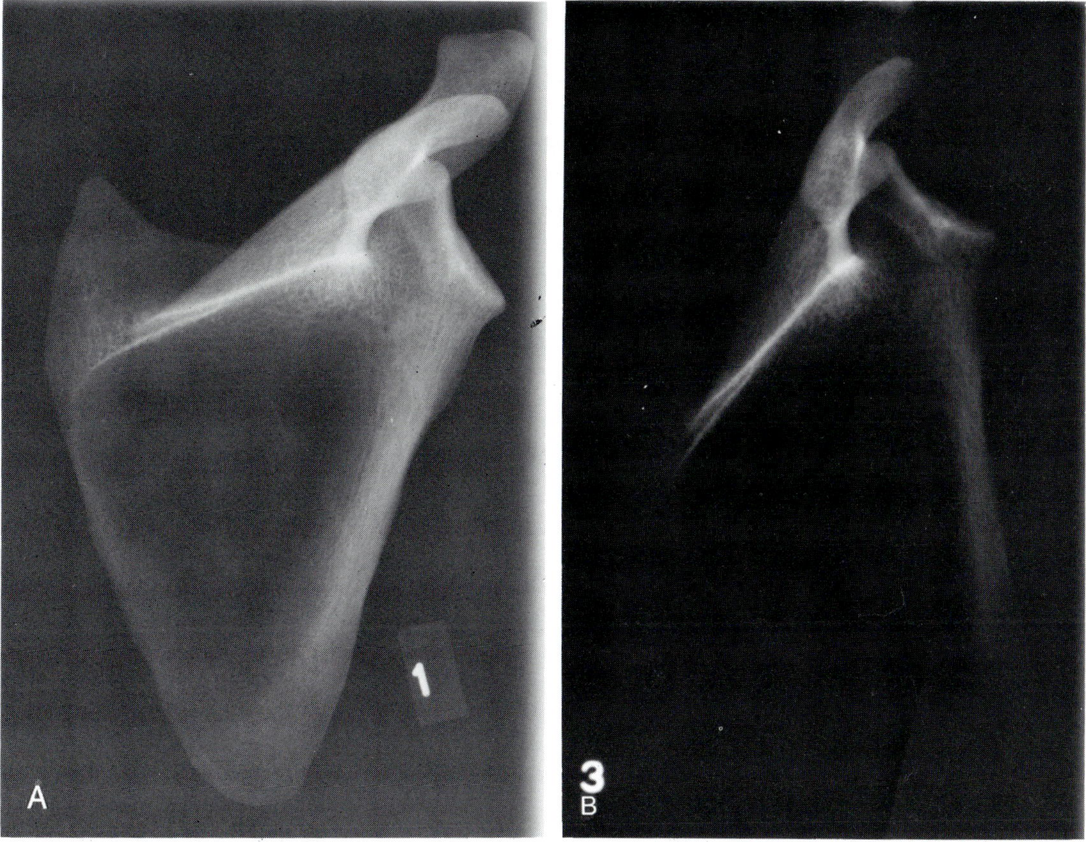


**FIGURE 5–14.** Rare earth phosphors are more efficient in converting x-ray photon energy to light than are calcium tungstate screens. *A,* Radiograph made using calcium tungstate screens with a relative speed of 100. *B,* Radiograph produced with rare earth screens rated with a speed value of 400. Radiographs made using rare earth screens require a significant reduction in the amount of exposure to produce the same amount of blackening on the film as exposures made with calcium tungstate screens.

image. Therefore, rare earth screens are faster and better suit the needs of the radiographer. Manufacturers are able to produce rare earth screens with different speeds (Fig. 5–14).

> RARE EARTH PHOSPHORS NEED LESS X-RAY ENERGY TO PROVIDE THE SAME ENERGY CONVERSION AS CALCIUM TUNGSTATE.

## Advantages of Rare Earth Screens

The use of rare earth screens results in lower exposure to the patient because less exposure is needed to produce a high-quality radiograph. Lower exposures are achieved because rare earth phosphors are more efficient in converting x-rays to light. The x-ray to light conversion for calcium tungstate is approximately 5%. This means that about 5% of the x-rays are converted to fluorescent light by the phosphor. This is not a very efficient system. Rare earth phosphors, on the other hand, have an x-ray to light conversion of 18 to 25%, which is four to five times greater than that of calcium tungstate.

> RARE EARTH SCREENS HAVE AN X-RAY TO LIGHT CONVERSION OF 18 TO 25%, WHICH IS FOUR TO FIVE TIMES GREATER THAN THAT OF CALCIUM TUNGSTATE.

Rare earth phosphors are more efficient in the kilovoltage range of 40 to 75. For kilovoltage levels lower than 40 and greater than 75, there is a gradual loss in the efficiency of the phosphor. At extreme ranges in kilovoltage settings, rare earth screens perform at speeds similar to calcium tungstate.

To obtain the best performance and for greatest efficiency with rare earth screens, one should ensure that kilovoltage remains constant and within the recommended range. When high kilovoltage settings are used with rare earth screens, quantum mottle may become a problem that decreases the sharpness of the image.

Since slightly lower kilovoltage selections are often used with rare earth screens, contrast is increased. An increase in kilovoltage will produce an increase in speed with calcium tungstate screens.

Because radiographers may also use shorter exposures with rare earth screens, motion does not become a major problem. Using less exposure allows for the frequent use of the small focal spot, which produces greater image sharpness. Over a long period of time, the smaller exposures will result in extended life of the x-ray tube.

The many advantages of using a rare earth system have overpowered the main disadvantage of rare earth screens, which is economic. Rare earth imaging systems are more expensive than calcium tungstate systems.

## SELECTION OF THE RADIOGRAPHIC IMAGING SYSTEM

The selection of accessories that compose the imaging system includes matching of the film type with the screen type. Blue-sensitive film should be matched with screens that emit a blue or blue-violet light. This will provide maximum speed efficiency for the system.

---

FILM AND SCREEN TYPES SHOULD BE MATCHED TO PROVIDE MAXIMUM SPEED EFFICIENCY.

---

When using a rare earth system with screens emitting a greenish light, one should select a green-sensitive film to provide maximum speed efficiency. A blue-sensitive system requires the use of a darkroom safelight in the orange-red color range, and a green-sensitive system requires a safelight in a darker red color.

## COMPARISON OF SPEED OF IMAGING SYSTEMS

Relative speed values have been assigned to allow effective comparison of screen/film imaging systems. The base for the assignment of relative speed values is calcium tungstate medium (par) speed screens with regular blue-sensitive film. The relative speed value is 100. High-speed calcium tungstate screens and blue-sensitive film combinations are given a relative speed value of 200. A relative speed value of 200 means the system is two times faster than a medium speed system with a speed value of 100. A higher speed value means that less exposure is needed to produce a radiograph while at the same time maintaining the same degree of darkening on the film.

---

A HIGH-SPEED VALUE MEANS LESS EXPOSURE IS NEEDED TO PRODUCE A RADIOGRAPH WITH ADEQUATE DENSITY.

---

A slower speed imaging system may have a relative speed value of 50. The lower speed value means the system is only one half as fast as a system with a speed value of 100 when producing a radiograph with the same degree of blackening. Systems of lower relative speed require greater amounts of radiation to produce radiographs and maintain adequate film blackening. On the positive side, slower systems usually have greater image sharpness. Table 5–1 provides relative speed system comparisons.

The table demonstrates examples of differences in efficiency between rare earth and regular calcium tungstate screens. Because specific film and screen types have not been used for the comparisons in Table 5–1, the examples listed above provide only a general comparison of imaging systems. Rare earth medium speed screens are three to five times faster, yet maintain the same high level of image sharpness and blackening on the film.

## SCREEN CONTACT

To achieve maximum image sharpness, the film and screen must be in complete contact across the

TABLE 5–1. IMAGING SYSTEM SCREEN-FILM COMPARISON

| Type of Screen | Type of Film | Relative Speed Value |
|---|---|---|
| Calcium tungstate (medium) | Blue-sensitive (regular) | 100 |
| Calcium tungstate (slow) | Blue-sensitive (regular) | 30–50 |
| Calcium tungstate (high-speed) | Blue-sensitive (regular) | 200 |
| Rare earth (slow—detail) | Green-sensitive (regular) | 100 |
| Rare earth (medium) | Green-sensitive (regular) | 300–500 |
| Rare earth (fast) | Green-sensitive (regular) | 800–1200 |

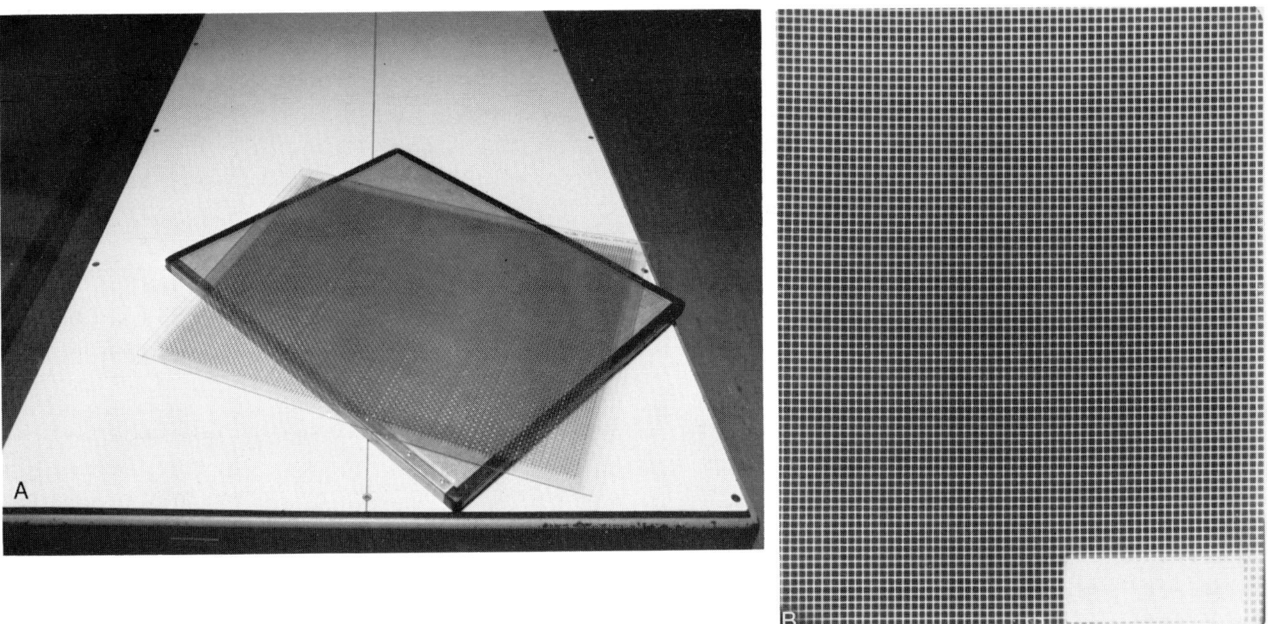

**FIGURE 5–15.** Film screen contact can be tested using a commercially produced wire mesh screen enclosed in plastic. *A,* The wire mesh screen is placed on top of the cassette to be tested. *B,* Radiograph produced using the testing device. The radiograph is evaluated for the overall density (blackening) and detail of the image of the wire mesh screen.

entire surface of the film. Poor screen-film contact will result in a loss of image sharpness, or "blurring" (Fig. 5–15).

---

THE FILM AND INTENSIFYING SCREEN MUST BE IN COMPLETE CONTACT ACROSS THE ENTIRE SURFACE TO ACHIEVE MAXIMUM IMAGE SHARPNESS.

---

To test for screen-film contact, load the cassette of interest with unexposed x-ray film. Place the cassette on top of the x-ray table. Lay a "wire mesh," designed for this purpose, on top of the cassette. Center the x-ray tube to the middle of the cassette and make an exposure. Process the film and exam-ine the finished radiograph for areas of blurring or changes in density. Blurring or areas of increased or decreased blackening may indicate areas of poor screen-film contact.

## CARE OF SCREENS

Intensifying screens are extremely important in the imaging process, and radiographers must practice good habits in the use of cassettes. Care must be taken not to cause abrasions or scratches on the screen surface while loading the film. Regular visual examinations of the screens should be made to reveal any dirt or specks. Screens should also be cleaned on a regular basis with an antistatic cleaner. Special cleaners may be purchased from the manufacturer.

# Processing the Radiograph

## CHAPTER OBJECTIVES

1. Describe the basic design and location of a radiographic darkroom.
2. Explain the advantage of using a passbox in darkroom design.
3. Describe the safety lock system needed for darkroom doors.
4. Name and describe two darkroom safelighting systems.
5. Discuss the term "safelight."
6. Describe the procedure for testing a safelight.
7. Define the term "processing system."
8. List the contents of developer and fixer, and explain their function.
9. From a diagram, label the parts of an automatic processor.
10. List the requirements for an automatic processing system.
11. Explain the importance of the time-temperature relationship for automatic processing.
12. Describe the advantages of the standardization of processing with the use of automatic processors.
13. List the five systems that are part of the processor and describe their function.
14. Describe the path of the film as it moves through the system, and explain what happens to the film at each point in the cycle.
15. Describe the maintenance procedures necessary to maintain processor consistency.
16. Explain the purpose of silver recovery.
17. Describe three methods for recovering silver from the fixer solution.
18. Define "daylight system."
19. List the advantages and disadvantages of the daylight processing system.

## KEY WORDS AND TERMS

Darkroom
Passbox
Electric safety lock
Darkroom illumination
Safelight
Safelight test
Processing system
Developing
Fixing
Washing
Drying
Automatic processor
Replenishment

Time-temperature relationship
Darkroom chemistry
Tackiness
Transport system
Recirculation system
Replenishment system
Turnaround rollers
Crossover rollers
Guideshoes
Squeegee assembly
Silver recovery
Daylight system

## RECOMMENDATIONS FOR GENERAL DISCUSSION QUESTIONS

1. Discuss the design, location, and need for the darkroom in radiography.
2. Compile a list of requirements for selecting a safelighting system.
3. Discuss the term "standardization" as it relates to processing of the radiographic image.
4. Describe each system within an automatic processor, and explain how each system contributes to the production of a high-quality radiograph.
5. Describe the silver recovery process, and explain why it is necessary.
6. Compare and contrast the traditional darkroom with the daylight system.

In radiography, x-ray film is exposed to x-radiation and fluorescent light from intensifying screens, producing the latent image. The latent image, as described in Chapter 5, is the image on the film; however, it is of no value to the radiographer until it has been processed to become visible.

## THE RADIOGRAPHIC DARKROOM

Processing of the latent image takes place in a darkroom, a room designed to be functional and convenient. The darkroom is designed for the handling and storage of x-ray film.

Radiography begins in the darkroom by loading the cassette with x-ray film and ends with the removal of the film, containing the latent image, from the cassette. The film is placed in the processor, where it becomes a visible and permanent image after proper developing and fixing of the film. The diagram in Figure 6–1 shows a sample radiographic darkroom.

The darkroom is a very busy place and must be designed for work. The location should be at a place in the department that requires the radiographer to walk as few steps as possible. Several wall-mounted passboxes, for passing cassettes in and out of the darkroom, should be strategically located to allow easy access without opening the main entrance door (Fig. 6–2).

A passbox allows cassettes to be passed to the darkroom personnel without opening doors. An interlock system prevents white light from entering the darkroom as cassettes are placed in the passbox.

---

THE PASSBOX ALLOWS CASSETTES TO BE PASSED TO THE DARKROOM WITHOUT OPENING THE DOOR AND EXPOSING THE ROOM TO LIGHT.

---

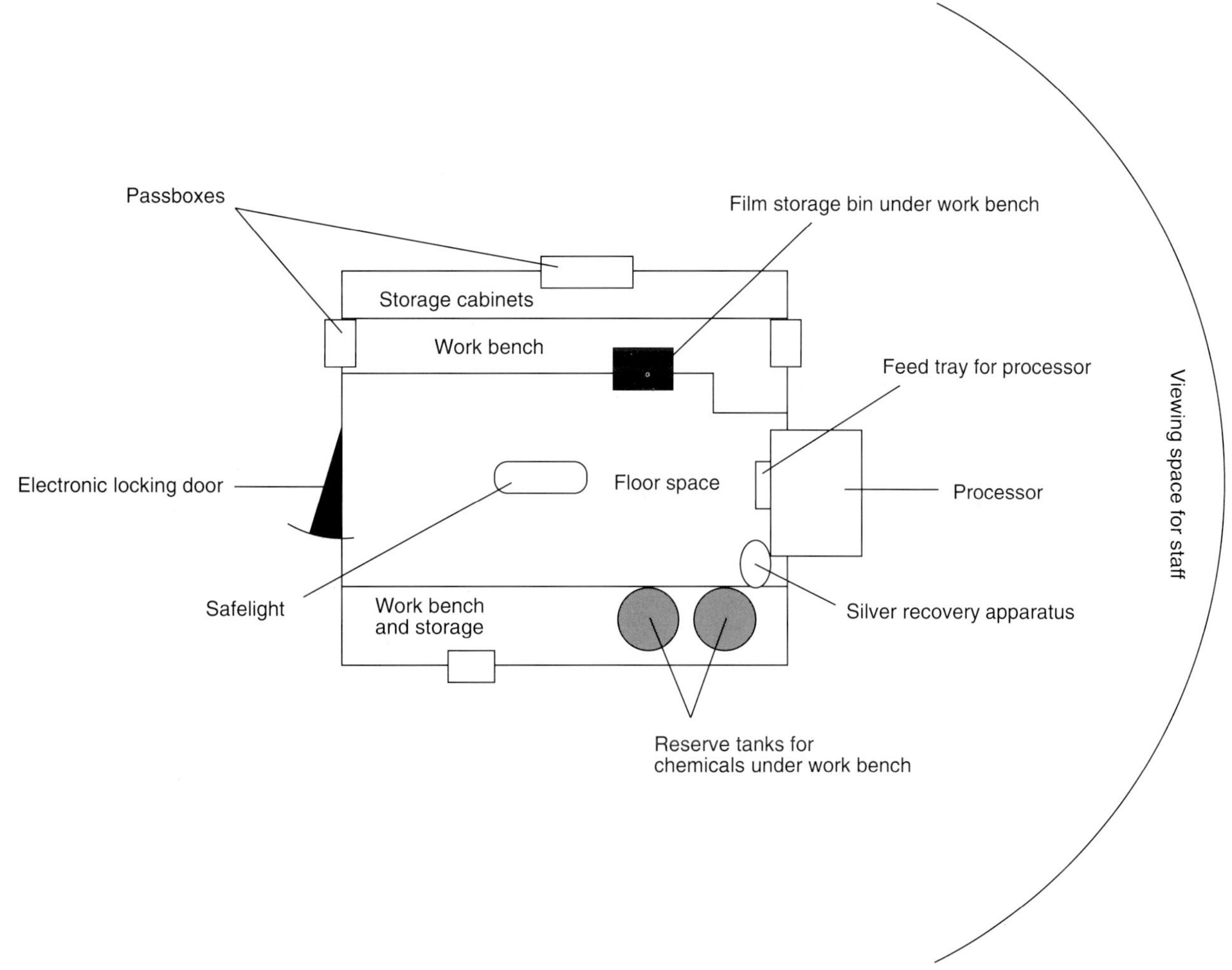


**FIGURE 6–1.** The radiographic darkroom is designed for efficiency. The feed tray for the automatic processor is near the work bench and film storage bin. Passboxes are located for easy access by the radiographers and darkroom personnel. Storage areas are needed for x-ray film and holders. Safelights and processor reserve tanks are strategically placed. The door must have a lock system to prevent accidental opening of the door.

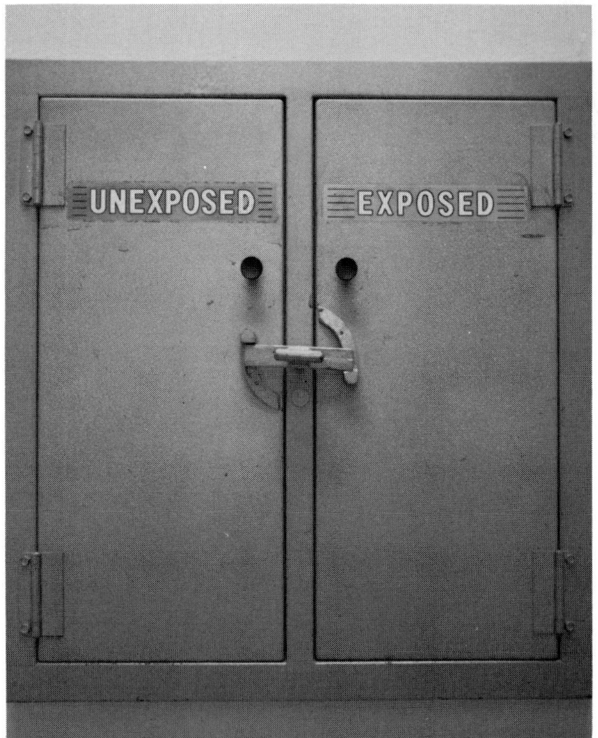


**FIGURE 6–2.** Passbox used in the design for radiographic darkrooms. There is an interlocking system in which the doors on one side cannot be opened until the doors on the opposite side are closed. As this photograph illustrates, exposed film is passed into the darkroom on the right side and the newly filled cassette is returned to the radiographer using the left side, marked Unexposed.

Entrances for darkrooms must be specially designed to prevent accidental opening of the door. Most radiographic darkrooms have doors with electric safety locks. When the lock is engaged, a safety lock will prevent the door from opening when the storage bin is open.

Other types of entrances include the "revolving door," maze, and double–door lock systems. The maze and double-lock systems require additional space. In newer radiology departments, these would not be the entrance of choice when space is at a premium.

Darkrooms require ventilation to prevent build-up of fumes from chemicals used in the processor system. Air from the dryer, which is part of the automatic processor, must be vented to the outside of the darkroom. The standard method may be to vent the warm air to the space immediately above the ceiling.

## Darkroom Illumination

Inasmuch as x-ray film is more sensitive after exposure to radiation and before processing takes place, attention to the lighting system for the darkroom is very important. Low or dim lighting is used with special filters to prevent exposure to x-ray film. Walls are generally a light gray or ivory color to provide reflection from the "safe" lighting system.

---

## X-RAY FILM IS MOST SENSITIVE AFTER EXPOSURE AND BEFORE PROCESSING.

---

The special illumination system used in the darkroom is called a "safelight" system. The term implies that a system should be "safe" for x-ray film to be removed from the storage bin, loaded in a cassette, and later removed for placement in the processor system without light fog becoming a problem. Calling the lights a safelight system means that the illumination will not affect the very sensitive emulsion of the x-ray film during normal handling of the film in the darkroom. No safelight is safe for indefinite periods of exposure. Examples are shown in Figure 6–3.

---

## THE SPECIAL ILLUMINATION REQUIRED FOR A RADIOGRAPHIC DARKROOM IS CALLED A SAFELIGHT SYSTEM.

---

Safelights use a filtering device to achieve the desired result of producing illumination in a partic-

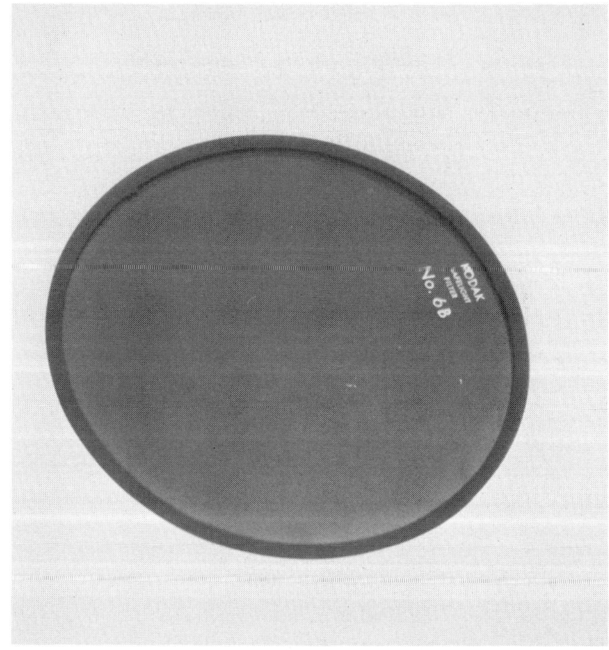

**FIGURE 6–3.** Kodak Wratten 6B filter used in the illumination of radiographic darkrooms.

ular energy range of the electromagnetic spectrum. Sodium vapor lights produce illumination in the orange-yellow range. The standard safelight system used in many departments is a 7.5- to 15-watt bulb with a Kodak Wratten 6B filter (shown in Fig. 6–3). The Kodak GBX all-purpose filter is more versatile and provides illumination in the darker red range. The versatility of the GBX allows for the use of green- and/or blue-sensitive x-ray film (Fig. 6–4).

Safelights of any type must be installed according to the manufacturer's guidelines and tested on a regular basis.

## Safelight Test

Safelights are only "safe" after they have been tested. Immediately following installation, each safelight must be tested. To test a safelight, a standard procedure should be followed.

**Procedure.** Load a cassette in the darkroom with all lights turned "off," including the safelights. Take the cassette to a radiographic room and expose it to a small amount of radiation. Return to the darkroom and with all lights remaining "off," remove the x-ray film from the cassette and lay it on a clean area of the work counter. Cover three quarters of the film surface and turn the safelight to be tested "on." It is important to test only one light at a time. Expose the film in this manner for approximately 60 seconds. With the safelight remaining "on," uncover another quarter of the film and hold again for

60 seconds. Continue this procedure, exposing one quarter of the film each time for a 60-second period.

As soon as the film has been exposed for 4 minutes, the safelight should be turned "off" and the film processed in the automatic processor. The finished radiograph should be evaluated using a densitometer, an instrument used to measure blackening on radiographs. If fog or blackening is present and/or increases in fog occur with continued exposure from the safelight, the safelight should be considered "unsafe."

## Darkroom Location

Radiographic darkrooms should be located in areas away from radiation, but this does not mean they should be out of the work area of the radiographers. The darkroom itself should be tested to assure that radiation exposure is *not* a problem. It must be radiation-proof. If it is located next to radiographic rooms, a layer of lead shielding must be added to the walls dividing the rooms. The lead shielding will absorb x-rays and prevent exposure to the film that is stored in the darkroom. The passbox must also be radiation-proof to prevent radiation exposure to x-ray film as cassettes are passed in and out of the darkroom.

---

THE DARKROOM SHOULD BE LOCATED IN AN AREA AWAY FROM RADIATION; SHIELDING IS OFTEN USED TO PROTECT THE DARKROOM.

---

## PROCESSING SYSTEM

Processing the exposed x-ray film changes the latent image to a visible image that is made permanent for handling, viewing, and storage. Processing of the x-ray film includes development, fixing, washing, and drying.

---

PROCESSING THE EXPOSED X-RAY FILM CHANGES THE LATENT IMAGE TO A VISIBLE IMAGE.

---

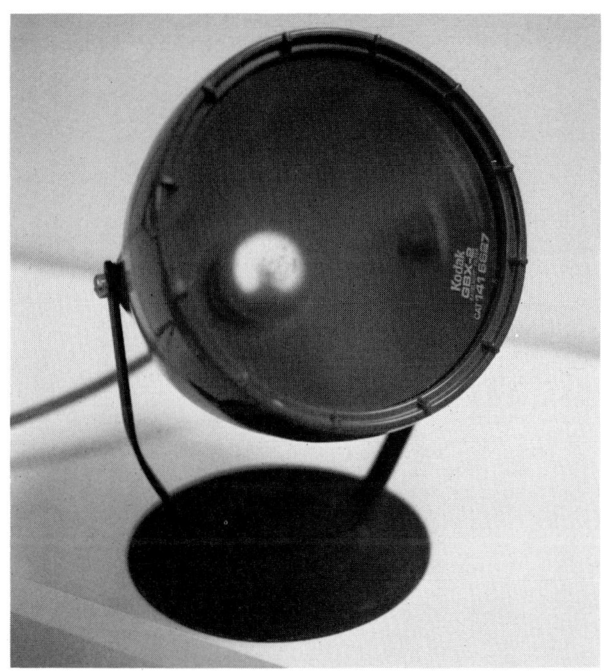

**FIGURE 6–4.** The more versatile Kodak GBX-2 filter provides illumination in the darker red range. Green-sensitive or blue-sensitive film can be used in the darkroom with this type of filter.

To process a film, first one places it in a development solution. As the image is developed, the chemicals cause the exposed silver halide crystals in the emulsion to change to a black metallic silver. Second, the film is placed in a solution called "fixer." The fixer solution stops development and hardens the emulsion so the film may be handled in white or bright light. The third step is washing of the film, which removes excess chemicals from the film surface. Finally, the film goes through a drying cycle to remove all moisture from the surface.

---

## TO PROCESS A FILM, ONE MUST DEVELOP, FIX, WASH, AND DRY IT.

---

Before radiography entered the high-tech arena, manual or hand processing was standard. The manual process involved hanging each film on a special metal hanger before the film could be passed from one tank to another. Each step was accomplished by a person in the darkroom lifting hangers from one tank to another. To process a single film by the manual method requires about 1 hour as well as excessive amounts of space. In addition, the results continue to be inconsistent and create a "wet mess." This practice is still available, even in this modern time, in private offices and remote small departments. For beginners, it is important to understand the steps in the manual process because they are the basics for automatic processor design and operation.

Automatic processors, sometimes referred to as "dry to dry" systems, were first made available in the 1950s. The first unit was designed by Eastman Kodak Company and required processing times in excess of 7 minutes for the film to enter the unit dry from the darkroom and exit as a dry radiograph ready for viewing by the radiographer. Figure 6–5 shows a diagram of a processor.

The advent of the automatic processor produced a significant advantage over the 1 hour required to process a film by hand. Today, automatic processors are available that reduce the processing time to as little as 45 seconds. A few of the newer models will allow the rate of film travel to be changed from one speed to another, for example, 45 seconds to 90 seconds.

## Requirements for a Processing System

For adequate processing of radiographs, rigid control of temperature is required, with only minor fluctuation permitted. Agitation or stirring of the chemical solutions is necessary to keep chemicals mixed thoroughly and in constant contact with the film.

---

## TO PROCESS RADIOGRAPHS, ONE MUST MAINTAIN RIGID CONTROL OF TEMPERATURE.

---

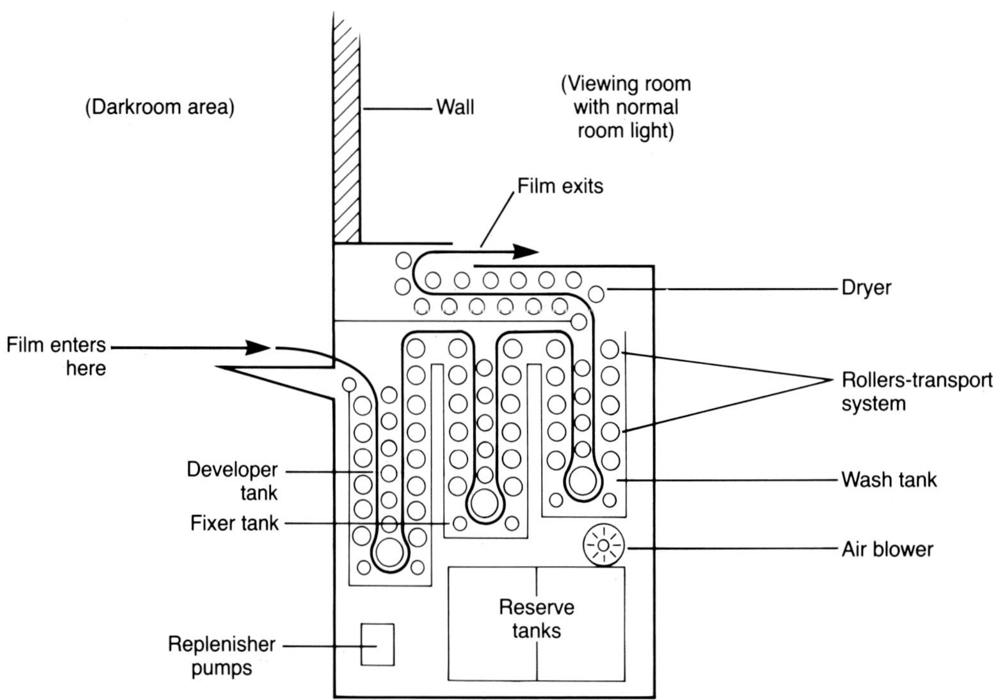


**FIGURE 6–5.** The design of automatic processors. The film enters from the feed tray in the darkroom and exits from the dryer as a completely processed radiograph.

As dry film is placed into solutions, replenishment is necessary to maintain volume and strength of the chemical solutions. In addition, the film must be moved from tank to tank with minimum spillage of chemicals.

---

REPLENISHER SOLUTION IS NEEDED TO MAINTAIN THE VOLUME AND STRENGTH OF DEVELOPER AND FIXER SOLUTIONS.

---

The time-temperature relationship is essential for consistency in the automatic processor. This means that the length of time the film stays in the developer and fixer depends on the temperature of the solution and the movement of the solution against the surface of the film.

---

THE TIME-TEMPERATURE RELATIONSHIP IS ESSENTIAL FOR CONSISTENCY IN THE PROCESSING OF RADIOGRAPHS.

---

In manual processing, the time-temperature relationship is 5 minutes at 68°F. The minimum fixing time is twice as long as required for the clearing of the unexposed silver crystals from the emulsion. As the temperature of the solutions increases, the time the film stays in the solution decreases, and vice versa.

In automatic processors, the time-temperature relationship is more precise and controlled by the multiple systems that make up the processor unit.

It is ideal for the processing system to use minimum space so multiple darkrooms can be placed throughout large radiology departments where work units exist. This prevents excessive walking for the radiographers.

Although the requirements and characteristics of automatic processors described above can be achieved by manual processing, it would be a difficult task, requiring several people and a tremendous amount of space. However, the automatic processing system is superior, enabling departments to operate with more consistency and quality control. Table 6–1 summarizes the requirements for automatic systems.

## AUTOMATIC PROCESSOR SYSTEMS

The automatic processor system consists of a processor unit containing individual systems operating

**TABLE 6–1. REQUIREMENTS FOR AUTOMATIC PROCESSORS**

| Requirement | Comment |
| --- | --- |
| 1. Control of temperature | Helps maintain adequate density and contrast |
| 2. Agitation of chemical solutions | Provides thorough mixing of chemical solutions |
| 3. Replenishment | Maintains volume and strength of solution |
| 4. Minimum spilling of chemicals as film moves from tank to tank | Reduces the contamination of chemicals |
| 5. Transportation of film through system remains constant | Controls length of time film is in developer and fixer |
| 6. Time-temperature relationship | Maintains consistency with all processor systems |
| 7. Compact in size | Requires very little space to operate |
| 8. Strategic placement | Reduces time spent by radiographers traveling to and from darkroom area |

in unison. The film enters by the entry tray located in the darkroom. Generally, the remaining part of the unit is outside of the darkroom in an area referred to as the "light room," a space set aside for viewing the radiographs as they exit the processor. As shown in Figure 6–6, only a small portion of the unit is actually located inside of the darkroom, thus allowing smaller darkrooms.

Automatic processor units provide consistency and efficiency. Temperature is controlled by thermostats, whereas agitation of the solutions is controlled by pumps and a roller transport system. Higher temperatures are used to increase the action of the processing chemicals.

---

AUTOMATIC PROCESSING UNITS STANDARDIZE THE PROCESSING OF RADIOGRAPHS WITH CONSISTENCY AND EFFICIENCY.

---

Special chemistry is required to be compatible with the emulsion and the high temperatures. Rigid control is also necessary for temperature, agitation, replenishment, and the speed of film movement through the system.

Each step in the process interrelates with others to become a controlled system (Fig. 6–7).

As the film enters the developer, the gelatin softens and swells. In the automatic system, excessive swelling causes the film to be slippery and tacky (sticky). Tackiness may cause the film to stick to the rollers of the transport system or fall through

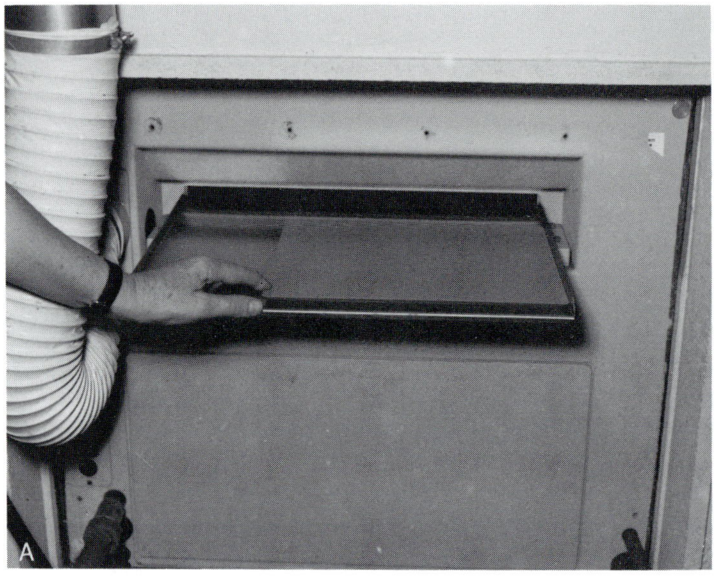

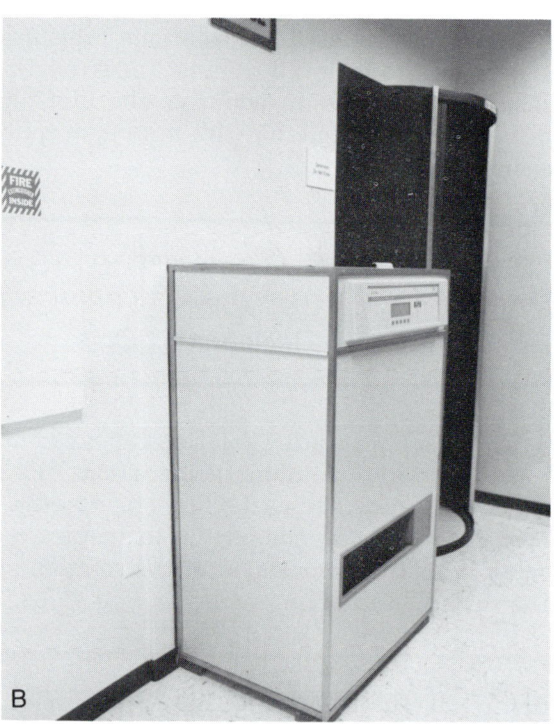

**FIGURE 6–6.** *A,* The processor feed tray is located inside the darkroom. *B,* The main processor unit is located outside the darkroom.

the rollers to the bottom of the tank. To correct the problem, one adds a special chemical hardener to control the swelling of the emulsion.

The solutions are warmed in order to work faster. (Remember the time-temperature relationship.) For example, the developer is warmed to approximately 92 to 94°F, with the time the film spends in the solution reduced to 22 to 24 seconds.

At the time a piece of film enters the processor unit, a replenishment pump will add replenisher to maintain the volume and strength of the solutions.

## Systems in the Processor Unit

The automatic processor is composed of five different systems that work together to become an integrated system. The five systems are transport, recirculation, replenishment, wash, and dry.

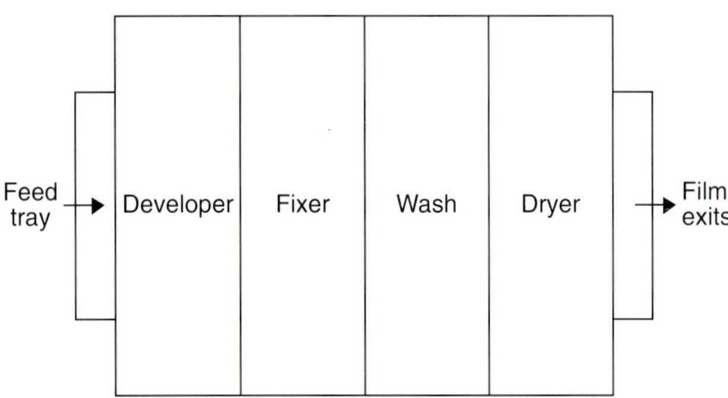

**FIGURE 6–7.** The film enters the processing cycle from the feed tray to the developer, fixer, wash, and dryer.

## Transport System

The transport system moves the film through the processor. It begins with the "rack" of rollers in the developer tank and moves the film from the feed tray into the developer, fixer, wash tank, dryer, and finally out of the processor into a receiving tray.

THE TRANSPORT SYSTEM MOVES THE FILM THROUGH THE PROCESSOR.

The film must turn around in the bottom of the tanks, and this is accomplished with a special component of the transport system called a "turn-around" (Fig. 6–8).

As the film rises to the top of the tank, it must be moved to the next tank or section. This is accomplished by the transport system with a "crossover" (Fig. 6–9).

Turnarounds and crossovers contain "guide-shoes," special devices that guide the film to change direction. Because the film does not curve naturally, the guideshoe must turn it around at the bottom of the tank and cross it over to the next section. Guideshoes are curved devices with small ridges that may cause a processing artifact called guide-shoe scratches if they are not properly adjusted.

As the film moves from the developer tank to the fixer tank, it must pass through the crossover sec-

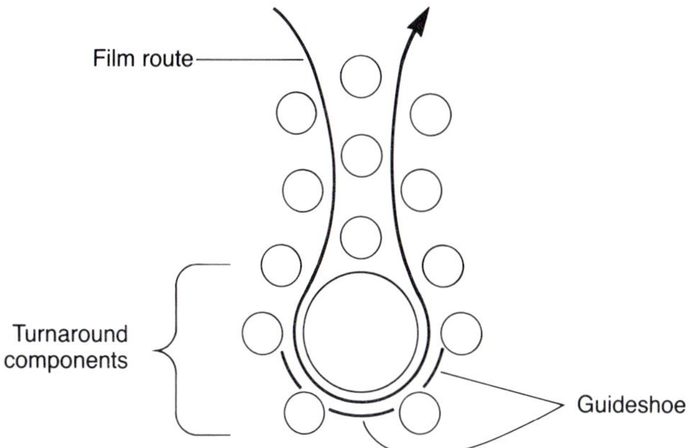



**FIGURE 6–8.** The turnaround is located at the bottom of the tank. As the film approaches the turnaround apparatus, the film is guided around the turn and moves up in a complete reverse of direction.

tion of the transport system. This part of the transport system contains a special "squeegee" assembly to squeeze the excess developer from the wet film emulsion. This step is very important to reduce the amount of developer carried into the fixer tank and to help maintain the strength and activity of the fixer chemicals.

The speed at which the transport rollers move the film through the processor unit is extremely important and must remain constant. The rate of travel determines how long the film remains in a specific tank or dryer. Rate of travel, along with the size of the tank, will determine the length of time for development, fixing, washing, and drying.

## THE SPEED AT WHICH THE FILM IS MOVED THROUGH THE PROCESSOR MUST REMAIN CONSTANT.

Because of constant movement, the transport system helps agitate the solutions and maintain constant temperature.

## THE TRANSPORT SYSTEM AGITATES THE SOLUTION AND HELPS MAINTAIN THE TEMPERATURE.

### Recirculation System

The purpose of the recirculation system is to provide continuous mixing of the chemicals. The continuous agitation and mixing play an important role in maintaining the proper temperature and strength of the solutions. The system is composed of a heater, thermostat, and filters. The filters serve to remove debris or other substances that may fall into the tanks.

## THE PURPOSE OF THE RECIRCULATION SYSTEM IS TO PROVIDE CONTINUOUS MIXING OF THE CHEMICALS.

### Replenishment System

The replenishment rate is one of the key elements to the successful use of automatic processors. The function of this system is to add solution to the developer and fixer tanks as each piece of x-ray film moves through the system.

## REPLENISHMENT IS THE ADDING OF SOLUTION TO THE DEVELOPER AND FIXER AS EACH FILM IS PROCESSED.

The replenishment system contains a pump controlled by a microswitch. In the darkroom, the film enters the processor by the feed tray. As the film moves between the rollers of the transport system, the microswitch activates the pump that sends replenisher solution into the tank. The length of time it takes for the film to enter the system determines how long the replenisher pump will operate. Once the film is completely in the transport system and in the developer tank, the microswitch stops the operation of the replenisher pump.

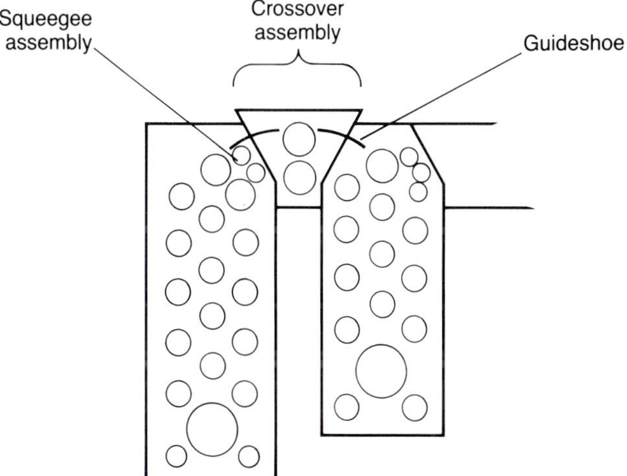



**FIGURE 6–9.** The crossover assembly moves the film from one tank to the next tank. The film moves between the squeegee roller and is directed around the curve by the guideshoe to the next tank.

The replenisher system serves to maintain volume and strength of the solutions in the developer and fixer tanks.

---

## REPLENISHMENT SERVES TO MAINTAIN VOLUME AND STRENGTH OF THE SOLUTIONS.

---

Adequate replenishment keeps the chemical activity stable and helps prevent tackiness of the film.

For high-volume processors, up to 50,000 films of mixed sizes can be processed before the chemicals must be changed if replenishment is adequate and consistent. Operators must adhere to manufacturer guidelines for replenishment rates.

As stated above, the length of time required for a film to enter the processor unit determines the amount of replenishment solution to be added. The direction of travel for a particular film size becomes an important key to control of replenishment. Manufacturer guidelines must be followed. Figure 6–10 provides a general guide for placement of film on the feed tray and movement into the processor unit.

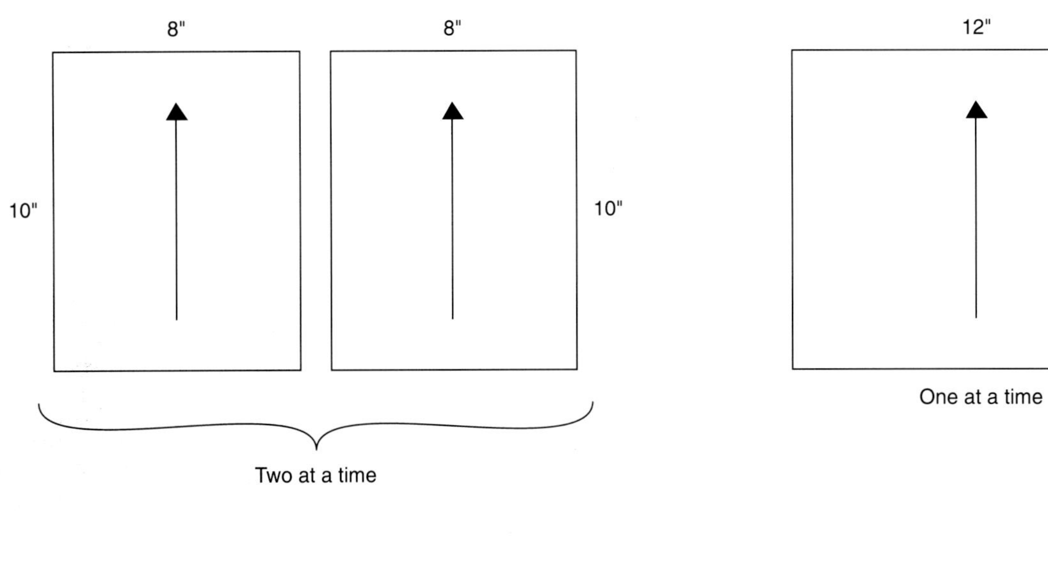


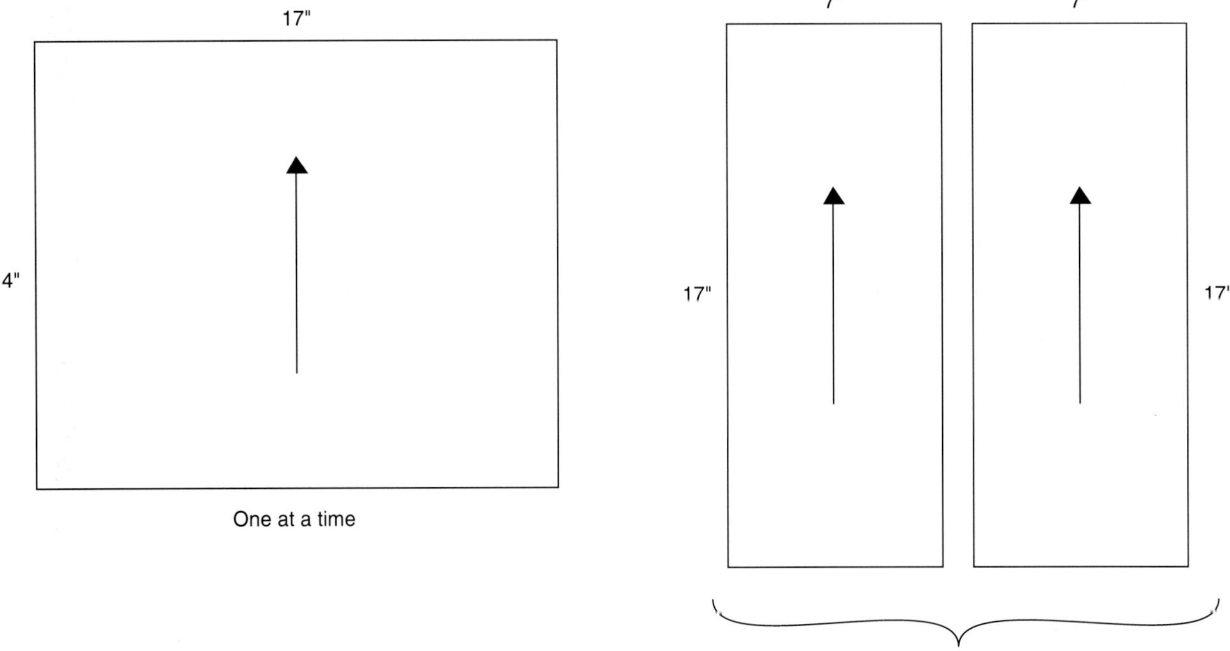


**FIGURE 6–10.** The recommended direction for film to be placed on the processor feed tray and fed into the system for processing. The direction must be consistent so as to control the amount of replenisher added to the tanks as each film enters the processor.

Consistency is important in the operation of the processor unit, and the direction of the film, as it moves across the feed tray into the processor, will have an important effect on replenishment. Whatever direction guidelines for film movement are determined to be for an individual department, they must be adhered to daily.

Small processors with low volume usually contain smaller replenishment tanks housed underneath the processor unit itself or next to the unit. High-volume units have separate and large replenishment tanks placed elsewhere in the darkroom area. The tanks are connected by tubing through which replenisher is pumped to the processor tanks. Filters are placed throughout the replenishment system. Cleaning of the filters and replacement must occur regularly to maintain clean solutions in the processor unit.

The replenisher rate should have periodic checks. Over-replenishment may result in a decrease in contrast and density on the film. Slight under-replenishment can result in an increase in contrast; however, a severe degree of under-replenishment contributes to a loss of both contrast and density. The manufacturer usually recommends a replenishment rate based on the volume of film expected to be processed during a daily or weekly period.

## Wash System

A thorough washing of the film as it moves out of the fixer tank is necessary to remove the excess chemicals. The finished film must contain only developed silver crystals. All excess chemicals must be washed away to prevent deterioration of the film after it is stored.

**WASHING OF THE FILM IS NECESSARY TO REMOVE EXCESS CHEMICALS.**

The film is washed as the transport system moves it into the wash tank. Water flows into the tank and a pump helps to keep clean water in contact with the film surface. Water flows continuously, with excess water flowing over the top of the tank and into a drainage system. Water also flows around the chemical tanks to help control temperature. Tap water is usually sufficient.

## Dryer System

To complete the processing cycle, the wet film must be dried for handling and storage. The dryer blows hot air across the surface of the film as the transport system moves it through the rollers of the dryer. The temperature of the air is held between approximately 110 and 120°F to remove surface moisture as rapidly as possible. The air is continually dried by a dehumidifier. Most of the dry hot air is recirculated; however, the dryer must be vented to release built-up air as new air is pulled into the system. The air from the dryer may be vented into the space immediately above the ceiling if a traditional vent system is not in place.

**THE DRYER BLOWS HOT AIR ACROSS THE SURFACE OF THE FILM TO ENHANCE DRYING OF THE SURFACE.**

## MAINTAINING THE PROCESSING UNIT

Automatic processor units will produce consistent high-quality radiographs daily only when regular maintenance procedures are in place. The maintenance procedures must include: (1) routine checks and cleaning of the transport rollers by lifting the racks out of the tanks; (2) careful examination and adjustment of guideshoes; and (3) cleaning and replacement of filters throughout the processor unit.

**REGULAR MAINTENANCE PROCEDURES ARE REQUIRED FOR CONSISTENCY IN THE PERFORMANCE OF PROCESSORS.**

Temperature readings, water flow, and drainage are to be checked as part of the daily maintenance procedures. The processor contains numerous filters that must be examined routinely. The replenishment rate and microswitch control for the replenisher pump must also be on the routine checklist.

## PROCESSING CHEMISTRY

The two chemical solutions in processing are the developer and fixer. The developer softens the gelatin and develops the latent image. The fixer removes the unexposed silver halide crystals and hardens the emulsion. After development and fixing, the film is washed and dried.

## Developer

The developer is an alkaline solution and contains an accelerator, restrainer, preservative, hardener (the hardener is not included in manual processing), and reducing agents. The chemicals are mixed with water as the solvent (Fig. 6–11).

The reducing agents, also called developing agents, change the latent image to a visible image.

As the dry film enters the developer, the wet solution causes the gelatin in the emulsion to soften and swell. The reducing agents seep into the emulsion and act on the metallic silver found around the sensitivity speck. As described in Chapter 5, the amount of metallic silver found at the sensitivity speck depends on the amount of exposure received by the silver halide crystal structure.

Phenidone and hydroquinone are the reducing agents. Figure 6–11 demonstrates how these agents work. Phenidone builds the grays and hydroquinone builds the blacks. As the chemicals act, the visible image begins to appear.

---

THE DEVELOPER CHEMICALS ACT ON THE EMULSION, CAUSING THE IMAGE TO BECOME VISIBLE.

---

The accelerator, sometimes called the activator, is sodium carbonate (Fig. 6–12). The accelerator controls the activity and alkalinity of the developer solution and accelerates the gelatin swelling and softening of the film emulsion.

The restrainer is potassium bromide, and it serves as an antifog agent. It restrains the chemicals from

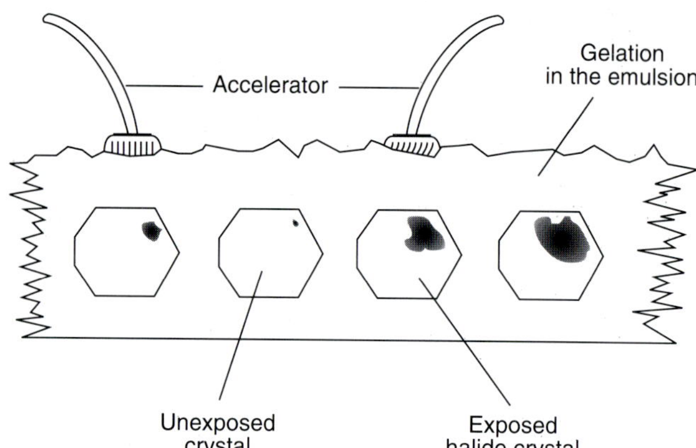


**FIGURE 6–12.** The accelerator controls the activity and alkalinity of the developer and accelerates the swelling of the emulsion. This facilitates the developing agents' penetration of the emulsion to reach the halide crystals.

overdevelopment or the developing of the unexposed silver halide crystals (Fig. 6–13).

The preservative is sodium sulfite, and it acts to reduce oxidation or deterioration of the developer solution (Fig. 6–14).

A hardener called glutaraldehyde is added to control the swelling of the gelatin. The temperature of the developer solution in a 90-second processor unit may be as high as 92 to 94°F. The high temperature results in significant swelling of the emulsion. Too much swelling will prevent the film from moving easily through the transport rollers. The hardener facilitates the movement of the film through the processing cycle. Table 6–2 summarizes the contents of the developer solution.

## Fixer

After the latent image has been developed, the film emulsion must be fixed to become permanent.

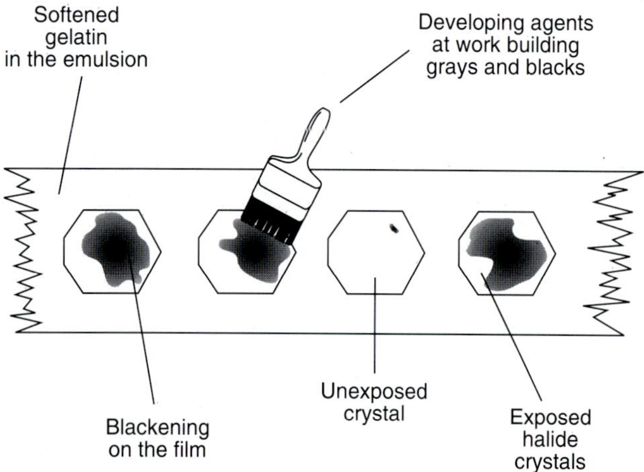


**FIGURE 6–11.** The developing agents (phenidone and hydroquinone) reduce the metallic silver to visible blackening on the film. The amount of blackening is dependent on the amount of exposure received by the film.

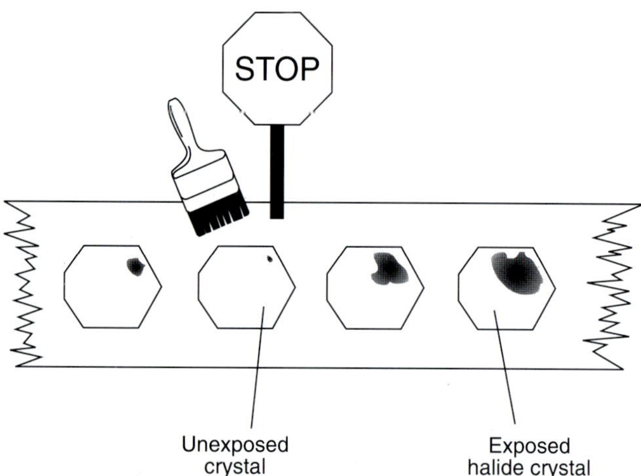


**FIGURE 6–13.** The restrainer serves as an antifog agent and restrains the developing agents from the development of the unexposed silver halide crystals.

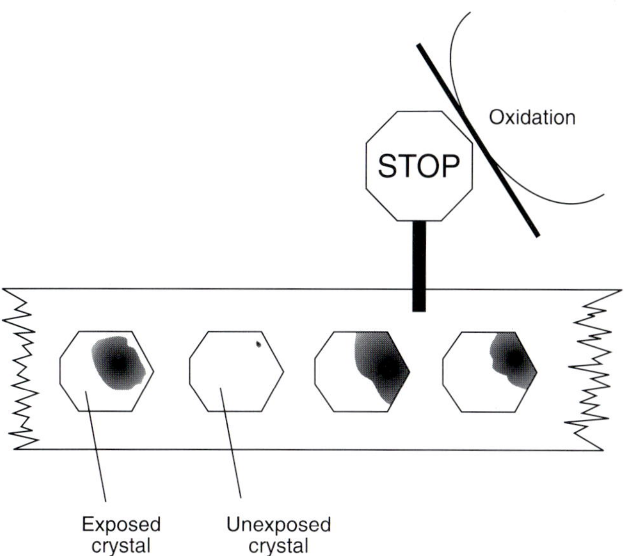



**FIGURE 6–14.** The preservative acts to reduce oxidation and extend the life of the developer.

**TABLE 6–2.** PROCESSOR SOLUTIONS

| Chemical | Function |
| --- | --- |
| ***Developer*** | |
| Phenidone | Reducing or developing agent. Builds gray tones |
| Hydroquinone | Reducing or developing agent. Builds blacks |
| Sodium carbonate | Accelerator. Facilitates the swell of the gelatin |
| Potassium bromide | Restrainer. Prevents overdevelopment |
| Sodium sulfite | Preservative. Reduces oxidation |
| ***Fixer*** | |
| Acetic acid | Acidifier. Neutralizes developer action |
| Ammonia thiosulfate | Clearing agent. Clears away unexposed halide crystals |
| Potassium alum | Hardener. Shrinks and hardens the emulsion |
| Sodium sulfite | Preservative. Prevents deterioration of chemicals and helps maintain chemical balance |

The fixer solution contains an acidifier, clearing agent, hardener, preservative, and water as the solvent for mixing the chemicals.

The fixer is an acid solution to counter the alkaline developer. Acetic acid is the acidifier used to neutralize the developer solution remaining in the wet emulsion. The immediate change in pH level stops further action by the reducing agents (Fig. 6–15).

because the dissolved silver is a polluting agent. The dissolved silver can be removed from the used fixer solution, after which the fixer may flow into a drainage system. See Table 6–2 for a summary of the fixer solution.

## THE FIXER SOLUTION NEUTRALIZES THE ACTION OF THE DEVELOPER AND HARDENS THE EMULSION.

The acidifier buffers the solution and enhances the action of the other chemicals in the fixer.

The unexposed silver halide crystals must be thoroughly cleared from the surface of the film to prevent further blackening as the film is later exposed to light for viewing. Ammonia thiosulfate is the clearing agent.

Potassium alum is the hardener that is added to shrink and harden the film emulsion.

The preservative is sodium sulfite. It is used to prevent deterioration of the clearing agent and maintain the chemical balance of the solution (Fig. 6–15).

The continuous use of the fixer causes a build-up of silver crystals that were dissolved and removed by the clearing agent. Replenishment brings fresh solution to the tank. Used fixer flows out of the tank; however, it cannot enter a drainage system

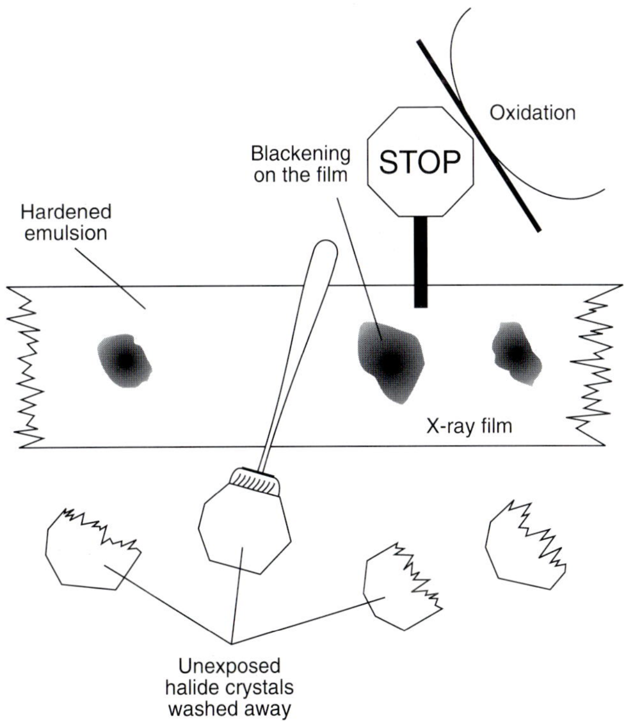



**FIGURE 6–15.** The fixer solution clears away the unexposed silver halide crystals and hardens the emulsion. After the film has been fixed, it is ready for drying.

## DAYLIGHT PROCESSING SYSTEM

A daylight processing system operates without the need for a conventional darkroom. The processor, with the attached film-loading device, operates in room light. It can be placed anywhere in the radiology department, ideally located next to the radiographic rooms.

DAYLIGHT SYSTEMS ELIMINATE THE NEED FOR CONVENTIONAL DARKROOMS.

Special cassettes are used to be compatible with the system. Unexposed x-ray film is stored in the

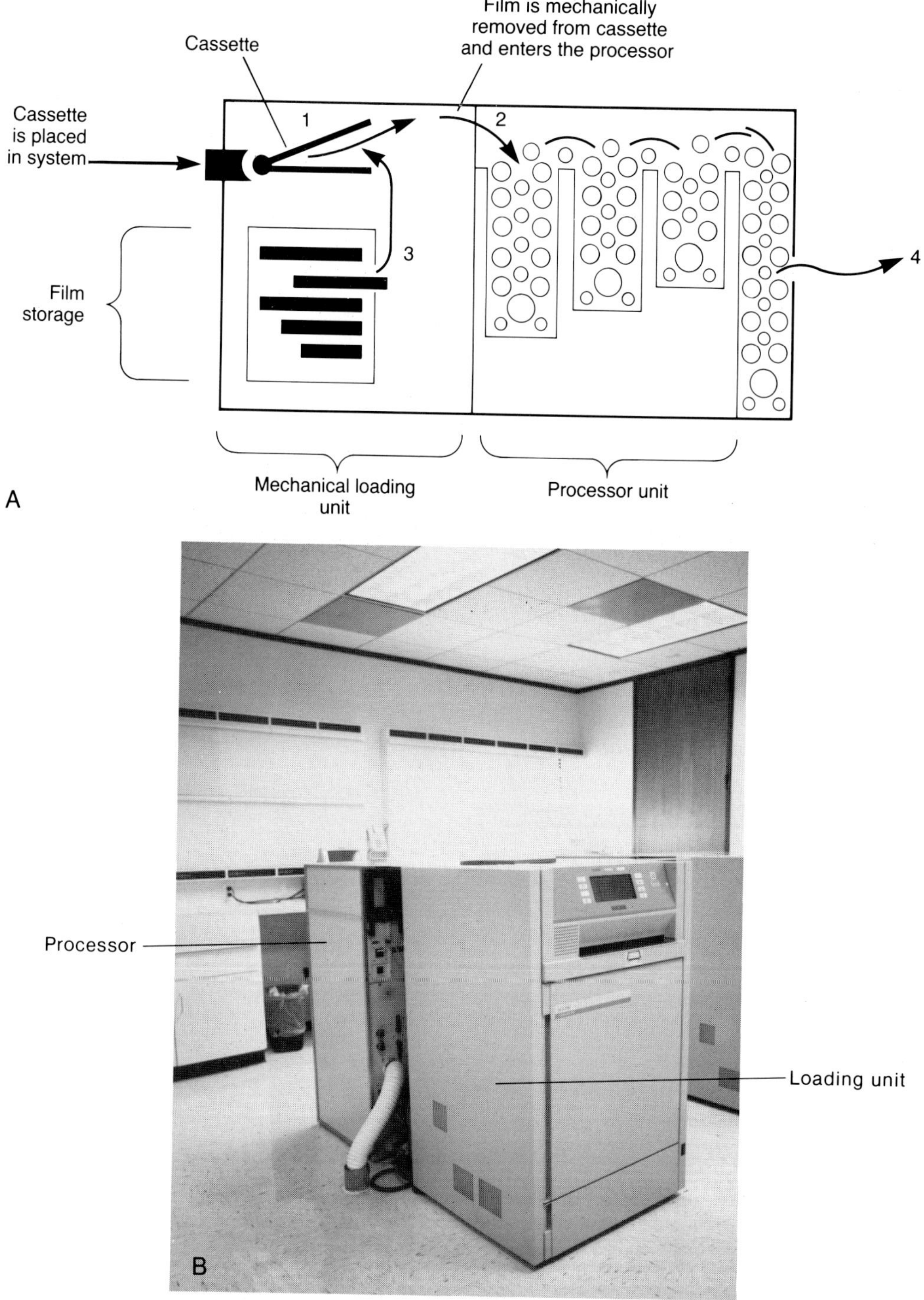



**FIGURE 6–16.** *A,* Daylight processing system. As the cassette is placed in the system, (1) the film is removed from the cassette. (2) The film moves by a transport device to the processor unit. (3) A new, unexposed film is placed in the cassette. (4) The finished radiograph exits the processor. *B,* Daylight system that includes the loading unit and the processor. As seen in this illustration, the daylight system can be located in the middle of the viewing area, using very little space and providing convenience for department personnel.

loading dispenser, as shown in Figure 6–16. The cassette is "fed" into the daylight system, where the film is mechanically removed and then an unexposed film is loaded into the cassette. The exposed film that was removed from the cassette is carried mechanically to the processor. After processing is complete, the film exits the system.

The daylight system eliminates the need for a darkroom with special safelights. The film is removed from the cassette and replaced with a new one without the aid of human hands.

The advantage is that a mechanical system attached to an automatic processor will remove the film from the cassette, load a new film, and move it into the processor without interaction by staff personnel. The system is more costly than a standard automatic processor; however, the need to build a conventional darkroom and train personnel is eliminated.

The disadvantages include mechanical breakdowns and artifacts caused by mechanical devices that move the film through the system.

## SILVER RECOVERY

Silver is a valuable substance that can be reclaimed from the fixer solution for recycling. It is also a polluting agent and must not be lost by allowing it to flow into a normal drainage system. The recovery of the dissolved silver from the used fixer makes silver available for recycling. This benefits the environment and serves as a supplemental financial resource for the radiology department.

---

SILVER IS A POLLUTING AGENT. THE RECOVERY OF SILVER FROM THE FIXER SOLUTION MAKES IT AVAILABLE FOR RECYCLING.

---

Special methods of recovery must be used because the silver has been dissolved by the clearing agent in the fixer. The amount of dissolved silver builds up in the fixer and, if it is not removed or reclaimed, the solution begins to lose its strength.

The two most commonly described methods for the recovery of silver are called electrolytic and chemical replacement. The electrolytic method uses an electric cathode, with a negative charge, immersed in a canister containing a positive charge. As the fixer solution passes through the canister, the positively charged silver ions are repelled by the canister and attracted by the cathode. The silver begins to separate from the solution and adhere to the cathode structure. The cathode structure must be removed from the canister frequently and the silver "chipped" off.

The reclaiming unit becomes part of the processing system. In a high-volume system, the used fixer is moved out of the processor by tubing into a holding tank, and from there it flows, at a constant rate, through tubes to the recovery unit. These units may be expensive to operate, and vendors provide a variety of services relating to the handling of the reclaimed silver.

Chemical replacement is the other, more common, method of recovering the silver from the fixer. This method uses a cartridge through which the fixer passes.

Inside of the cartridge is a canister with iron in the form of a very fine steel wool or a very fine screen mesh. As the dissolved silver flows through, it is attracted to the iron material and begins to build up on the mesh. Finally, the layers of the silver substance begin to break off and fall to the bottom of the tank, forming "sludge."

After a recommended volume of fixer passes through the cartridge, the inside canister is removed and replaced. The silver is recovered from the sludge. The cartridge is the more economic method for a recovery system.

# Technical Factors in Radiography

## CHAPTER OBJECTIVES

1. Define "technique."
2. List the four technical factors used to produce a radiographic image.
3. Define: kilovoltage (kV), milliampere (mA), milliam"pereseconds (mAs), time, and distance.
4. Explain the function of kilovoltage in the production of x-rays.
5. Discuss how kilovoltage affects wavelength and penetration of the x-ray photons.
6. Define kilovoltage peak (kVp).
7. Explain how kilovoltage affects the energy of the primary x-ray beam.
8. Describe the 15% rule, and explain how it will affect exposure to the film.
9. Describe the criteria to evaluate a radiograph for adequate penetration.
10. Explain how changes in kVp and mAs can be used to control the amount of exposure to the film.
11. Explain how mA and mAs contribute to the production of x-rays.
12. Explain how kilovoltage influences the production of scatter radiation.
13. Discuss mA and mAs as quantitative terms in x-ray production.
14. Define "focal spot blooming."
15. Calculate mAs with mA and time values.
16. Describe the relationship between mA and time.
17. Calculate mathematical problems using mA and time formula.
18. Describe the reciprocity law.
19. Explain how distance (FFD) affects exposure to the film.
20. Define the inverse square law.
21. Calculate mathematical problems using the inverse square law and mAs-distance formulas.
22. Differentiate between the inverse square law formula and mAs-distance formula, and explain how each is used by the radiographer.

## KEY WORDS AND TERMS

| | |
|---|---|
| Technique | Scatter radiation |
| Technical factors | Milliamperes |
| Sine wave | Milliam"pereseconds |
| Kilovoltage | Focal spot blooming |
| Kilovoltage wave pattern | Time (seconds) |
| Wavelength | Qualitative factor |
| Penetration | Quantitative factor |
| 15% rule | mA-time relationship |
| Underpenetration | mAs-distance relationship |
| Direct/proportional relationship | Reciprocity law |
| Inverse relationship | Distance (FFD) |
| Overexposure | Inverse square law |

# RECOMMENDATIONS FOR GENERAL DISCUSSION QUESTIONS

1. Name the technical factors in radiography, and describe how these factors contribute to the production of high-quality radiographs.
2. Outline the characteristics of kilovoltage, and explain how each factor affects the production of x-rays.
3. Describe mAs and its contribution to the production of x-rays.
4. How does kilovoltage influence the production of scatter radiation?
5. Explain the mathematical relationship of:
    - mA-time formula
    - mAs-distance formula
    - Inverse square law formula

Radiography is an art and a science. To produce radiographs, the radiographer operates equipment that will produce x-rays. To do so, the radiographer must be skilled in the use of "technique" factors that consistently produce good radiographs.

"Technique" is the systematic procedure used by the radiographer to accomplish the task of producing a high-quality radiograph. This systematic procedure includes the ability to select appropriate factors to produce an x-ray beam that will adequately penetrate the body part and provide the appropriate level of blackening (density) and subject contrast on the radiograph.

## TECHNIQUE IS THE SYSTEMATIC PROCEDURE USED TO PRODUCE A HIGH-QUALITY RADIOGRAPH.

To produce a radiograph, the radiographer selects and manipulates four significant factors—kilovoltage, milliamperes, exposure time, and distance. The knowledge of how all of these factors interrelate and combine with each other to produce a diagnostic radiograph is the science of radiography. Radiographers must understand how each factor functions in the production of x-rays, penetration of the human body parts, and absorption by body tissue, and how each factor produces changes in film density and subject contrast.

## KILOVOLTAGE

Kilovoltage is defined as the force applied to accelerate (push) the electrons from the cathode to the anode at the time of the exposure. If it was appropriate to select one factor, kilovoltage would be the most significant factor in the production of x-rays and radiographs. The selection of a particular kilovoltage setting affects the speed at which electrons travel from the cathode to the anode in the x-ray tube at the time of the exposure. In turn, the force behind the stream of electrons determines the speed at which the electrons "slam" into the focal spot (Fig. 7–1).

## KILOVOLTAGE IS THE FORCE THAT ACCELERATES THE ELECTRONS FROM THE CATHODE TO THE ANODE.

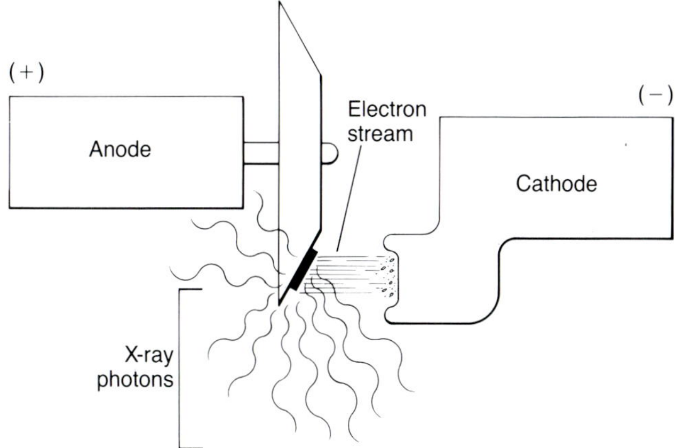


**FIGURE 7–1.** The kilovoltage selection determines the force or rate of acceleration of the electrons as they move to strike the target during the exposure. The greater the force of the electrons as they hit the target, the greater the percentage of high energy x-ray photons that will be produced.

Kilovoltage has a significant effect on the quality of the photons in the x-ray beam. The energy of the x-ray beam is determined by the kilovoltage peak selection made at the control panel.

## THE ENERGY OF THE X-RAY BEAM IS DETERMINED BY THE KILOVOLTAGE SELECTION.

The force produced by the voltage applied between the cathode and anode can be graphed, as illustrated by the wave pattern shown in Figure 7–2. The wave pattern produced by a single-phase x-ray generator at the time of the exposure is graphed in Figure 7–2C.

The waveform shows that as soon as voltage reaches its peak, it falls to zero. Only a portion of this waveform is useful in producing a radiograph. The highest level of energy, or crest of the waveform representing x-ray photon energy, is referred to as the kilovoltage peak, or kVp.

## THE KILOVOLTAGE PEAK IS THE CREST OF THE WAVEFORM THAT REPRESENTS PHOTON ENERGY.

The energy of the x-ray photons as they come from the focal spot can be illustrated by the concept of wavelength. As the x-ray photons travel through matter, they travel in wave-like fashion, as illustrated in Figure 7–3.

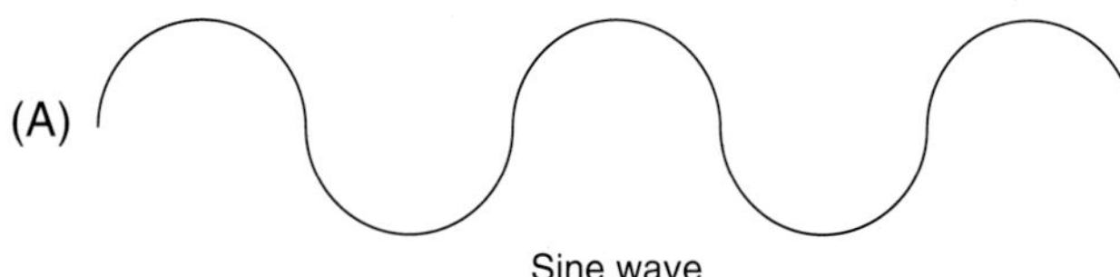

Sine wave

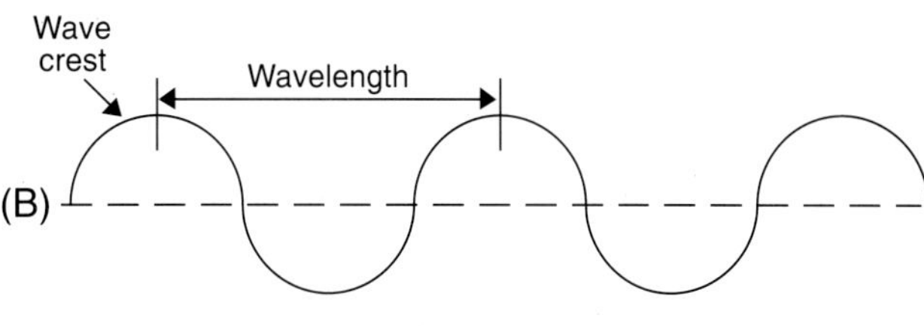

Wavelength measurement

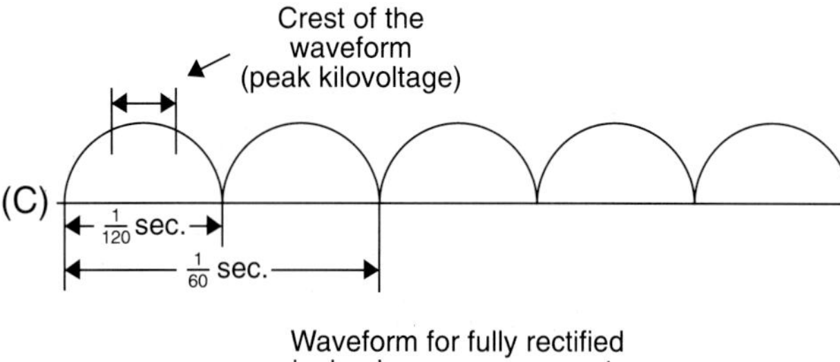

Waveform for fully rectified
single-phase x-ray generator

**FIGURE 7–2.** *A,* Sine wave representing kilovoltage. *B,* Wavelength measurement. Wavelength is measured from the crest of one wave to the crest of the next wave. As the kilovoltage increases, the wavelength is shorter. *C,* A waveform representing kilovoltage during an exposure using a fully rectified, single-phase x-ray generator. The useful portion of the wave is the crest or peak, called the kilovoltage peak, or kVp.

## X-RAY PHOTONS TRAVEL THROUGH MATTER IN WAVE-LIKE FASHION.

Wavelength describes one full wave pattern or cycle, as shown in Figure 7–3. Wavelength is the distance measured from the crest (or peak) of one wave to the crest of the next wave.

## WAVELENGTH IS THE DISTANCE FROM THE CREST OF A WAVE TO THE CREST OF THE NEXT WAVE.

As the energy of the x-ray photons increases, the crests of the waves are closer together, producing shorter wavelengths. Therefore, an increase in kilovoltage will produce x-ray photons of shorter wavelength.

## AN INCREASE IN KILOVOLTAGE WILL PRODUCE X-RAY PHOTONS OF SHORTER WAVELENGTH.

The kilovoltage selection determines the wavelength of the x-ray photons (refer to the diagram in Fig. 7–3 to review the concept of wavelength and energy). An increase in kilovoltage will produce shorter wavelength x-ray photons with greater ability to penetrate body tissue.

Kilovoltage is the factor that determines the energy of photons in the beam and the penetrating power of the beam. Figure 7–4 demonstrates how kVp affects penetration of thick and thin parts.

The illustration shown in Figure 7–4*A* and *B* demonstrates a low-energy x-ray beam. The radio-

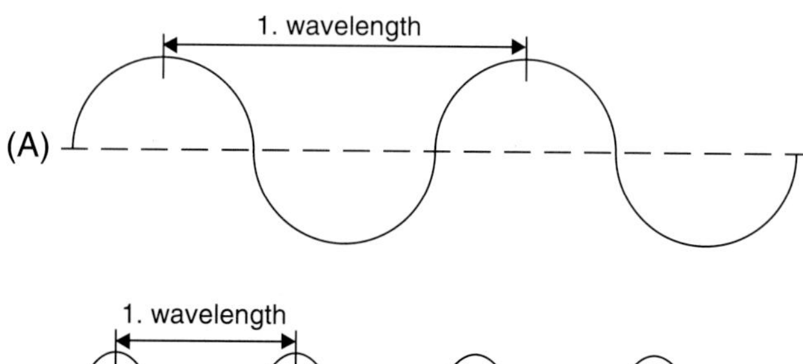

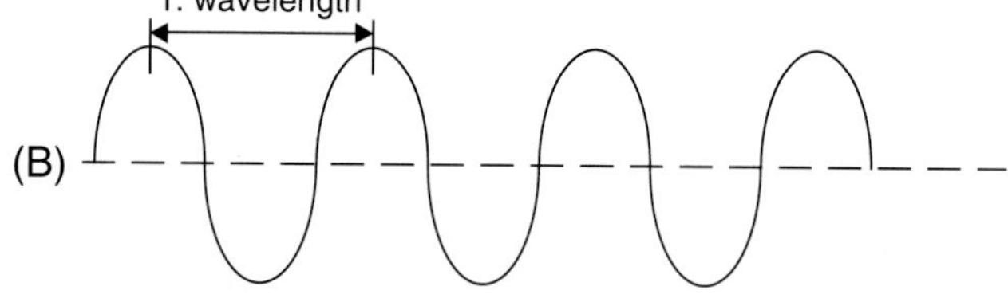

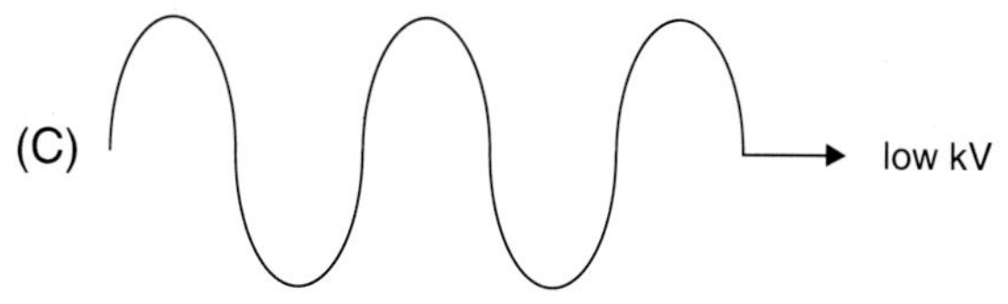

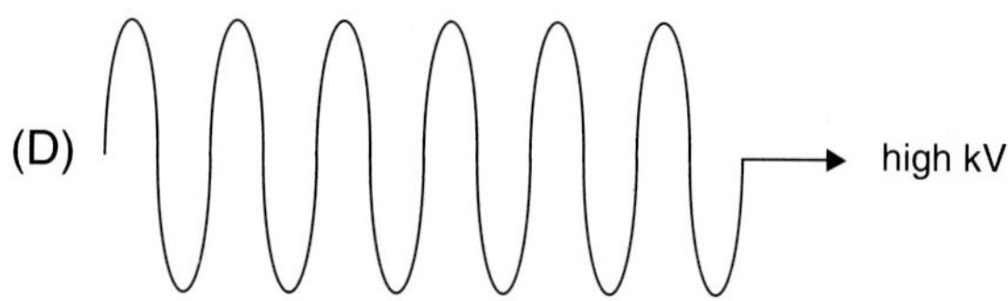

**FIGURE 7–3.** X-ray photons travel through matter in wavelike fashion. Changes in photon energy can be illustrated by wave patterns, as shown here. *A,* Long wavelength. *B,* Short wavelength. The kilovoltage selection will determine the wavelength of the x-ray photon. *C,* X-ray photon energy for lower kilovoltage selections. *D,* Wave pattern created by high kilovoltage. As kVp is increased, the wavelength decreases and the energy of the photon will be greater. Photons with shorter wavelength have greater energy and are more likely to penetrate the part to be imaged.

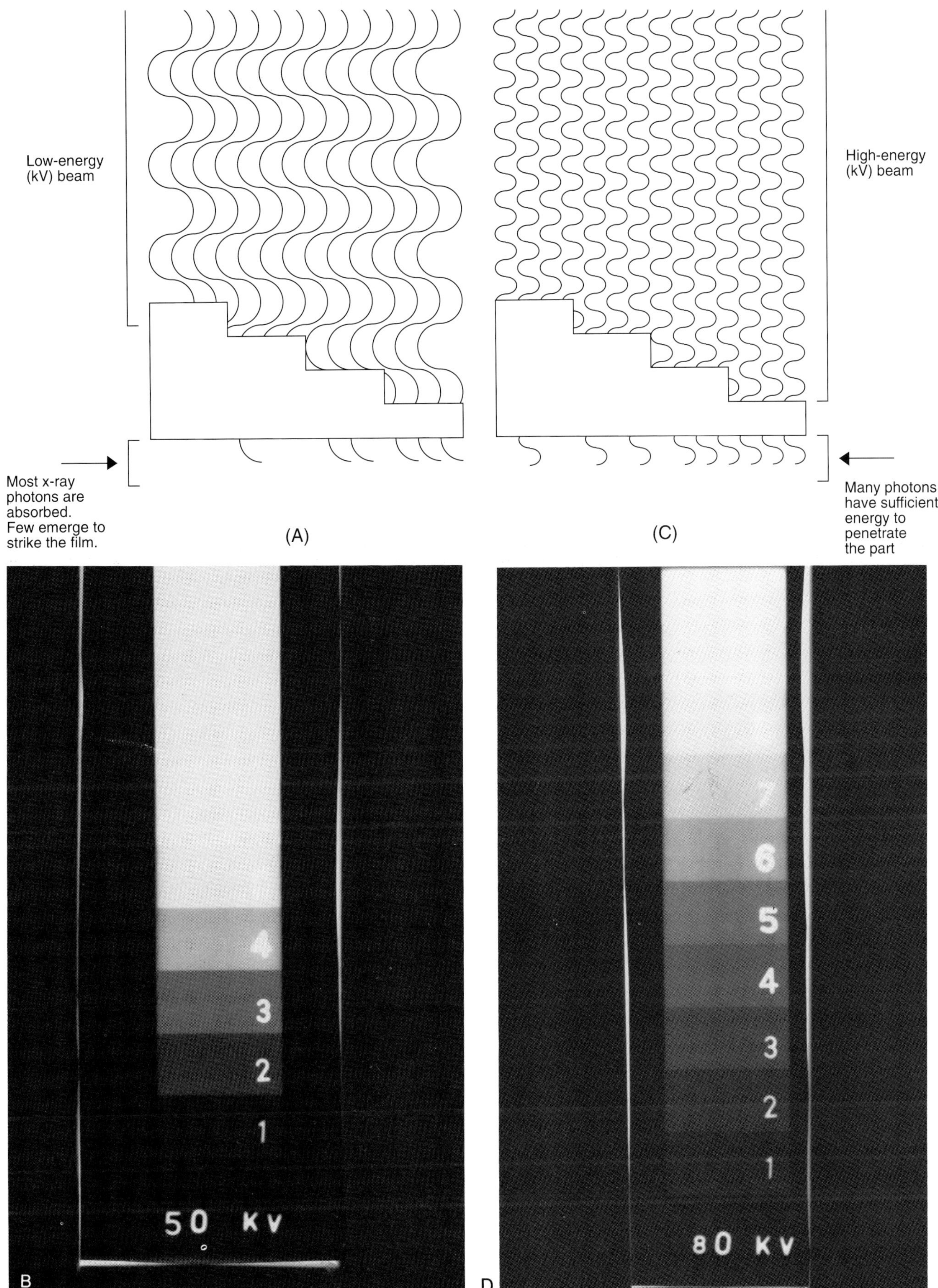


**FIGURE 7–4.** The kilovoltage selection determines the energy of the beam. *A* and *B*, A lower kV x-ray beam. The photons have a longer wavelength with less penetrating capability. *C* and *D*, A beam using higher kVp. The wavelength is shorter and more photons have penetrated the part.

graph of the penetrometer demonstrates that few areas have been completely penetrated. This situation results from an x-ray beam that has insufficient energy to penetrate the part. Figure 7–4C and D demonstrate how a higher energy (kVp) beam will penetrate more areas of the penetrometer.

Kilovoltage affects the intensity of the beam. As kilovoltage is increased, the intensity of the beam will increase. An increase in kVp results in more photons that have higher energy levels.

---

AN INCREASE IN KILOVOLTAGE PRODUCES MORE X-RAY PHOTONS THAT HAVE HIGHER ENERGY LEVELS.

---

## Fifteen Percent Rule

The effects of kVp on a radiograph are complex. An increase in kVp will increase the intensity of the beam and its penetrating ability. The increase in photon energy and beam intensity will result in an increase in the amount of radiation reaching the film. This will produce more blackening on the film.

For practical purposes, it is important to realize that an increase in kVp does not produce more x-rays to increase the blackening on the film. The increase in kVp increases the energy of the x-ray photons. It is this increase in energy that permits more x-rays to penetrate the body part, producing increased blackening on the film.

---

AS KILOVOLTAGE INCREASES, THE ABILITY OF THE X-RAY PHOTONS TO PENETRATE THE PART WILL INCREASE.

---

As a general rule, it has been considered that a 15% increase in the kilovoltage will result in doubling the amount of blackening on the film. The 15% rule is demonstrated in Figure 7–5.

---

AN INCREASE IN KILOVOLTAGE BY 15% WILL RESULT IN DOUBLING THE AMOUNT OF BLACKENING ON THE FILM.

---

With the use of the 15% rule, radiographers are able to control the overall blackening levels on the film when it is necessary to make changes in the kVp selection.

---

EXAMPLE:

A radiograph is made using 70 kVp. After the radiograph has been reviewed, the decision is made to increase the blackening on the film. A second exposure is made using a 15% increase in kVp. The new selection would be 81 kVp.

To calculate:

15% is written as 0.15
15% of 70          $0.15 \times 70 = 10.5$
Add 10.5 to the original kVp
$70 + 10.5 = 80.5$ kVp

The reduction of kVp by 15% will reduce the blackening on the film by approximately one half.

---

A DECREASE IN KILOVOLTAGE BY 15% WILL REDUCE THE BLACKENING ON THE FILM BY ONE HALF.

---

EXAMPLE:

15% of 70          $0.15 \times 70 = 10.5$
Subtract 10.5 from original kVp
$70 - 10.5 = 59.5$ kVp

The 15% rule is a nonlinear and nonproportional relationship; however, it serves the radiographer well as a practical application tool when changes in kVp are necessary in order to control the amount of exposure to the film (Fig. 7–5).

Caution must be exercised by the radiographer when kVp is the factor of choice used to decrease the amount of blackening on the film. A significant reduction in kVp may result in the energy of the x-ray photons becoming inadequate to penetrate the body part of interest. The kilovoltage selected must be adequate to penetrate the part.

## Penetration of the Part

The phrase "penetration of the part" must be clearly understood in the application of kVp principles. Penetration of the part means the kVp selected is adequate for producing x-ray photons that have sufficient energy to pass through the part and emerge as remnant radiation to strike the film. Figure 7–6 represents an example of underpenetration compared with adequate penetration.

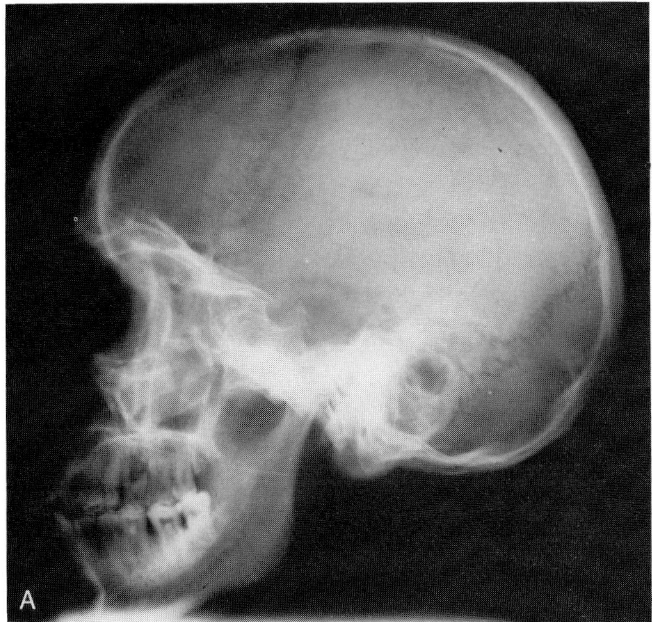 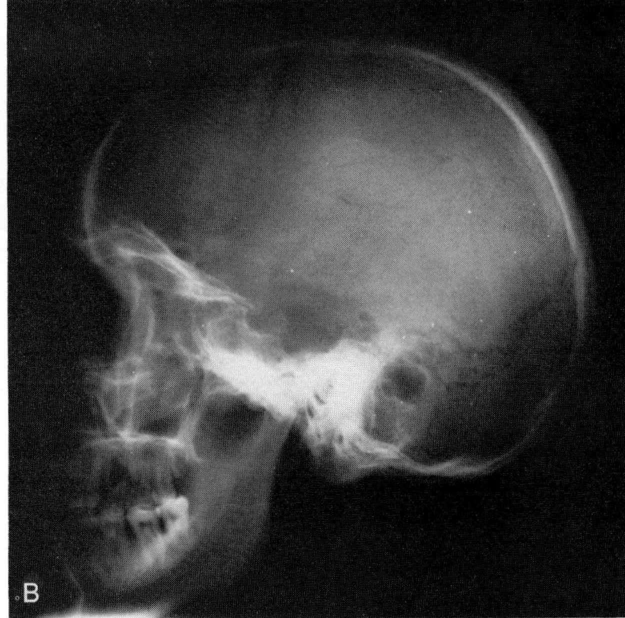

**FIGURE 7–5.** An increase in kVp of 15% will double the amount of blackening on the film. *A*, Radiograph using 70 kVp. *B*, Radiograph made with a 15% increase in kilovoltage (or 81 kV). The amount of blackening on the film (density) increases with an increase in kilovoltage.

PENETRATION OF THE PART MEANS THE X-RAY PHOTONS HAVE SUFFICIENT ENERGY TO PASS THROUGH THE PART AND EMERGE AS REMNANT RADIATION.

Selections below 60 kVp may not be adequate to penetrate the part, and the fine markings of the skeletal tissue that comprise the bones of the knee would not be visible. Hairline fractures would be overlooked if penetration of the object were not adequate.

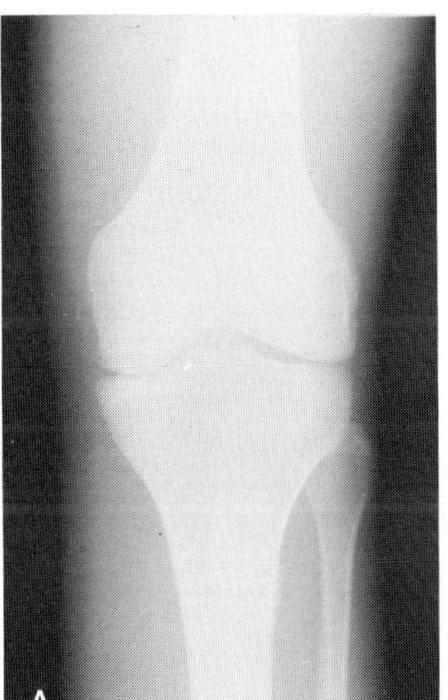 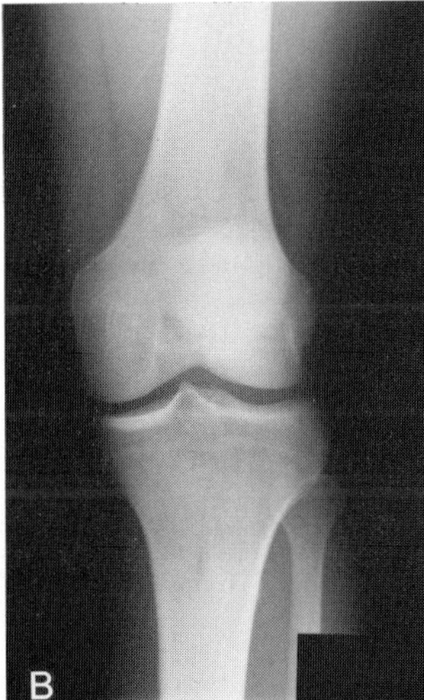

**FIGURE 7–6.** *A*, Inadequate penetration of the part is demonstrated. *B*, Radiograph of the knee with adequate penetration.

In many situations, kVp would not be the factor of choice to control blackening on the film. Once adequate penetration is achieved for the average thickness of a body part, kVp remains essentially the same even if the thickness and volume of body tissue are less than or more than average. The mA or mAs would serve as the major controlling factors for blackening on the film. Conditions for the radiographer at the time of exposure are not always optimal. Alternatives in the use of the technical factors must be available.

## Relationship Between Kilovoltage Peak and Milliamperseconds

When adjustment of the technique factors is necessary, a decrease in kVp can be compensated for by an increase in milliamperseconds (mAs), and vice versa. The general rule for the mAs and kVp relationship is: A decrease in kVp by 15% may be compensated for by doubling the mAs; or an increase in kVp by 15% may be compensated for by decreasing the mAs by one half (Fig. 7–7).

A DECREASE IN KILOVOLTAGE BY 15% WILL DECREASE THE BLACKENING ON THE FILM IN THE SAME MANNER AS REDUCING THE MILLIAMPERESECONDS BY ONE HALF.

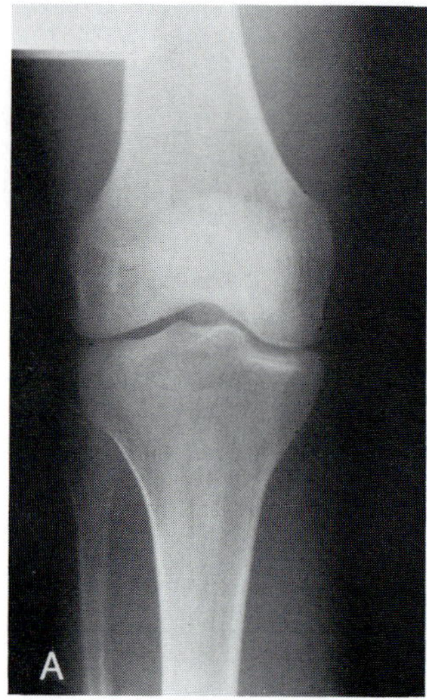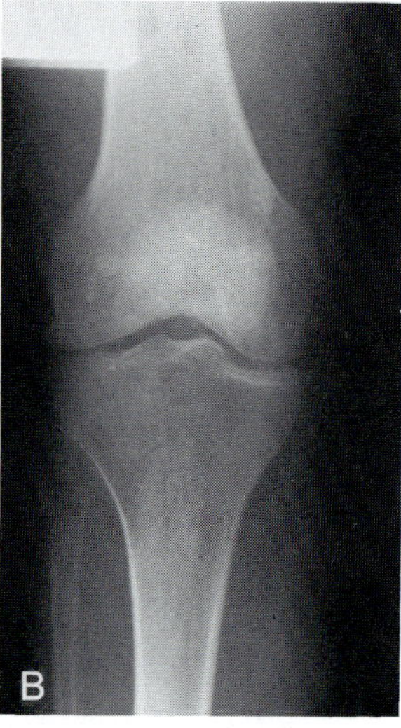

**FIGURE 7–7.** The kVp-mAs relationship is demonstrated in these two radiographs. *A*, Radiograph made using 70 kVp and 20 mAs (100-speed system). *B*, Radiograph produced using 80 kVp and 10 mAs (100-speed system). Although there is a small visible difference in the gray tones, the overall density is approximately the same.

AN INCREASE IN KILOVOLTAGE BY 15% WILL INCREASE THE BLACKENING ON THE FILM IN THE SAME MANNER AS DOUBLING THE MILLIAMPERESECONDS.

EXAMPLE:

A radiograph is made using 80 kVp and 100 mAs. A request is made to make a second exposure with lower kVp but to maintain the same overall blackening on the film.

Change kVp by 15%
15% of 80       $0.15 \times 80 = 12$
$80 - 12 = 68$ kVp
Double the mAs
$100 \times 2 = 200$ mAs
New factors are 68 kVp and 200 mAs

When using these practical rules, it must be understood that increases in the mAs *do not* result in an increase in the penetration of the x-ray beam. An increase in the mAs cannot compensate for inadequate kVp selection.

Kilovoltage selections that are too high do not produce "overpenetration." To penetrate means to break through the object. Therefore, the x-ray photons that hit an object and pass on through have penetrated the object. If sufficient energy is not present, the photon weakens and becomes absorbed by the object. Either the part is adequately penetrated by the x-ray photons or underpenetration is present. If the amount of blackening on the film is excessive, the film has been "overexposed," as demonstrated in Figure 7–8B.

## Scatter Radiation

Kilovoltage is a factor in the production of scatter radiation. As x-ray photons strike the body part, interactions take place. In diagnostic radiology, two predominant interactions occur—Compton scattering and the photoelectric effect. The specific details of these complex atomic interactions are beyond the scope of this textbook.

Generally, as kVp is increased, the probability of Compton interactions increases. A Compton interaction results in an x-ray photon undergoing a change in direction. If sufficient energy exists, the scattered x-ray photon may strike another object. Because of the interaction at the atomic level, the photon may exit the body part traveling in a direction different from its original straight-line path.

Radiation produced as a result of Compton interactions is called scatter (Fig. 7–8).

Scatter radiation exits the body traveling in many different directions and with different energies.

SCATTER RADIATION EXITS THE BODY AND TRAVELS IN DIFFERENT DIRECTIONS WITH MANY ENERGY LEVELS.

Scatter radiation is a danger to the patient and the radiographer, and a detriment to film quality. The object being imaged becomes the source for scatter radiation. For this reason, radiographers must be shielded from the patient when exposures are made.

SCATTER RADIATION IS A DANGER TO THE PATIENT AND THE RADIOGRAPHER, AND IT BECOMES A DETRIMENT TO FILM QUALITY.

Reduction in kilovoltage will reduce Compton interactions; however, another type of interaction called the photoelectric effect may occur. The pho-

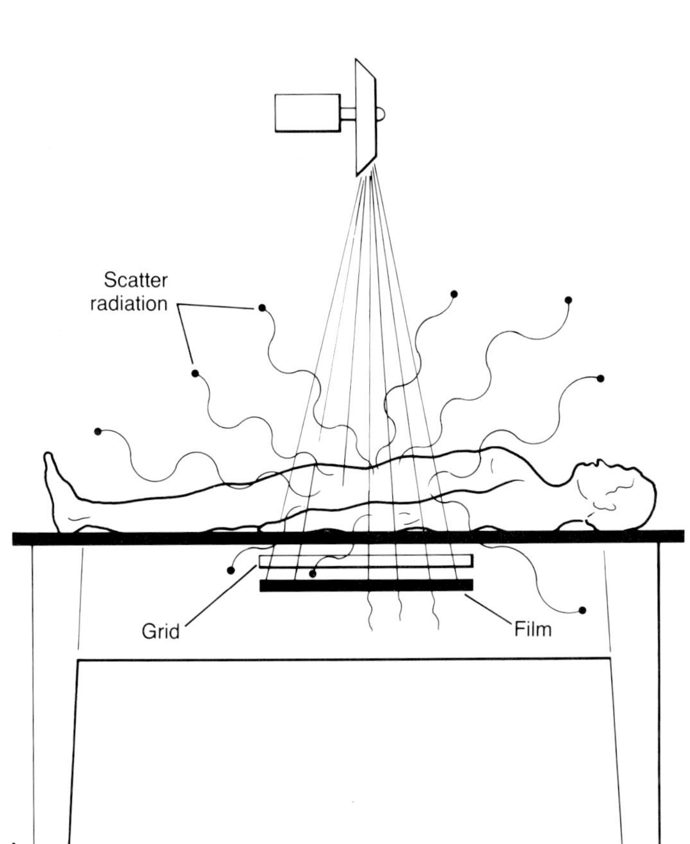
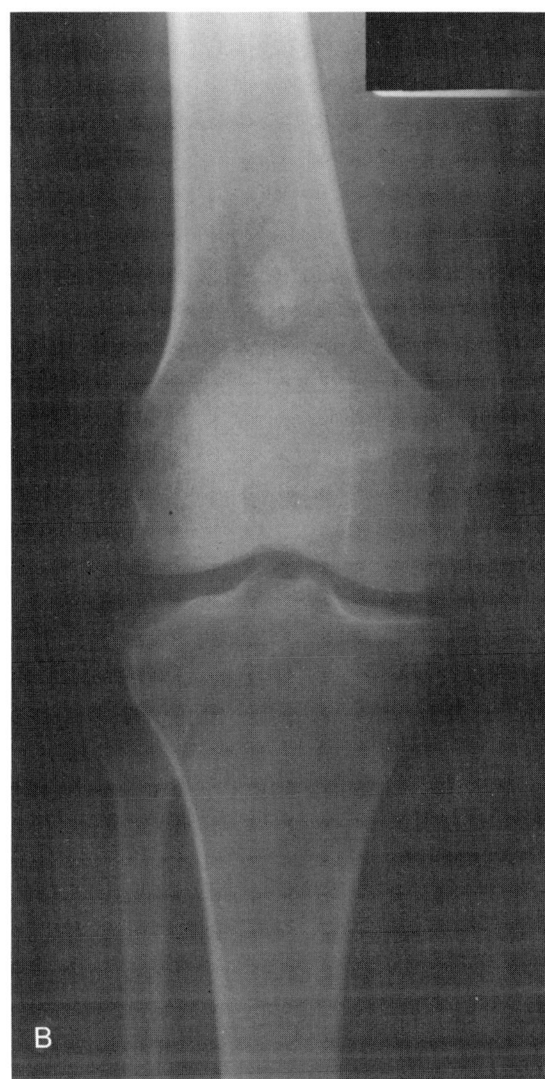



**FIGURE 7–8.** *A,* As the x-ray photons interact with the body, scatter radiation is produced traveling in many directions and with different energies. *B,* Radiograph of the knee produced with a kVp selection of 85. The film is overexposed; in addition, the beam was not adequately restricted. An overall gray tone is present, resulting from excessive scatter radiation reaching the film.

toelectric effect becomes more prominent when lower energy x-ray photons are present.

When a photoelectric interaction occurs, the x-ray photon involved does not have sufficient energy to penetrate the body part. The photon is absorbed by the body tissue. This description is oversimplified, but an atomic interaction takes place that produces a change in the electron configuration at the atomic level. The result is a free electron and the production of a low energy x-ray photon called characteristic radiation. Again, the patient is the source. The characteristic radiation produced by the photoelectric effect has very little effect on film quality. It is primarily absorbed by the patient. An increase in the photoelectric interactions increases the amount of exposure to the patient, as shown in Figure 7–9.

## THE CHARACTERISTIC RADIATION PRODUCED BY THE PHOTOELECTRIC EFFECT IS MOSTLY ABSORBED BY THE PATIENT.

Characteristic and scatter radiation, produced as x-rays interact with body tissue, become major factors in the practice of radiography. Radiographers stand behind walls or glass containing lead that shields them from scatter radiation. The lead serves as a protection device by absorbing the x-rays. There are many accessories and techniques that are used to control the effects of scatter radiation, and these will be discussed in later chapters of this book.

A minimum of exposure to the patient and the

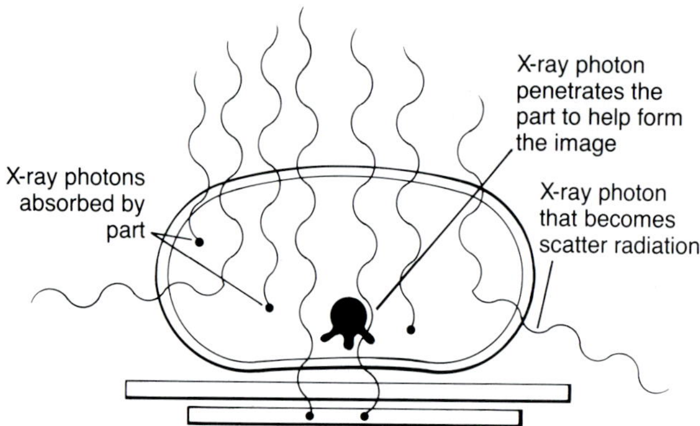


**FIGURE 7–9.** To help form the image, the x-ray beam interacts with the body by (1) absorption, (2) production of scatter radiation, and (3) penetration.

highest quality radiograph are the key objectives in the selection of technique factors. The kVp selection will affect the amount of scatter and characteristic radiation produced and the amount of radiation absorbed by the patient. In general, higher kVp settings reduce the amount of x-ray photons absorbed by the patient, and lower kVp settings increase the amount of radiation absorbed by the patient. Higher kVp selections will also increase the amount of scatter radiation exposing the film. The energy of the scatter radiation will be greater, increasing the chance that it will exit the patient and reach the film.

---

AS KILOVOLTAGE INCREASES, THE AMOUNT OF RADIATION ABSORBED BY THE PATIENT IS REDUCED.

---

### Film Quality

When one evaluates film quality, one recognizes kVp as the controlling factor of radiographic contrast. Increases in kVp produce more scatter radiation that will affect the film adversely. Increased scatter produces more fog on the film, and contrast is reduced. Some scatter is necessary for adequate film blackening. Scatter photons may account for as much as 50 to 80% of the photons exposing the film.

A decrease in kVp increases the probability of photon absorption. With lower kVp, there will be less fog on the film, resulting in an increase in radiographic contrast.

---

KILOVOLTAGE IS THE CONTROLLING FACTOR OF RADIOGRAPHIC CONTRAST.

---

## MILLIAMPERES

The second important technique factor is milliamperes (mA). Milliampere is defined as the current flow through the cathode filament at the time of the exposure. As described in Chapter 3, the amount of mA selected at the time of the exposure controls the current flow through the cathode filament. An increase in mA will increase the current flow, and the temperature of the filament will rise. As the filament temperature rises, the number of electrons released from the filament (thermionic emission) will increase.

---

MILLIAMPERES REPRESENTS THE CURRENT FLOW THROUGH THE CATHODE FILAMENT AT THE TIME OF THE EXPOSURE.

---

An increase in mA yields a greater number of electrons in the space charge available for producing x-ray photons. The increase in mA will increase the amount of x-ray photons produced at the anode target. An increase or decrease in mA is represented as a quantitative factor. It is important to understand that an increase in mA does not affect the energy of the photons produced at the target. The purpose of increasing mA is to increase the number of electrons available to travel from the cathode to the anode, producing more x-ray photons.

---

AN INCREASE IN MILLIAMPERES WILL INCREASE THE NUMBER OF X-RAY PHOTONS IN THE PRIMARY BEAM.

---

In the evaluation of radiographs, one can expect to see a proportional relationship between film blackening and the mA selected. If the mA is doubled, for example from 200 to 400, the amount of blackening on the film is doubled (Fig. 7–10).

---

A DOUBLING OF THE MILLIAMPERES WILL DOUBLE THE AMOUNT OF BLACKENING ON THE FILM.

---

If the mA is changed from 200 to 100, the amount of blackening on the film is reduced by one half. Changes in the amount of blackening on the film

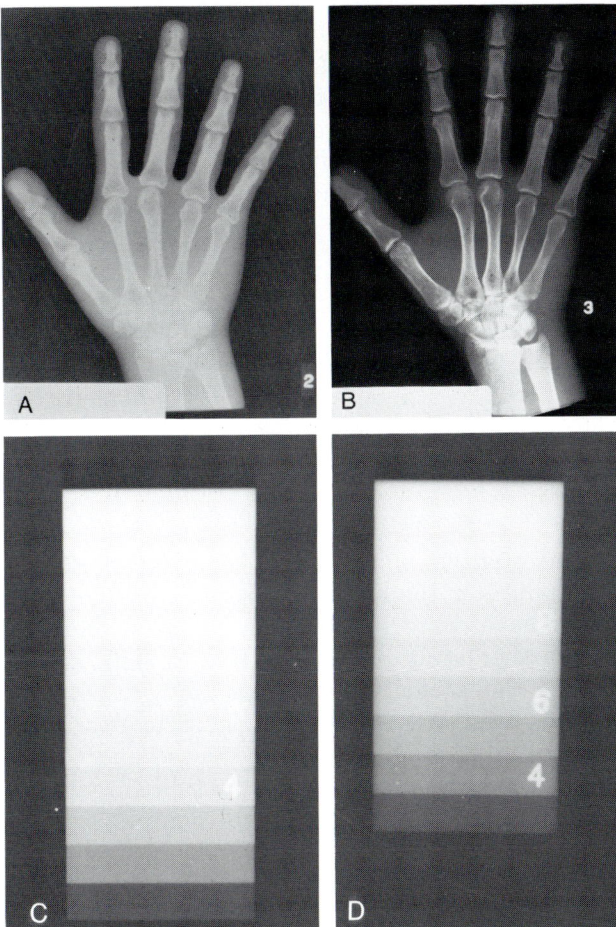

**FIGURE 7–10.** An increase in mA will result in an increase in the number of photons in the beam. *A* and *B* were made using a hand phantom. *A* was exposed using 5 mAs and *B* was exposed using 10 mAs. The radiograph shown in *B* has increased density as a result of the increase in mAs. *C* and *D* represent the change in the x-ray beam as mAs is increased. As the mAs is increased, the number of photons in the primary x-ray beam will increase proportionally.

can be subtle. Therefore, the increase or decrease in mA must be great enough to produce a visible change in the amount of blackening on the film. Generally, a change of at least 30 to 35% must be made to see a change in blackening on the film.

Milliamperes is the factor of choice to control the amount of blackening on the film. The mA can be manipulated to control blackening without producing significant changes in scatter radiation. However, an increase in the mA will generally increase the amount of exposure absorbed by the patient.

## Focal Spot "Blooming"

Milliampere and kilovoltage selections may affect the function and size of the focal spot. The "blooming" effect is an increase in the actual focal spot size with an increase in tube current. Significant

increases in the mA may produce focal spot blooming.

FOCAL SPOT BLOOMING IS AN INCREASE IN THE FOCAL SPOT SIZE WHEN THE TUBE CURRENT INCREASES.

The actual focal spot size will decrease slightly with an increase in kVp. Focal spot size is a factor in producing a high-quality radiograph; therefore, blooming caused by high tube currents may affect the radiograph adversely. Focal spot blooming can be reduced by lower mA and higher kVp settings.

## TIME

Exposure time (S) is the technical factor that sets the length of the time for an exposure. It is also a quantitative factor that, when combined with mA, determines the exposure rate.

TIME IS THE FACTOR THAT CONTROLS THE LENGTH OF THE EXPOSURE.

$$\text{Milliamperes} \times \text{Time} = \text{Milliampereseconds}$$
$$\text{mA} \times \text{S} = \text{mAs}$$

Once the radiographer understands the basic concepts related to mA and time, the factors are combined as mAs and recognized as a single quantitative factor. An increase in mAs increases the amount of x-ray photons exposing the film.

The mA and time relationship is inversely proportional. Because mAs is considered as one value in the selection of exposure factors, the two factors relate to one another inversely. This means that an increase in mA requires a decrease in the exposure time. This would be necessary to maintain the same exposure value and essentially the same amount of blackening on the film.

mAs and time relationship:

$$\frac{\text{mA}_1}{\text{mA}_2} = \frac{\text{S}_2}{\text{S}_1}$$

$S_1$ and $mA_1$ represent factors of the first or original exposure; $S_2$ and $mA_2$ represent the factors for the new exposure. The mAs in the two exposures must remain the same.

EXAMPLE:

A radiograph is made with the following factors: 200 mA, 0.2 S, 90 kVp. A second radiograph must be made with the same mAs and kVp, but with 500 mA. What will be the new exposure time?

Calculate:

$$\frac{200}{500} = \frac{X}{0.2}$$

$$500X = 40.0$$

$$\frac{500X}{500} = \frac{40}{500}$$

$$X = \frac{40}{500}$$

$$X = 0.08 \text{ S}$$

The new factors are 500 mA and 0.08 S (80 milliseconds).

In the example given above, both exposures have the same quantity of radiation in the primary beam because both are made with 40 mAs. This principle is expressed in the reciprocity law first described by the late Arthur Fuchs. The reciprocity law states that blackening on the film remains constant as long as the total energy exposing the film is constant. Proper calibration of the equipment is necessary to produce dependable results when time and/or mA changes must be made. Fast film-screen systems such as rare earth would also affect the results.

---

THE RECIPROCITY LAW INDICATES THAT BLACKENING ON THE FILM REMAINS CONSTANT AS LONG AS THE TOTAL ENERGY EXPOSING THE FILM IS CONSTANT.

---

The mA-time relationship, as described by the reciprocity law, fails with screen exposures of less than 10 milliseconds and more than 6 or 7 seconds.

Time, like mA, has no effect on the penetrating ability of the photons. It is considered a quantitative factor. Short exposure times are necessary to prevent body motion during the exposure. Longer exposures increase the risk of motion, which is detrimental to film quality.

## DISTANCE

Distance is measured from the focal spot to the recording medium (x-ray film) and is called the focal-film distance (FFD). The FFD is also called the source-to-image distance (SID). In most diagnostic departments, the FFD is standardized for all procedures. In general radiography, the FFD is 40 to 42 inches, and in radiography of the structures of the thoracic cavity, the FFD is usually 72 inches (Fig. 7–11).

---

DISTANCE REPRESENTS THE LENGTH OF SPACE FROM THE FOCAL SPOT TO THE RECORDING MEDIUM.

---

The intensity of the x-ray beam is affected by the changes in the FFD. As described in Chapter 4, x-rays have characteristics similar to visible light. The farther away one moves from a light source, the less the intensity becomes as the light is spread over a larger area. The same characteristics exist with x-radiation. X-rays are produced at the focal spot of the x-ray tube and exit the tube through the tube port. As the photons travel from the focal spot to the film, the intensity becomes less and they diverge from the point of origin. The relationship

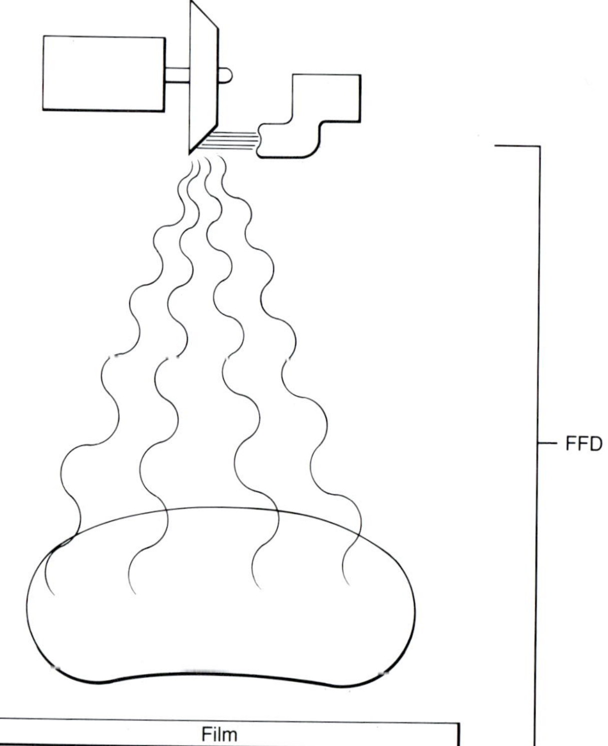


**FIGURE 7–11.** The distance from the focal spot to the film or other recording medium is the focal-film distance (FFD).

can be explained by the inverse square law. When the distance is doubled, the same number of photons is spread over an area four times as large, resulting in an intensity, at any given point, that is now one fourth the original intensity (Fig. 7–12).

---

WHEN THE FFD IS DOUBLED, THE SAME NUMBER OF PHOTONS IS SPREAD OVER AN AREA FOUR TIMES THE ORIGINAL AREA, AND THE INTENSITY OF THE BEAM IS REDUCED TO ONE FOURTH OF THE ORIGINAL INTENSITY.

---

## Inverse Square Law

The inverse square law is the guide for understanding how changes in focal-film distance affect the intensity of the x-ray beam. The law states that radiation intensity will vary inversely with the square of the distance from the source. This means that as the distance increases, the beam intensity will decrease in proportion to the square of the distance. When this law is applied to the process of producing radiographs, arbitrary changes in the FFD will affect the amount of exposure to the film. An increase in FFD will result in less exposure to the film, and a decrease in FFD will result in more exposure to the film. The FFD should be standardized for all procedures, or the results will vary, often resulting in a radiograph that is not acceptable because of the lack of diagnostic value.

Inverse square law formula:

$$\frac{I_1}{I_2} = \frac{D_2{}^2}{D_1{}^2}$$

where:

$I_1$ = the original beam intensity
$I_2$ = the new intensity
$D_1{}^2$ = the original distance squared
$D_2{}^2$ = the new distance squared

Note: beam intensity is measured in roentgens (R).

---

EXAMPLE:

A radiographer makes an exposure using the standard FFD of 40 inches. An ionization chamber measures the radiation at 40 inches to read 5R. The same exposure is made with the measurement taken at 45 inches from the focal spot. What is the radiation intensity (R) at 45 inches FFD?

Calculate:

$$\frac{5R}{X} = \frac{45^2}{40^2}$$

$$\frac{5R}{X} = \frac{2025}{1600}$$

$$2025X = 8000$$

$$\frac{2025X}{2025} = \frac{8000}{2025}$$

$$X = \frac{8000}{2025}$$

$$X = 3.95R$$

The result demonstrates that as the distance from the source increases, the beam intensity will decrease. Although understanding these changes in the beam intensity is important, the application in the radiographic room must be more practical. The radiographer needs to know how and which changes in the exposure factors must be made when variations in the FFD occur. This becomes an important concept in mobile radiography, where the FFD often cannot be standardized.

The inverse square law provides a means to understand how the amount of exposure to the film can be affected when there is a variation in the distance between the focal spot and the film. A practical adoption of this concept can be used in the mAs and distance formula.

mAs and distance relationship:

$$\frac{mAs_1}{mAs_2} = \frac{D_1{}^2}{D_2{}^2}$$

where:

$mAs_1$ = the mAs for the original exposure
$mAs_2$ = the mAs for the new exposure
$D_1{}^2$ = original FFD squared
$D_2{}^2$ = new FFD squared

This formula shows a relationship where the mAs needed for an exposure is directly proportional to the square of the FFD. As the distance (FFD) is increased, the mAs must also increase to maintain adequate blackening on the film.

---

AS THE DISTANCE INCREASES, THE mAs MUST ALSO INCREASE TO MAINTAIN ADEQUATE BLACKENING ON THE FILM.

---

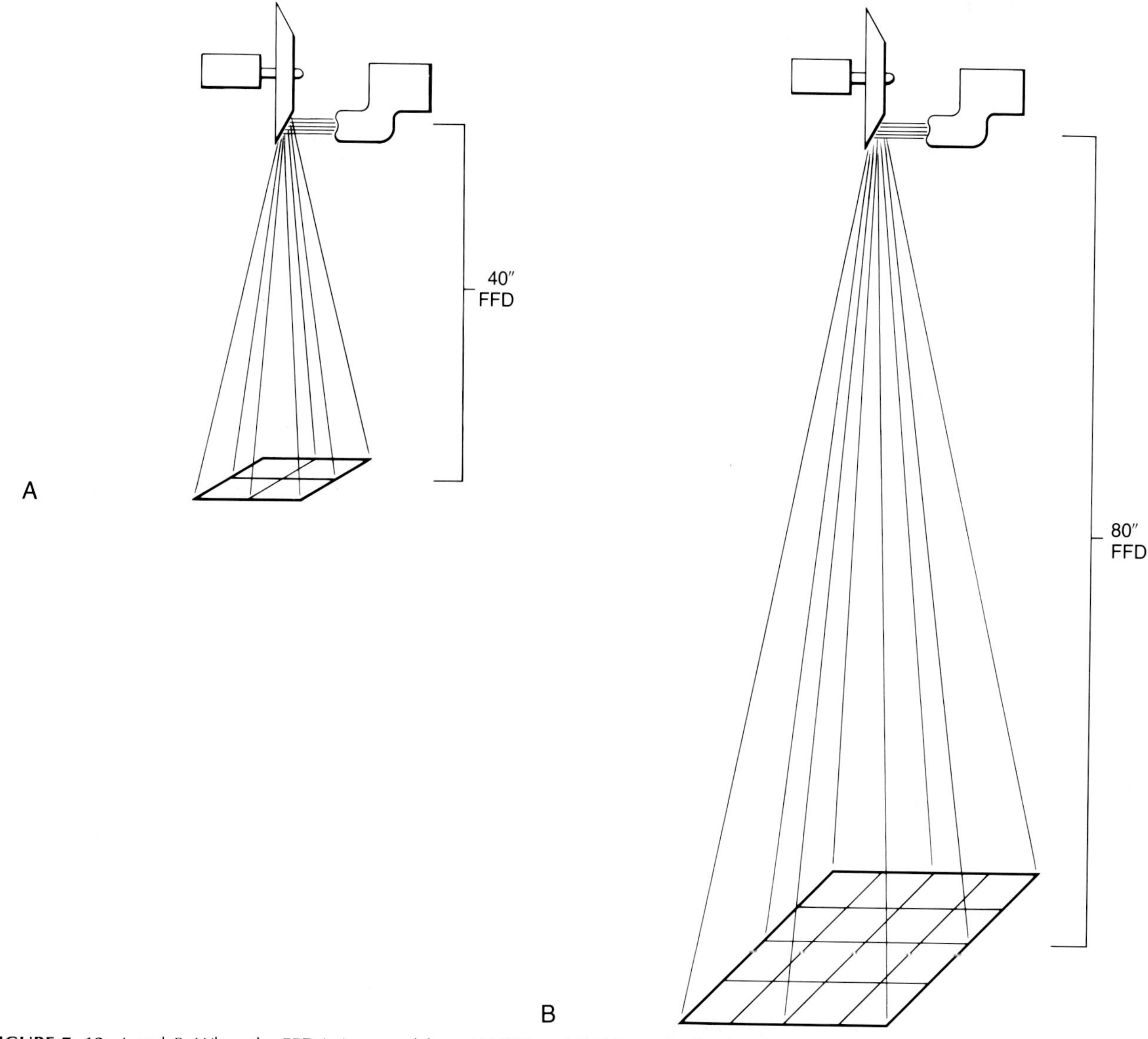



**FIGURE 7–12.** *A* and *B,* When the FFD is increased from 40" FFD to 80" FFD (with all other factors remaining the same), the same amount of radiation is spread over an area that is four times the area covered at 40" FFD. At 80" FFD, the beam intensity is one fourth the intensity of the beam at 40" FFD. As the FFD increases, the beam intensity will decrease.

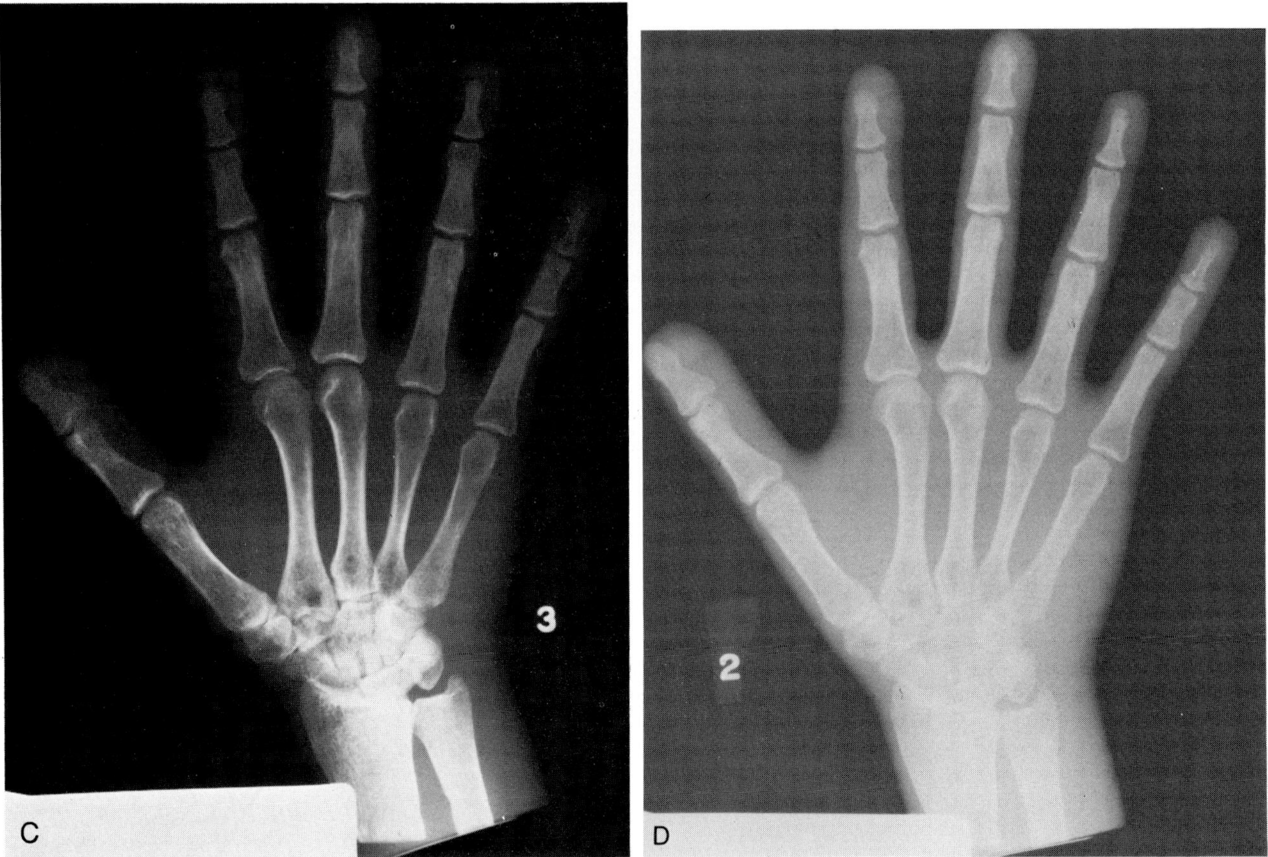

**FIGURE 7–12** *Continued C,* Radiograph exposed using a 36″ FFD. *D,* The same hand phantom exposed using a 72″ FFD without an increase in the exposure factors. The result reveals that the film made at 72″ FFD has one fourth the density of the radiograph exposed at 36″ FFD.

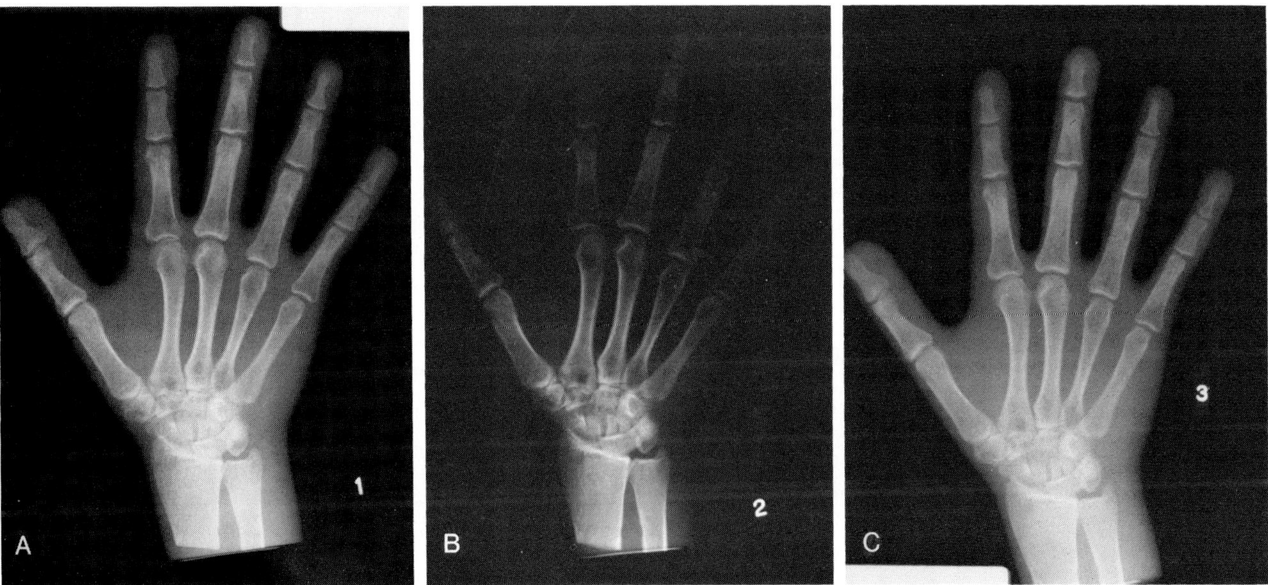

**FIGURE 7–13.** The mAs-distance relationship is an important concept in understanding how to change exposure factors when the FFD must be changed. *A,* Radiograph exposed using 72″ FFD and 10 mAs. *B,* Radiograph made by adjusting the x-ray tube to produce an FFD of 36″ with no change in the exposure factors. *C,* Another radiograph of the hand made with 36″ FFD; however, the mAs was reduced to one fourth of the original mAs (2.5 mAs).

EXAMPLE:

A radiographer exposes a patient's chest at bedside in the PA projection using 3 mAs, 75 kVp, and 72-inch FFD. A second radiograph is required, but as a result of a change in the patient's condition, only a 54-inch FFD can be used because the radiography must be performed with the patient in the supine position. What is the new mAs for the second exposure?

Calculate:

$$\frac{3 \text{ mAs}}{X} = \frac{72^2 \text{ FFD}}{54^2 \text{ FFD}}$$

$$\frac{3}{X} = \frac{5184}{2916}$$

$$5184X = 8748$$

$$X = \frac{8748}{5184}$$

$$X = 1.69 \text{ mAs}$$

With the application of the mAs-distance formula, the radiographer is able to adjust the mAs and maintain control of the photon quantity to produce excellent radiographs when distance must be modified, as demonstrated in Figure 7–13.

The inverse square law and the mAs-distance formula are important concepts in radiography. If a 40-inch FFD is doubled to an 80-inch FFD, the intensity of radiation at the 80-inch FFD is one fourth the intensity at a 40-inch FFD. At the 80-inch FFD, the radiographer must increase the mAs four times the amount at the 40-inch FFD to maintain the same amount of film blackening. The inverse square law describes a physical characteristic of the x-ray beam, whereas the mAs-distance formula is the radiographer's tool used to control changes in film blackening with changes in the FFD.

Distance also affects other qualitative factors, which will be discussed in greater detail in the following chapters.

Table 7–1 provides a summary for each technical factor.

**TABLE 7–1.** SUMMARY OF TECHNICAL FACTORS IN RADIOGRAPHY

| Factor | Characteristics |
| --- | --- |
| Kilovoltage (kV) | Force that accelerates electrons from cathode to the anode<br>Controls energy of the x-ray beam<br>Determines penetrating ability of photons<br>Determines wavelength of photons<br>Affects blackening on the film by the 15% rule<br>Affects the production of scatter<br>Controls radiographic contrast<br>Affects exposure to the patient |
| Milliamperes (mA) | Current flow through the cathode filament<br>Number of electrons in space charge<br>Determines the number of x-ray photons in primary beam<br>Controls blackening on film<br>Influences focal spot blooming |
| Time (S) | Length of the exposure<br>Number of photons exposing the patient with mA-time relationship |
| Distance (D) | Distance from focal spot to recording medium<br>Affects blackening on the film<br>Inverse square law<br>mAs-distance relationship |

# Overview of Radiographic Quality

## CHAPTER OBJECTIVES

1. Define "radiographic quality."
2. Differentiate between "high-quality" and "poor-quality" radiographs.
3. List the four qualitative factors.
4. Define: density, contrast, definition, and distortion.

## KEY WORDS AND TERMS

Quality radiograph

Density

Contrast

Definition

Distortion

## RECOMMENDATIONS FOR GENERAL DISCUSSION QUESTIONS

1. Explain the concept of film qualitative factors.
2. How does each of the factors listed below affect the quality of the image?

Density

Contrast

Definition

Distortion

Quality relates to the characteristics of an object and indicates the degree of excellence that the object may exhibit. A high-quality radiograph is a radiograph with all factors at optimum. Quality identifies the amount of information available for reviewing the radiograph.

Radiographers must be able to evaluate the quality of a radiograph by visual inspection. To many radiographers, quality is often too abstract and hard to measure. The "art" of radiography is the ability of the radiographer to work with concepts and characteristics present on a finished radiograph in order to measure the degree of excellence.

A high-quality radiograph is one that demonstrates the specific anatomic part of interest with a sharp image and with the appropriate amount of blackening (density) distributed over the film. It is a radiograph with a sufficient distribution of film blackening that provides excellent subject contrast. The image has been recorded with the least possible magnification and distortion of the actual size and shape of the anatomic part. Fig. 8–1 shows two radiographs, one with poor quality and one with excellent quality.

A HIGH-QUALITY RADIOGRAPH MUST HAVE A SHARP IMAGE WITH ADEQUATE DENSITY AND CONTRAST.

To evaluate the degree of quality, a radiographer must be able to assess density, contrast, definition, and distortion. The factors are controlled and affected by the selection of technique components and the use of radiographic accessories.

## DENSITY

Radiographic density is the blackening on the finished radiograph (Fig. 8–2). It is produced by development of exposed silver halide crystals in the film emulsion. The prime factor that controls film density is milliamperseconds (mAs). As discussed in the previous chapter, film density is also affected by the kilovoltage (kVp) selection.

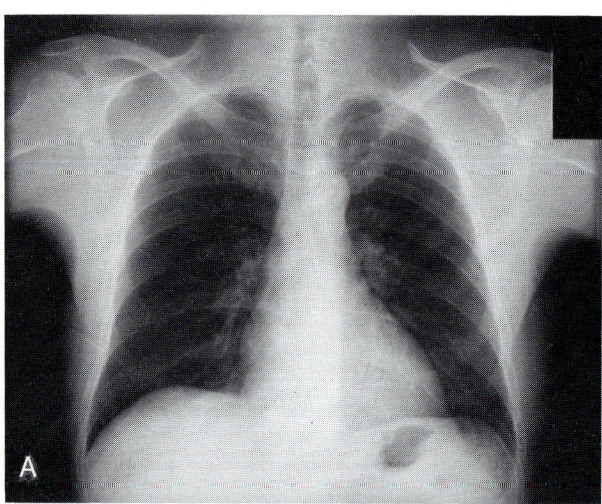
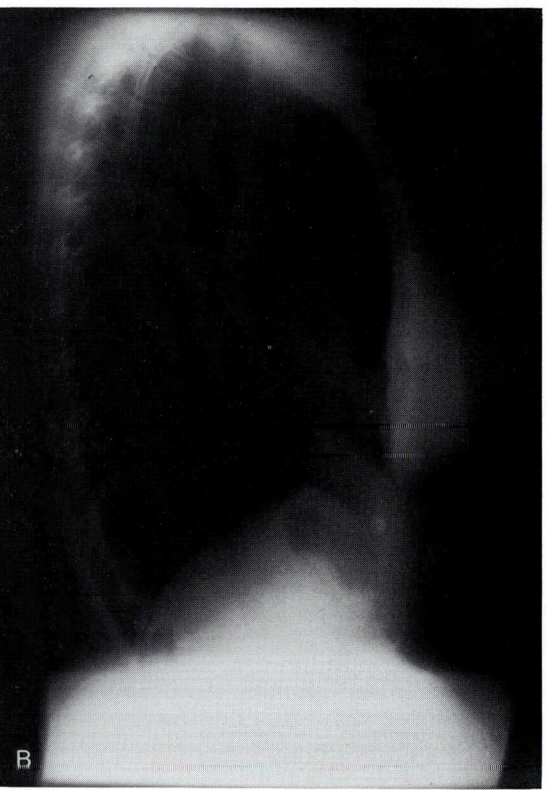

**FIGURE 8–1.** Radiographers must be able to evaluate the quality of radiographs and make corrections when necessary. *A,* A high-quality radiograph. Penetration is adequate and the overall density and contrast are very good. *B* was overexposed, producing a poor-quality radiograph. There is too much blackening across the film, preventing accurate visualization of anatomic parts.

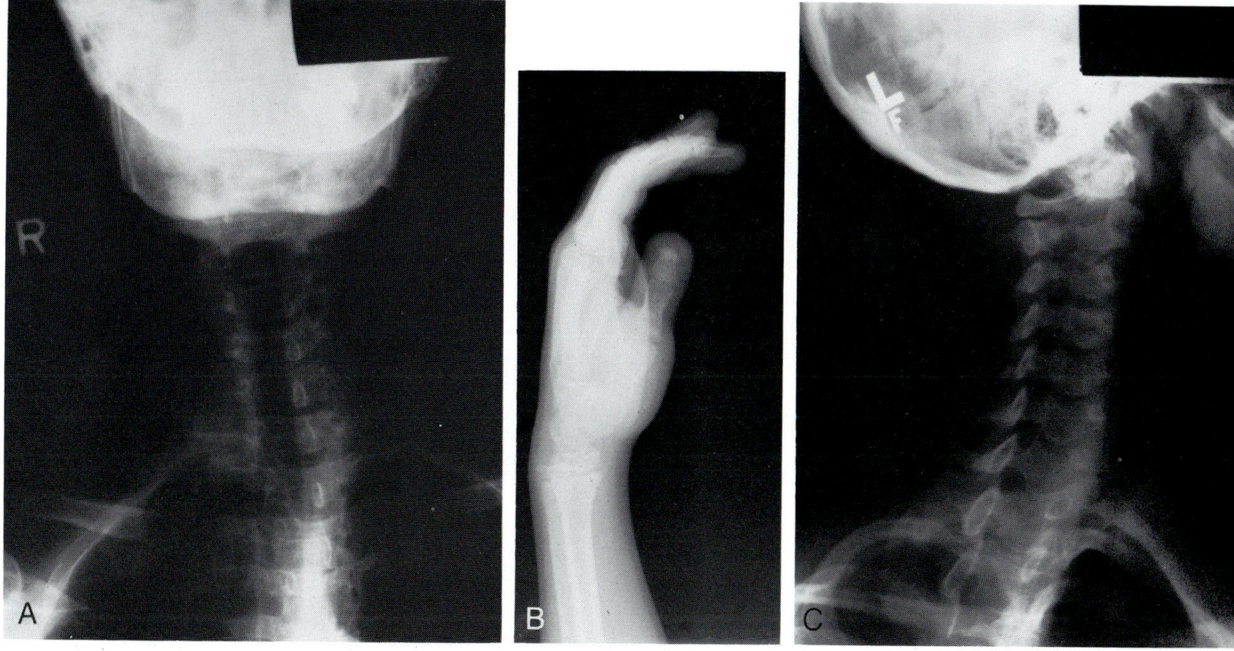

**FIGURE 8–2.** *A,* A radiograph with too much density; *B,* too little density; *C,* good density levels to allow for visualization of the anatomic parts.

RADIOGRAPHIC DENSITY IS THE OVERALL BLACKENING ON THE FILM. DENSITY IS CONTROLLED BY mAs.

## CONTRAST

Radiographic contrast is the second quality factor. Contrast represents a variation in density levels across the film and serves to make anatomic detail visible. Contrast is also described as a distribution of different density values. The function of contrast is to make structural detail visible.

CONTRAST MAKES DETAIL VISIBLE.

Contrast also refers to a range of density levels that can range from very dark (black) to areas on the radiograph with little or no density (clear or white). The prime factor that controls contrast is kVp (Fig. 8–3).

CONTRAST IS THE VARIATION IN DENSITY LEVELS THAT MAKES DETAIL VISIBLE. CONTRAST IS CONTROLLED BY KILOVOLTAGE.

## DEFINITION

The third quality factor is definition. Definition refers to the clarity and distinctness of the fine structural lines or borders of anatomic parts. To produce a radiograph with good definition, one must give careful attention to these aspects: selection of the focal-film distance (FFD); focal spot size; placement and alignment of the tube, part, and film; the amount of exposure to the film; and the use of adequate kVp and accessories that help control the amount of scatter radiation reaching the film. Each of the factors mentioned above contributes to the production of a radiograph with good definition (Fig. 8–4).

DEFINITION REFERS TO THE CLARITY AND SHARPNESS OF THE STRUCTURAL LINES OF THE ANATOMIC PARTS.

## DISTORTION

The fourth quality factor is distortion. This factor indicates an undesired change in the size and/or shape of the anatomic part has occurred in the process of imaging the part. Distortion misrepre-

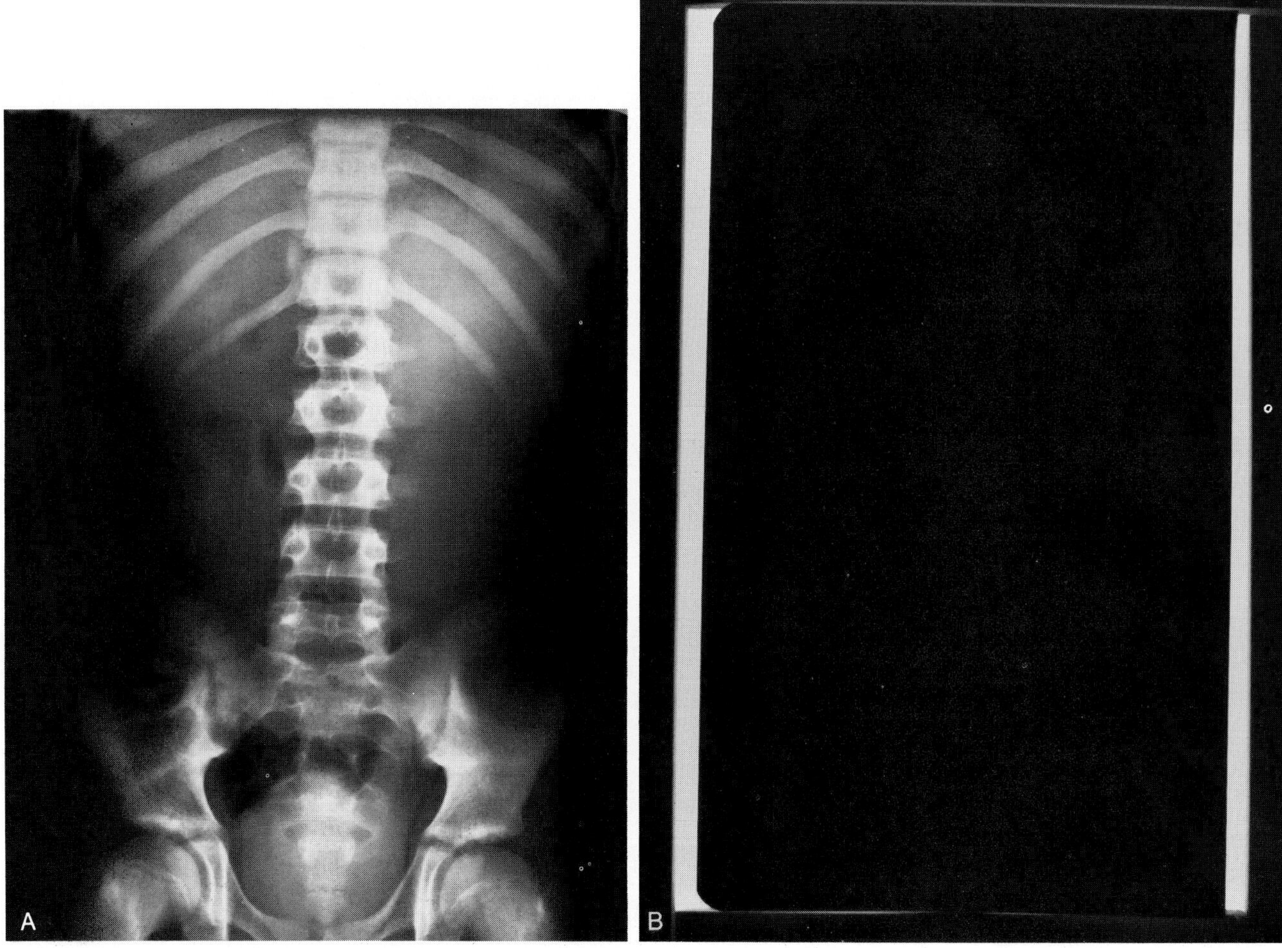

**FIGURE 8–3.** Radiographs with and without contrast. *A,* A radiograph of the abdomen. Contrast is present, with different density levels making the anatomic parts visible. *B,* A radiograph that is completely black across the entire surface of the film. Although density is present, there is no variation in the density level and no contrast is present.

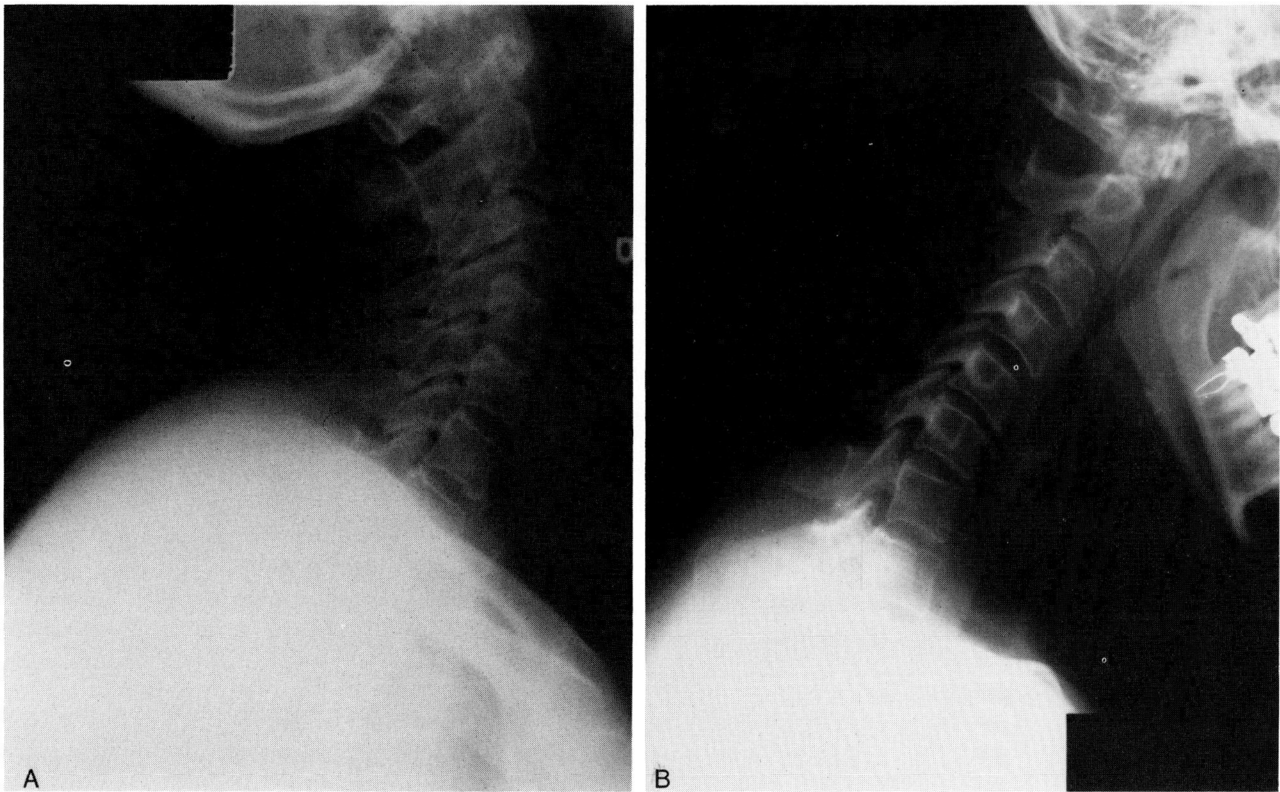

**FIGURE 8–4.** Two radiographs of the cervical spine. *A* shows the cervical vertebrae; however, the borders of the individual vertebrae are blurred and unsharp. In *B*, the borders of the individual vertebrae are very clear and sharp. *B* is a radiograph with good definition.

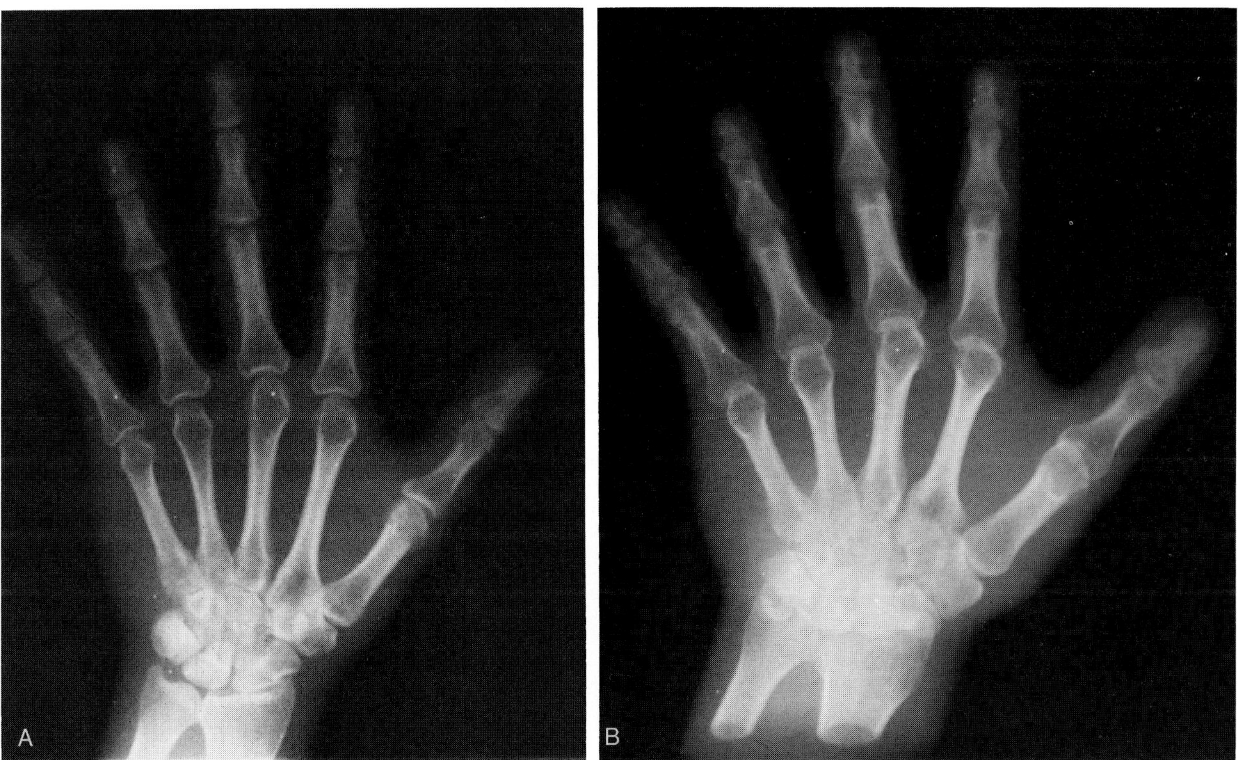

**FIGURE 8–5.** *A*, A radiograph of the hand with minimal distortion. *B* was produced with the hand tilted, resulting in distortion of the image. The fingers appear shorter and the bones of the wrist are superimposed over one another.

**TABLE 8–1.** THE RELATIONSHIP OF QUALITATIVE AND TECHNICAL FACTORS

| Quality Factor | Related Technical Factor | |
| --- | --- | --- |
| | *Control* | *Influence* |
| Density | mAs | kVp |
| | | FFD |
| Contrast | kVp | |
| Definition | FFD | kVp |
| | | mAs |
| Distortion | FFD | |

**TABLE 8–2.** RADIOGRAPHIC QUALITY

| | Definition | |
| --- | --- | --- |
| *Recorded Detail* | *Distortion* | *Visibility of Detail* |
| Focal spot size | Alignment of: | Density (mAs) |
| Focal-film distance (FFD) | part | Contrast (kVp) |
| Object-film distance (OFD) | film | Scatter radiation |
| Motion | tube | Grids |
| Screens | FFD | Beam restriction |
| | OFD | |

sents the size and/or shape of the object, and the degree of distortion can be great or small. The prime factors associated with distortion are placement of the tube, the part, and the film (Fig. 8–5).

DISTORTION IS THE MISREPRESENTATION OF THE SIZE AND/OR SHAPE OF THE ANATOMIC PART OF INTEREST.

Table 8–1 represents a summary of the four quality factors and their relationship to the technical factors.

Understanding the relationship between quality and the technical factors is essential for radiographers. To successfully practice their skills, radiographers work with technical and quality factors and the combination of these factors.

To many radiographers, quality is an abstract term. Understanding the quality factors gives radiographers the tools to evaluate radiographs. To better understand the quality concept, review Table 8–2. As demonstrated in this table, the umbrella for radiographic quality is definition. All factors support the process of producing high-quality radiographic images. The concept of radiographic quality is described in detail in the following chapters.

# Radiographic Density

• • • • • • •

## CHAPTER OBJECTIVES

1. Define radiographic density.
2. Write the formula that expresses radiographic density.
3. Describe the difference in density for areas on a radiograph that are black and clear.
4. Explain how exposure to the film affects density.
5. Differentiate between radiographic film density and tissue (object) density, and explain the relationship.
6. Define densitometer and describe its function.
7. Identify the optical density range for medical radiography.
8. Define attenuation.
9. Explain how attenuation of the primary x-ray beam affects density.
10. Name the major technical factors that control density.
11. Explain the relationship between mAs and density.
12. Explain how kVp affects density.
13. Describe how the following will affect density:

| | |
|---|---|
| Distance (FFD) | Tissue characteristics |
| Anode heel effect | Pathology |
| Filters | Equipment calibration |
| Processing | Grids |
| Film-screen systems | Beam restriction |
| Fog | |

14. Evaluate radiographs to determine if adequate density is present.


## KEY WORDS AND TERMS

| | |
|---|---|
| Density | Attenuation |
| Opaque | mAs-distance relationship |
| Blackening on the film | Density-distance relationship |
| Tissue density | kVp-density relationship |
| Pathology | Anode heel effect |
| Foreign body density | Equipment calibration |
| Contrast media density | Screen conversion factor |
| Densitometer | Filters |
| Density formula | Compensating filters |
| Optical density range | |

## RECOMMENDATIONS FOR GENERAL DISCUSSION QUESTIONS

1. Define radiographic density with the formula:

$$D = Log_{10}\frac{L_I}{L_T}$$

2. What criteria should a radiographer use to evaluate radiographic density?
3. Explain attenuation and how it affects the formation of the image.
4. Name the factor used to control density, and provide supporting information.
5. Identify and discuss at least 10 factors that will affect the amount of density recorded on the film.

Radiographic density is the opacity of the radiograph or its inability to be penetrated by light. As described in previous chapters, radiographic density is defined as the blackening on the film. Radiographs are like overhead transparencies used in classroom instruction. Clear areas allow light to shine through, and more opaque areas absorb light and prevent the light from coming through (Fig. 9–1).

---

**RADIOGRAPHIC DENSITY IS THE OPACITY OF THE RADIOGRAPH, ALSO DESCRIBED AS THE AMOUNT OF BLACKENING ON THE FILM.**

---

After a radiograph has been processed, it is examined by placing it on a viewbox (Fig. 9–2). The viewbox is a wall-mounted or portable device with fluorescent light bulbs that is covered with white transparent material. The transparent cover causes the light to be diffused evenly across the viewing surface.

The degree of optical opaqueness on the radiograph is *density*. When a radiograph is placed on the viewbox, the light can be seen coming through in some areas where less density (blackening) is present, and some areas are found with little or no density (clear/white). Little or no light will come through the areas with more density. The increase in density on the film causes these areas to be more opaque.

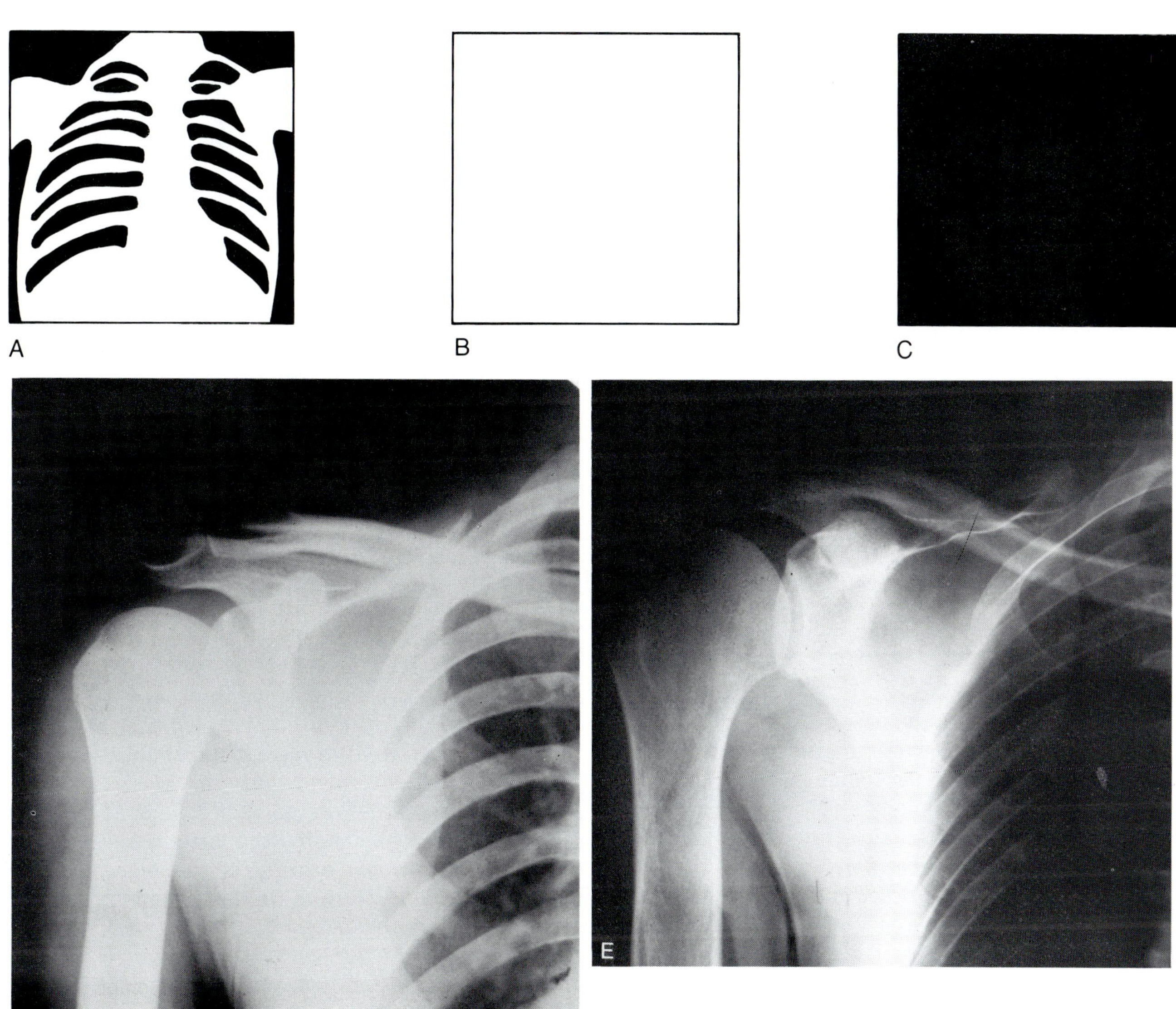

**FIGURE 9–1.** Density is blackening on the film. *A,* Different densities are distributed across the film, producing an image of the thorax. *B,* A processed film with no density present; *C,* a film with the density level the same across the entire surface of the film. The radiograph in *D* has too little density to visualize the part of interest, and *E* represents a radiograph with sufficient density.

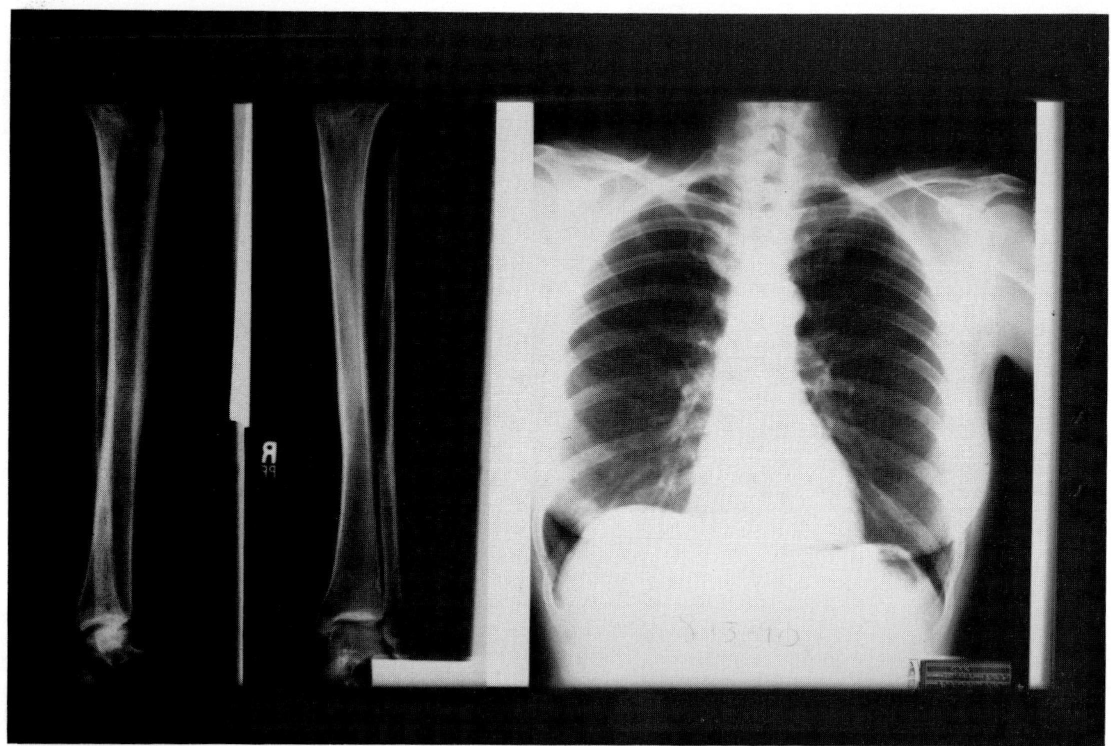

**FIGURE 9–2.** Radiographs on a lighted viewbox. The areas with less density allow more light to pass through.

Density is given a general definition of the blackening on the radiograph. The blackening is the result of processing the latent or invisible image into a visible image. The amount of exposure from x-rays and the light from the intensifying screen determine the amount of blackening that is present after development of the image.

THE AMOUNT OF EXPOSURE REACHING THE FILM DETERMINES THE AMOUNT OF DENSITY ON THE FINISHED RADIOGRAPH.

Density is the characteristic of the radiograph that is described as a photographic or optical quality. A radiograph is a permanent photographic record. The presence of density and the many different density levels across the surface of the film make the image visible. Because density defines the completeness of the image, it becomes the key to radiographic interpretation. The part of interest must be visualized with the appropriate levels of density to make it visible. Other quality factors depend on the presence of proper density. Without the proper density, the other factors of definition may lose their significance because the film is useless.

WITHOUT PROPER DENSITY, OTHER FACTORS MAY LOSE THEIR SIGNIFICANCE.

## RADIOGRAPHIC FILM DENSITY VERSUS TISSUE DENSITY

It is important to differentiate the word density as it is used in the medical sciences. Density is also used to describe the nature of tissue, such as bone, characteristics of contrast media, and foreign bodies. The bones of the skeleton are more dense than muscle. Teeth are more dense than bone, and lung tissue is much less dense than either bone, teeth, or muscle (Fig. 9–3). Contrast media, such as barium, will change tissue density and increase attenuation of the beam. Foreign bodies, such as metallic objects, will also change the attenuation of the beam, producing an outline of the object on the radiograph. The study of anatomy and physiology is necessary to be able to discern tissue density levels throughout the body.

Tissue density is important in radiography in the recording of proper radiographic density. As stated earlier, radiographic density is necessary to make the image visible. Tissues of greater density, such

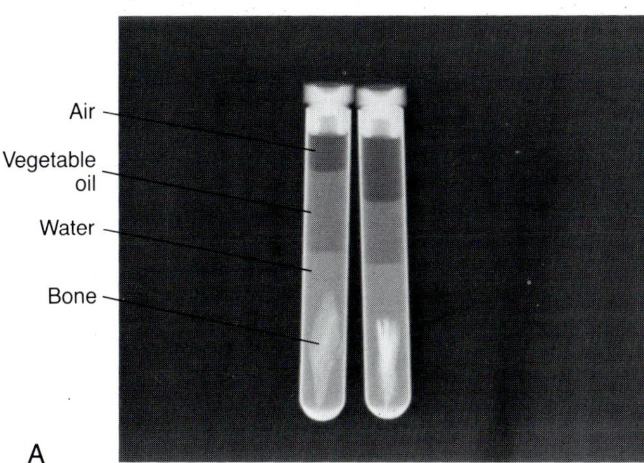


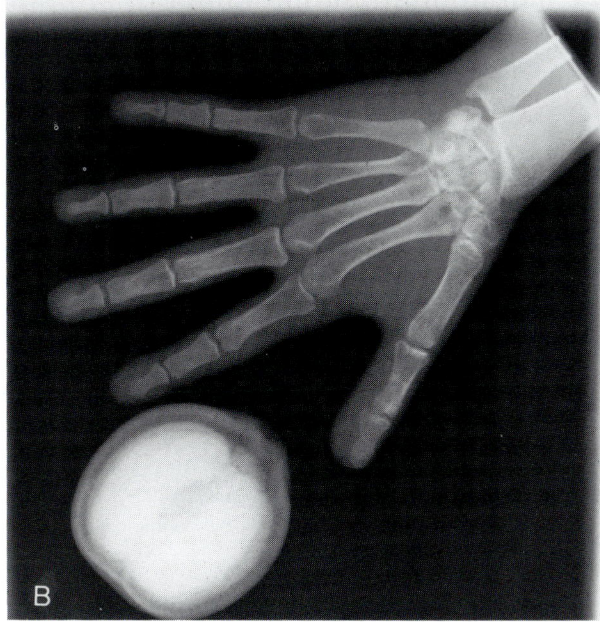


**FIGURE 9–3.** A radiograph made with test tubes filled with a small bone sample, water, fat (vegetable oil), and air. This example shows the variation in tissue density for the four basic tissue components of the body. *B,* A radiograph made with an orange and hand phantom.

as bone, require more exposure in order to visualize the markings and characteristics on the radiograph. In radiography, we categorize tissue into five major groups: aerated tissue, fatty tissue, water, bone, and teeth.

As shown in Figure 9–3, aerated tissue such as the lungs has the least tissue density and requires a small amount of exposure to record the appropriate level of density. Fatty tissue is the next to lowest level of tissue density. Third is tissue with a high water content such as muscle. Bones and teeth are the most dense tissue in the body and require the greatest amount of exposure to record appropriate density levels on the radiograph. Fig. 9–3B shows a radiograph of a hand phantom and an orange. The hand phantom demonstrates a greater variation in tissue densities than the orange.

## MEASUREMENT OF DENSITY

Radiographic density is a quality factor that can be measured with an instrument called a densitometer (Fig. 9–4).

THE DENSITOMETER IS AN INSTRUMENT USED TO MEASURE DENSITY.

The densitometer contains a light source with a known amount of illumination. The light source is covered with a translucent material containing a very small pinhole. The pinhole allows light to pass through the cover without hitting any absorbing material. The area of interest on the radiograph to be measured is placed over the pinhole, and a reading probe is placed exactly on the area for measurement. The instrument then reads the amount of light passing through the radiograph at the specific point of interest. The readings are recorded in logarithms (Fig. 9–5).

For measurement purposes, radiographic density is defined as the logarithm (base 10) of the ratio of light hitting the film to the amount of light transmitted through the film. $L_I$ represents the light

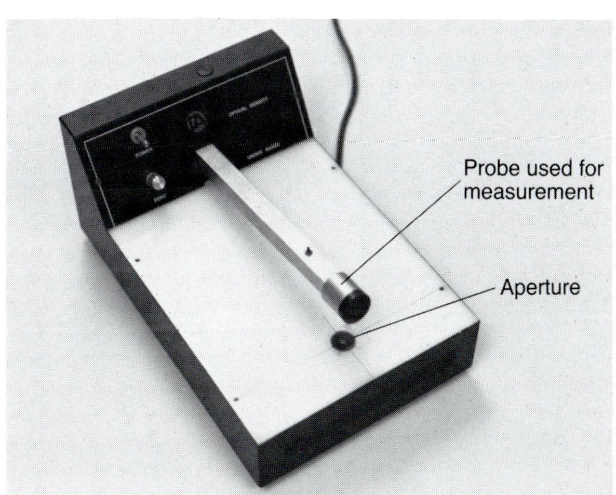


**FIGURE 9–4.** Densitometer used to measure radiographic density.

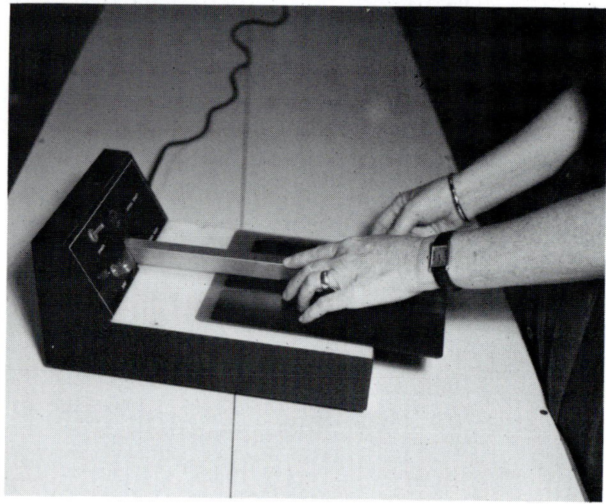

**FIGURE 9–5.** Measuring density levels using the densitometer. The area of interest is placed over the aperture. The probe is placed against the film. The optical density reading is given in a logarithm.

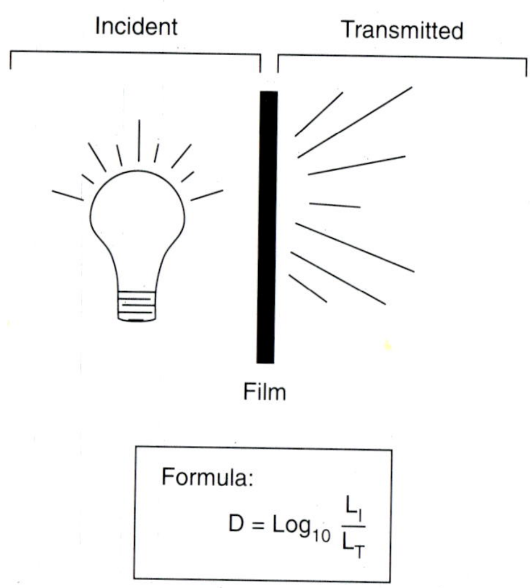



$$D = \mathrm{Log}_{10}\frac{L_I}{L_T}$$

**FIGURE 9–6.** Measuring density on the radiograph.

hitting the film and is a known standard. $L_T$ represents the amount of light transmitted (Fig. 9–6).

With the use of a densitometer, one may measure density levels on any area of the radiograph.

In medical radiography, optical density readings are most useful between 0.25 and 2.00. (Remember, these numbers are logarithms, so the range is actually very broad.) A reading of 0.25 is an area that is almost clear, with very little blackening. An area with a 2.50 reading is an area that is almost too black for one to be able to visualize many structures.

> IN RADIOGRAPHY, DENSITY READINGS ARE MOST USEFUL BETWEEN 0.25 AND 2.00.

## ATTENUATION AND DENSITY

Attenuation means a reduction in strength or force. As the x-ray photons travel through the body, they are attenuated (absorbed) by tissue structures.

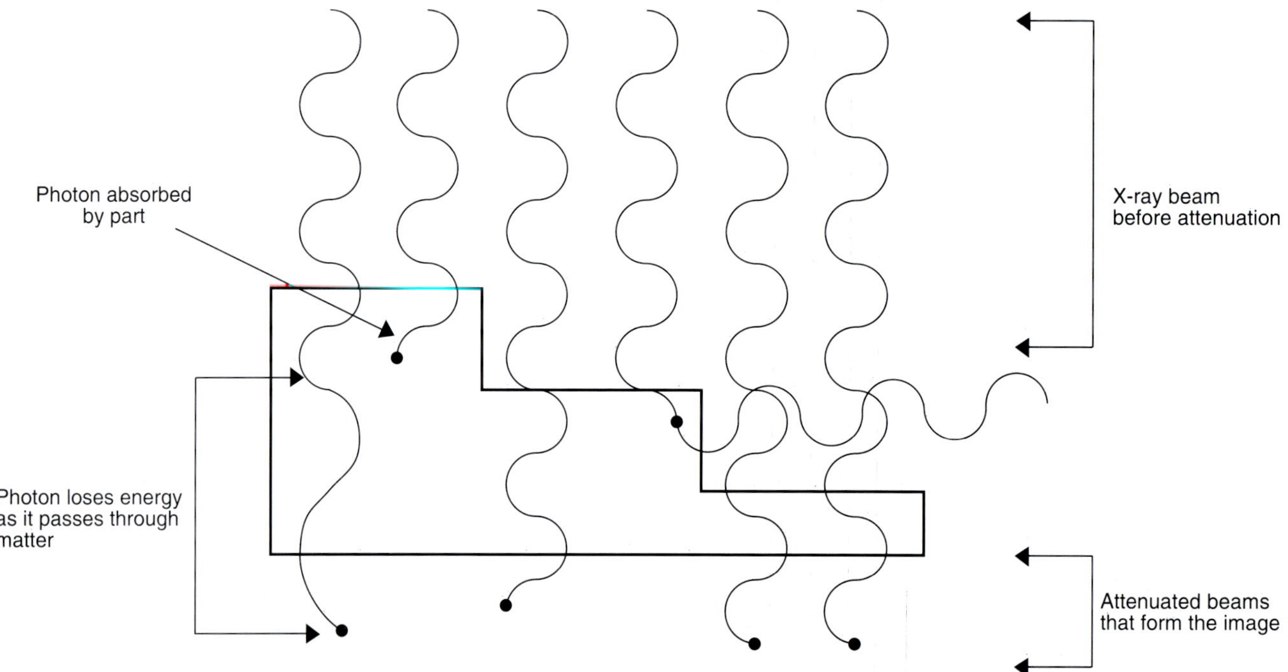



**FIGURE 9–7.** Attenuation of the x-ray beam as it passes through an object causes the beam to weaken and lose energy. Because the beam is attenuated more by thicker parts, less photon energy is present to expose the film. Areas of the film under thicker body parts have less density.

As the photon beam emerges from the body to strike the film, it is no longer a uniform beam like the primary beam. Areas of the beam with almost complete attenuation produce very little radiographic density and the parts of the beam with very little attenuation produce areas of greater optical density on the finished radiograph.

## ATTENUATION IS THE REDUCTION IN STRENGTH OR FORCE.

Attenuation causes the radiograph to represent the body part in terms of different density levels. Without attenuation, the end result would be a film with the same density level across the entire surface (Fig. 9–7).

## ATTENUATION OF THE BEAM CAUSES DIFFERENT DENSITY LEVELS TO BE PRESENT ON THE RADIOGRAPH.

The degree to which body parts attenuate the beam affects density. Bone attenuates the beam more than muscle or fatty tissue. Areas of the film under bone receive very little exposure and therefore have less radiographic density. Bones are demonstrated by light areas on the radiograph. Lung tissue and gas in the intestinal tract attenuate the beam much less and are demonstrated by darker areas on the radiograph (Fig. 9–8).

## CONTROLLING FACTORS FOR DENSITY

Density on a radiograph is primarily controlled by the milliamperseconds (mAs). Distance (focal-film distance [FFD]) can also be used to control density; however, distance variables are eliminated as much as possible to help produce consistent results. Distance (FFD) is standardized in most radiology departments and eliminated as a controlling factor for density. Changing the distance (FFD) is not practical because the image definition would also be affected. This concept is explained in Chapter 11.

Changing the mAs is the radiographer's prime method used to control the blackening on the film. The mAs is the factor that controls the number of photons in the x-ray beam (Fig. 9–9).

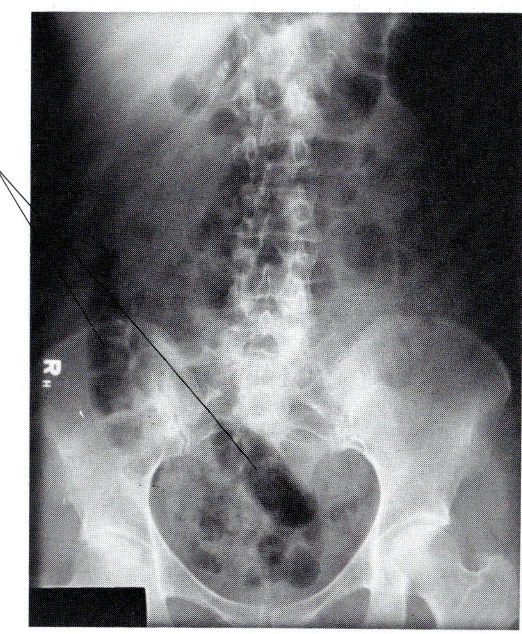


**FIGURE 9–8.** Air or gas in the gastrointestinal tract attenuates the beam less than does skeletal tissue. As illustrated here, gas shadows are present in the small and large intestine as areas of increased density.

## DENSITY IS CONTROLLED BY mAs.

The relationship between mAs and density is directly proportional. If the mAs is doubled, the amount of density recorded on the film is doubled. If the mAs is reduced by one half, the amount of density recorded is reduced by one half.

## THE RELATIONSHIP BETWEEN mAs AND DENSITY IS DIRECTLY PROPORTIONAL.

The more photons available as the beam exits the body, the more exposure the film receives. As the mAs is increased, the x-ray film receives more exposure. The sensitivity specks in the film emulsion will attract more silver ions, and when the film is developed, the amount of black metallic silver deposits will increase. This produces an increase in blackening on the film.

## AS THE mAs IS INCREASED, THE FILM RECEIVES MORE EXPOSURE.

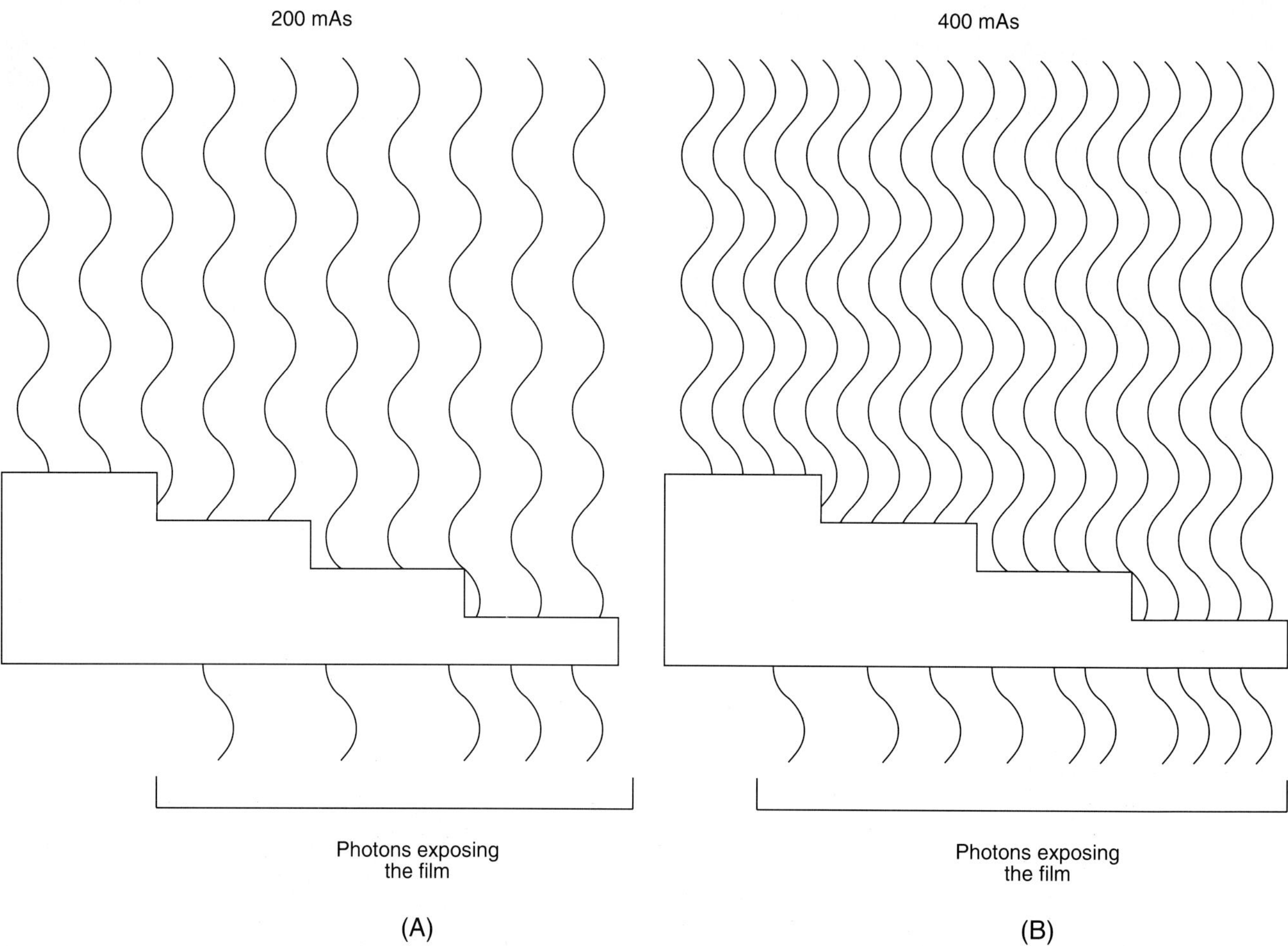



**FIGURE 9–9.** Changing the mAs from 200 to 400 will double the density on the film. The number of photons exposing the film will increase, producing more blackening on the film.

The maximum density level that is photographically useful is 2.00. Measurements of 3.0-plus may be obtained, but at this level, it is not important to the radiographer. The naked eye can not differentiate density levels in this range. Once total blackness on the film occurs, all silver in the emulsion has been changed to black metallic silver. To continue the exposure will have no advantage on optical density because the maximum optical density has previously been achieved. In the photographic range, to see a visible difference in density on a radiograph, one must increase the mAs by at least 30 to 35%.

---

TO SEE A VISIBLE CHANGE IN DENSITY, ONE MUST INCREASE THE mAs BY AT LEAST 30 TO 35%.

---

## KILOVOLTAGE AND DENSITY

It is important to understand that although mAs is the primary factor used to control density, kilovoltage changes can also significantly affect density on the film. An increase in kilovoltage peak (kVp) will result in an increase in density recorded on the film. The relationship between kVp and radiographic density is not one of proportion.

An increase in kVp increases the penetrating ability of the beam. The density distribution changes, producing a radiograph with a different appearance as a result of the different density levels.

The 15% rule is used to predict changes in density levels with kVp. An increase in kVp by 15% will approximately double the overall density on the film. By using this rule, a change of more than 10 kVp would be needed at higher kVp settings, whereas at lower kVp settings, small changes of only 4 to 5 kVp may be needed (Fig. 9–10).

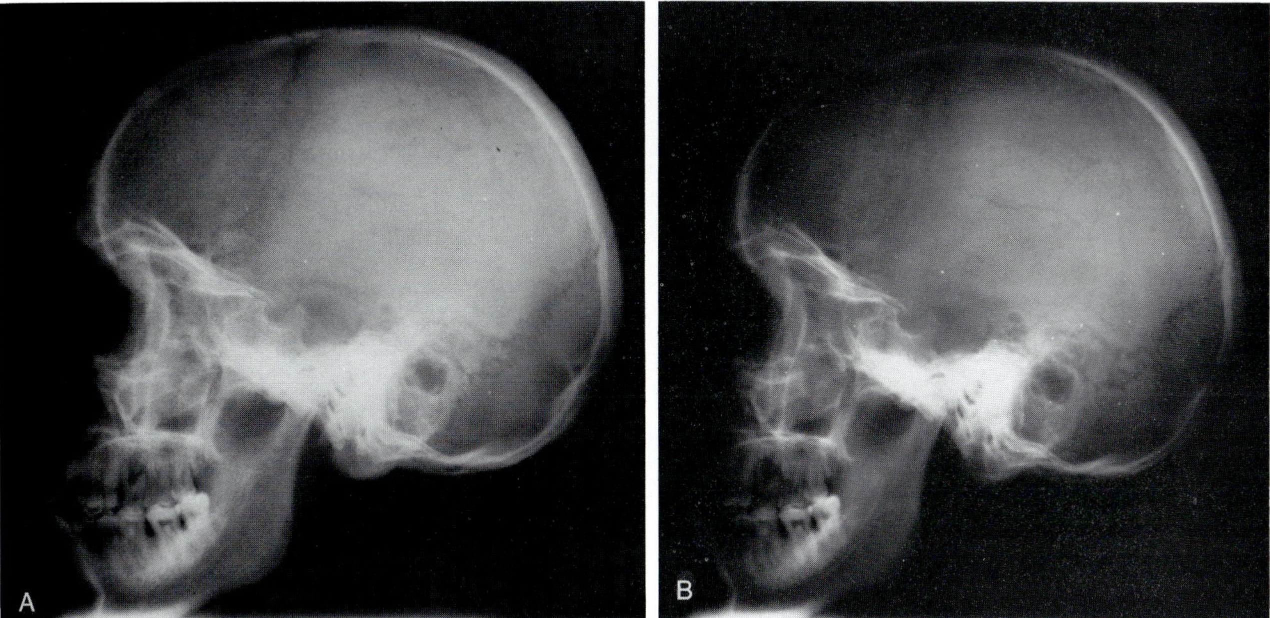

**FIGURE 9–10.** Kilovoltage changes will affect density. *A* and *B*, Density level is changed as the kilovoltage is increased by 15%. *A* was produced using 70 kVp and *B* was produced using 81 kVp (all other factors remained the same). The density level in *B* is greater as a result of the increase in kilovoltage.

A 15% INCREASE IN kVp WILL APPROXIMATELY DOUBLE THE DENSITY ON THE FILM.

When kVp is increased, more scatter radiation is produced, which adds density on the film. Scatter will also produce more fog across the film. When only a change in density is required to improve a radiograph, the most effective factor is milliampereseconds.

AS kVp INCREASES, MORE SCATTER RADIATION IS PRODUCED AND EXPOSES THE FILM, THUS INCREASING DENSITY.

## SECONDARY FACTORS THAT AFFECT DENSITY

Milliampereseconds (mAs) is the major factor used to control density. In addition, kVp changes also have a significant effect on recorded density. Other factors that affect density are the anode heel effect, equipment calibration and operation, proc-

essing of the latent image, film type, screen type and speed, characteristics of the part to be radiographed, filters, Potter-Bucky diaphragm (grids), beam restriction, and fog (all types).

### Anode Heel Effect

X-rays originate from the focal spot area and travel in all directions. In radiography, the useful beam consists of those photons exiting from the focal spot area and traveling through the tube port or window. The physics of x-ray production demonstrate that a variation in intensity is present when one measures the intensity on the anode and cathode side of the x-ray beam. The intensity of the beam is less on the anode side of the beam. Figure 9–11 demonstrates the anode structure. The lowermost portion of the anode is described as the heel.

THE ANODE HEEL EFFECT CAUSES THE BEAM INTENSITY TO BE LESS ON THE SIDE OF THE ANODE.

Photons move from their origin through the target to become part of the primary beam. The loss in intensity is a result of traveling further through

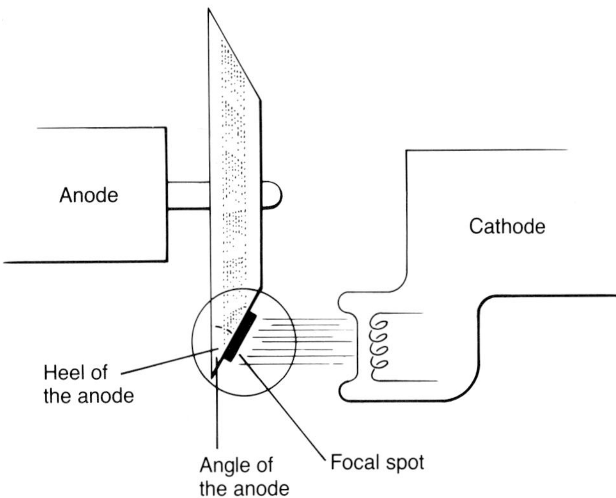


**FIGURE 9–11.** Anode structure. The lowermost portion of the anode target is the area of the heel. The angle of the anode refers to the lower edge of the target and identifies the size of the angle. Anode angles range from 8 to 20 degrees.

the anode heel portion of the target. This is called the anode heel effect and results in photons with slightly lower intensity on the anode side.

Measurement of the primary beam on the cathode and anode sides will demonstrate this phenomenon. Radiographers must recognize the anode heel effect and act to overcome any possible effects on the film. A larger field size and a shorter FFD will produce a more noticeable anode heel effect on the finished radiograph.

The angle of the anode structure will also affect the presence of the anode heel effect. The heel effect will increase with a decrease in the anode angle (Fig. 9–12).

To overcome the density changes that result from the anode heel effect, the radiographer places the thicker body parts under the cathode side of the tube, with thin body parts under the anode side, as shown in Figure 9–13. Longer focal-film distance (FFD) and smaller field sizes will reduce the consequences of the anode heel effect.

---

LONG FFD AND SMALL FIELD SIZE WILL REDUCE THE CONSEQUENCES OF THE ANODE HEEL EFFECT.

---

## Equipment Calibration and Operation

Maintenance of the x-ray equipment is necessary for consistency in exposure. Density can be severely affected (plus or minus) by poorly calibrated equip-

ment. Proper selection of factors and proper operation are also essential. Radiographers must understand how to select exposure factors, especially the use of time and milliampere (mA) factors. At the time of exposure, radiographers must be able to determine if full exposures are obtained. The recording of proper density depends upon the knowledge and skill of the radiographer in the use of the x-ray equipment.

## Processing of the Latent Image

The time-temperature relationship is important in processing radiographs to show optimum density. Solution temperatures that are too hot will increase density, and temperatures that are too low will produce radiographs with insufficient density. Contaminated processing chemicals and improperly prepared chemicals can also affect density levels by increasing fog levels, which are undesirable on the film.

## Film Type

Film types that contain increased amounts of silver halide crystals will increase density. Care must be taken by the radiographer to prevent overexposure or too much density. Slower film types build less density and require an adjustment in the exposure factors. Radiographers must be aware of the film type that they are using to produce the radiograph.

## Screen Type

Intensifying screens increase density on the film by intensifying the action of the x-rays. As the screen speed increases, the density will increase; therefore, less exposure will be needed to keep density at the appropriate level. Speed of the screen and its impact on density are important factors with the rare earth systems, which are much faster than calcium tungstate screens (compare the examples of speed factors as given in Table 5–1). The reduction in exposure necessary with rare earth screens greatly reduces the amount of radiation exposure to the patient.

## Characteristics of Tissue

The structure and composition of body tissue may affect density by changing attenuation. More dense

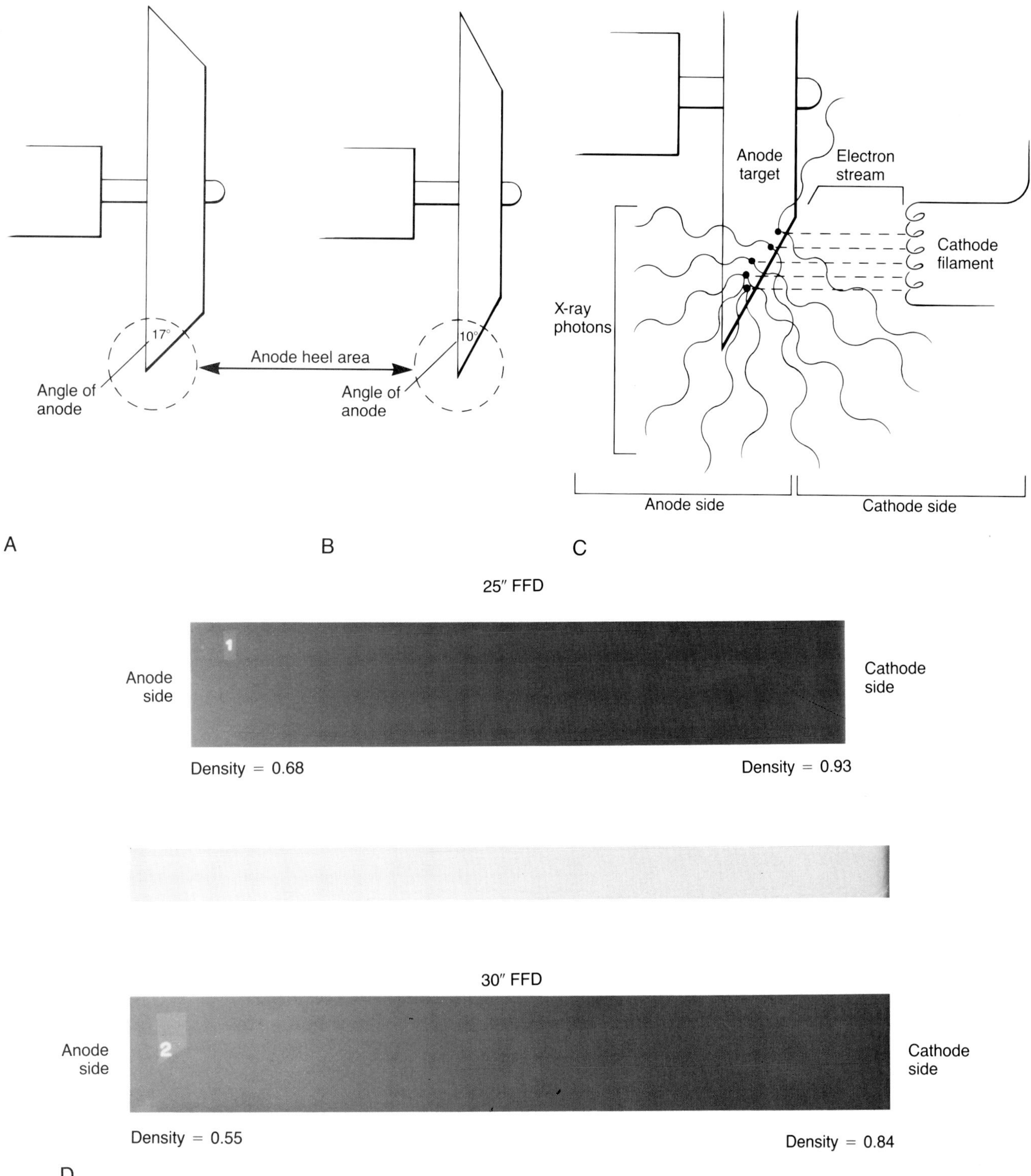



**FIGURE 9–12.** *A* and *B* represent anode targets with 17° and 10° angles. *C* illustrates how the x-ray photons produced as the electrons strike the focal spot area travel in all directions. The heel effect results from a decrease in photon intensity as photons travel further through the heel of the anode before they exit the target. The primary beam has slightly lower intensity on the anode side. The angle of the anode will also influence the anode heel effect, with a decrease in the angle of the anode increasing the heel effect. The heel effect will be greater with a 10° anode angle than with a 17° anode angle. *D,* Radiographs demonstrating the anode heel effect. The top exposure (#1) was made using a 25″ FFD. The collimator was opened as wide as possible with the long axis of the tube. The transverse shutters of the beam restrictor were limited to produce an image about 3″ wide. The anode is located to the left and the cathode to the right. The density measurements are 0.68 on the anode side and 0.93 on the cathode side. The lower image (#2) was produced using the same beam restriction technique but with a 30″ FFD. The density measurement on the anode side of the exposure is 0.55. On the cathode side, the density reading is 0.84. A closer examination reveals an image with increased density on the cathode side of the exposure.

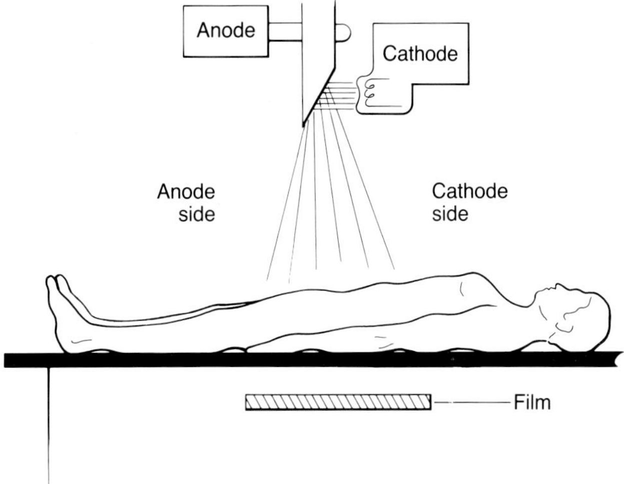



**FIGURE 9–13.** Density changes caused by the anode heel effect may be overcome by placing the thickest part under the cathode side of the x-ray tube, as illustrated here.

or compact structures will absorb more of the x-ray photons as they pass through the tissue. Less radiation will exit the part to strike the film, and density will be decreased. Soft tissue, such as the anatomic parts of the gastrointestinal tract, will absorb less radiation, and these areas may appear darker (or show more density) than the areas representing bone.

## THE STRUCTURE AND COMPOSITION OF BODY TISSUE MAY AFFECT DENSITY BY CHANGING THE ATTENUATION OF THE BEAM.

Pathologic processes may also affect the recording of density on the film. For example, destructive processes of the skeleton may be demonstrated by increased density readings. Bone tissue that has been destroyed by a disease process, resulting in less radiation absorption, will be demonstrated by an area of increased density on the radiograph. Figure 9–14 demonstrates examples of density changes as a result of pathology changes. Radiographers must study pathologic processes in order to understand how diseases change body tissues. To compensate, exposure factors must be decreased for destructive diseases such as emphysema or osteoporosis, and exposure factors must be increased for diseases that cause an increase in tissue density.

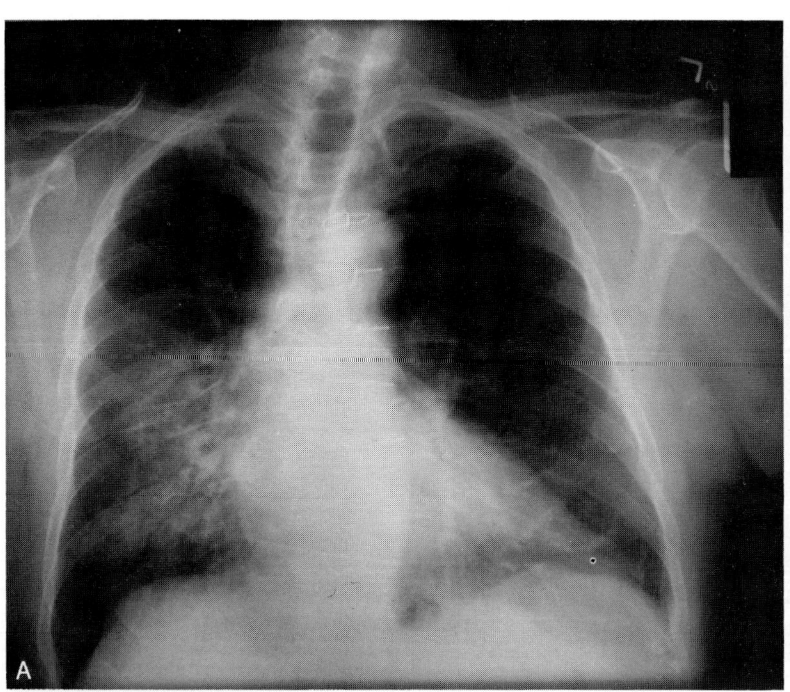

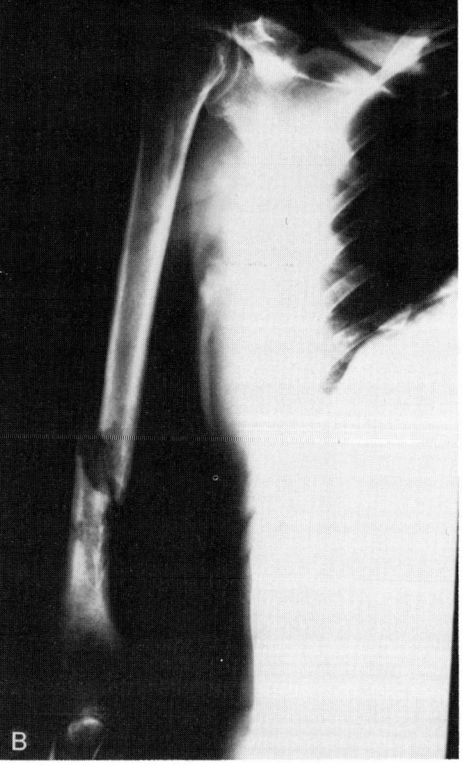

**FIGURE 9–14.** Pathologic changes in tissue can influence density on radiographs. *A* shows an area of increased tissue density in the right lung as a result of disease. Radiographic density is decreased owing to the increase in tissue density. *B* shows a pathologic fracture of the humerus. Around the fracture are areas of decreased tissue density that are a result of the disease. The radiographic density increased owing to the decrease in tissue density.

Adjustment of the exposure factors is necessary to maintain proper density on the radiograph.

CHANGES IN TISSUE DENSITY DUE TO PATHOLOGIC PROCESSES MUST BE COMPENSATED FOR WITH A CHANGE IN THE EXPOSURE FACTORS TO MAINTAIN ADEQUATE DENSITY.

## Filters

Filters are thin aluminum or metal devices that are located between the x-ray tube and beam restriction device. The purpose of filtration is to absorb the low-energy x-ray photons in the beam as they exit the tube. The low-energy photons contribute nothing to the radiograph; however, these low-energy photons greatly increase the patient's skin dose of absorbed radiation. To protect the patient, filtration is required.

Compensating filters are an added filtration to provide a more overall uniformly exposed radiograph. For example, the femur with surrounding tissue is a body part that is usually significantly thicker at the proximal end. With the use of a wedge-type filter (Fig. 9–15), the exposure to the film will be more evenly distributed. For a detailed discussion of filters, refer to Chapter 12.

COMPENSATING FILTERS ARE ADDED TO PROVIDE A MORE UNIFORMLY EXPOSED RADIOGRAPH.

Compensation filters can be very effective when one is imaging body parts with great variation in tissue thickness.

## Grids (Potter-Bucky Diaphragm)

Grids are used to absorb some of the scatter and secondary radiation produced by the body part. The grid is placed between the patient and the film. Scatter and secondary radiation account for up to 50 to 90% of the density on a radiograph. Grids improve the quality of the film by absorbing scatter radiation. The absorption of radiation causes a reduction in the total amount of radiation reaching

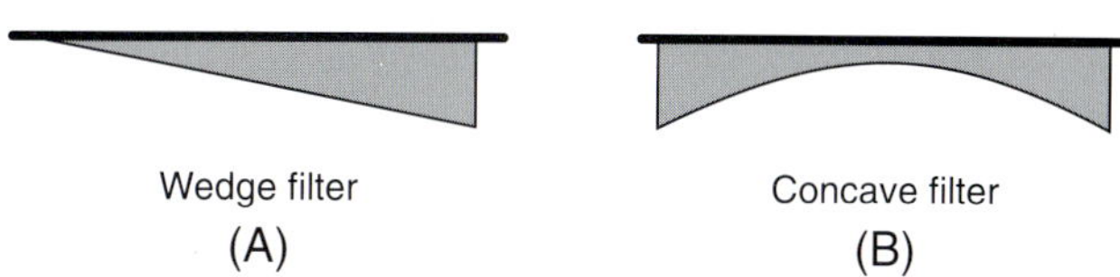


**FIGURE 9–15.** Compensating filters are added to produce a primary beam that will provide a more uniform exposure to the film. *A,* The wedge filter can be used with the thick part placed over the thin part of the anatomy. *B,* The concave filter would be useful in radiography of the thorax.

the film. In other words, the addition of a grid will reduce density. The use of a grid requires an increase in exposure factors to maintain adequate density levels on the radiograph. For example, to change from a non–grid exposure to a grid exposure requires approximately four times the original exposure to keep film density constant. A more detailed discussion of grids is found in Chapter 14.

GRIDS ARE USED TO DECREASE THE DENSITY ON THE FILM PRODUCED BY SCATTER RADIATION.

## Beam Restriction

Beam restriction devices are used to restrict the beam field size to the size of the part. Collimators are the most common type of beam restriction. Cones and aperture diaphragms are alternate types of beam restriction. Beam restriction devices reduce the field size and the actual area exposed on the patient by the primary radiation beam. As the field size decreases, smaller areas are exposed and less scatter radiation is produced. The result is less

**TABLE 9–1.** FACTORS AFFECTING DENSITY

| Controlling Factor | Influencing Factor |
| --- | --- |
| Milliamperseconds (mAs) | Kilovoltage (kVp) |
| | Tissue thickness |
| | Tissue density |
| | Foreign bodies |
| | Contrast media |
| | Distance (FFD) |
| | Scatter radiation |
| | Anode heel effect |
| | Processing |
| | Equipment operation |
| | Film-screen systems |
| | Filters |
| | Grids |
| | Beam restriction |
| | Fog |

density recorded on the film. Compensation of exposure factors is necessary to maintain the proper density level on the radiograph. For example, if the field size is reduced from a 14 × 17 film size to a 10 × 12 film size, the mAs must be increased approximately 35% to keep the density constant.

---

BEAM RESTRICTION DECREASES DENSITY ON THE FILM BY REDUCING THE AMOUNT OF SCATTER RADIATION.

---

## Fog (All Types)

Fog is increased or unwanted density on the radiograph. It is undesirable and a detriment to the quality of the film. The main source of fog on radiographs is scatter radiation. Table 9–1 summarizes the factors that control and influence density.

---

FOG IS INCREASED DENSITY ON THE RADIOGRAPH.

---

# Radiographic Contrast

## CHAPTER OBJECTIVES

1. Define radiographic contrast.
2. Explain the relationship between density and contrast.
3. Explain how tissue absorption affects contrast.
4. Describe how attenuation affects contrast.
5. Identify the major technical factor that controls radiographic contrast.
6. Describe the function of contrast.
7. Discuss the relationship between mAs and contrast.
8. List two types of contrast in radiography.
9. Describe how contrast media and pathologic processes affect contrast.
10. Discuss the inherent factors that affect film contrast.
11. Differentiate between long scale and short scale of contrast.
12. Differentiate between high contrast and low contrast.
13. Write the terms that refer to long scale of contrast.
14. Write the terms that refer to short scale of contrast.
15. Explain how the kVp selection affects long scale, short scale, high degree or high contrast, and low contrast.
16. Define the phrase "moderate scale of contrast."
17. List the disadvantages for a scale of contrast that is too long or too short.
18. Describe the criteria for evaluating a radiograph for adequate contrast.
19. Explain how the following will affect contrast:

    Film-screen systems    Grids
    Rare earth screen      Beam restriction
    Processing             Tissue compression

20. Evaluate radiographs to determine if adequate contrast is present.

## KEY WORDS AND TERMS

Radiographic contrast
Tissue contrast
Film contrast
kVp-contrast relationship
Penetration of the part
Underpenetration of the part
Long scale of contrast
Short scale of contrast
High contrast

Low contrast
High degree of contrast
Low degree of contrast
Exposure latitude
Moderate scale of contrast
Grids
Beam restriction
Pathologic conditions

# RECOMMENDATIONS FOR GENERAL DISCUSSION QUESTIONS

1. What is the function of contrast?
2. Discuss the importance for adequate film density to achieve optimal contrast on the film.
3. How does beam attenuation affect contrast?
4. Create an outline for explaining the terminology associated with contrast using the following:

| | |
|---|---|
| Long scale | High contrast |
| Short scale | Low contrast |
| High degree | More contrast |
| Low degree | Insufficient contrast |

5. Explain how each characteristic of contrast identified in #4 is achieved by manipulation of technical factors and/or accessories.
6. What are the criteria for the evaluation of a radiograph for optimal contrast?

The second important quality factor and property of a radiograph is contrast. Density must be present in order for one to visualize contrast. Is it possible to have density on a radiograph without the presence of contrast? The answer is "yes." If the entire surface of the film has been exposed to a uniform amount of x-radiation and/or fluorescent light from the intensifying screens, the result will be a radiograph that has the same density level over the entire surface of the film (Fig. 10–1).

## DENSITY MUST BE PRESENT IN ORDER FOR ONE TO VISUALIZE CONTRAST.

Is it possible to have contrast present on a radiograph without the presence of density? The answer is "no." Contrast on a radiograph depends on the presence of density.

Contrast is the difference in density between two structures. Contrast can be high with sharp differences in dark and light areas, or low with very little differences between densities. The presence of contrast means that different density levels are visible on the radiograph. The density levels on a radiograph are multiple, ranging from light (almost clear) to dark areas (black) (Fig. 10–2).

Contrast can also be identified as the ratio of radiation intensity as it exits a specific type of tissue to radiation intensity exiting an adjacent type of tissue. For example, the amount of radiation striking the film as it exits the area of the lung tissue measured 20 milliroentgens (mR) and the amount measured as the radiation exits the area of the heart is 8 mR. In this generalized example, the lungs would have more exposure and would be shown to be a darker area when compared with the adjacent heart shadow, where less remnant radiation exited the part to strike the film. Contrast is present, and the radiologist would then be able to distinguish the heart shadow from the surrounding lung tissue (see Figure 10–1C).

Contrast is important on a radiograph because it functions to make structural detail visible. The radiologist must be able to see detail with visible borders present. Contrast is the factor that makes the borders of the anatomic structures visible as well as the fine details within the object.

## THE FUNCTION OF CONTRAST IS TO MAKE DETAIL VISIBLE.

Radiographic contrast can also be described as a variety of density levels distributed across the film. In reviewing Figure 10–1, we see that *A* shows a radiograph with no contrast present. The level of density is uniform across the entire surface of the film. Figure 10–1*B* and *D* show radiographs with two and three density levels present. A block of paraffin wax, which has a uniform composition, was radiographed, producing an image with basically two levels of density. Contrast is present inasmuch as the block of paraffin is readily visible with a darker density border. The radiograph in Figure 10–1*C* shows a routine posterior-anterior chest radiograph with many different levels of density distributed across the film. Contrast is present, which permits the visualization of the lungs, heart, ribs, diaphragm, etc.

## ATTENUATION AND CONTRAST

Attenuation is a reduction in strength or force as a result of absorption and interactions. As the x-ray photons travel through body tissue, they are attenuated. The result is an x-ray beam that is no longer uniform.

## ATTENUATION OF THE BEAM IS A REDUCTION IN STRENGTH OR FORCE DUE TO ABSORPTION AND INTERACTIONS.

Contrast is the result of attenuation and the differential absorption of tissue. Without beam attenuation, contrast would not be present because a uniform density level would be present. When no absorber has been placed in the beam, the density levels will not change. Figure 10–1 shows how contrast results from beam attenuation. *A* represents a beam with no attenuation, whereas *C* represents an attenuated beam with different degrees of absorption as a result of the many different tissue densities. *C* represents differential absorption of the tissue of the thorax. As you can see, the heart attenuates the beam more than lung tissue.

## CONTRAST IS THE RESULT OF ATTENUATION AND THE DIFFERENTIAL ABSORPTION IN TISSUE.

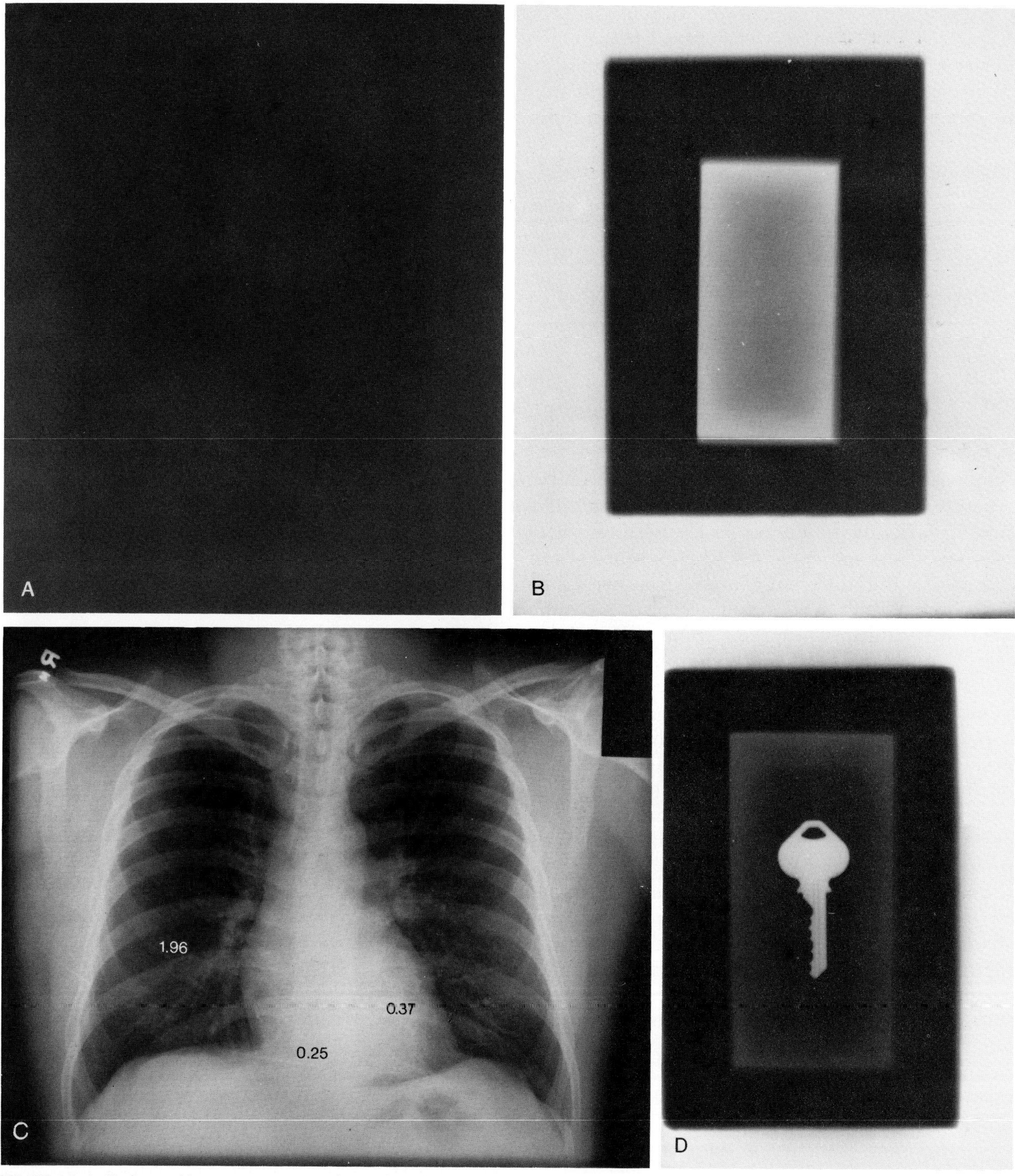

**FIGURE 10–1.** Radiographic contrast. *A,* A radiograph with no contrast. Density is present; however, because there is no variation in the density level, no contrast is present. *B,* A radiograph produced by placing a block of paraffin wax on the cassette. Two levels of density are present, producing contrast. *C,* A radiograph of the chest. Because multiple levels of density are present, contrast is present. Density readings are shown for the areas of the lower thoracic vertebrae (0.25), lung (1.96), and heart (0.37). *D,* This radiograph was produced with a block of paraffin wax and a key. Because of the variation in density levels, the block of wax and the key are visible. There must be a variation in the density levels to produce contrast.

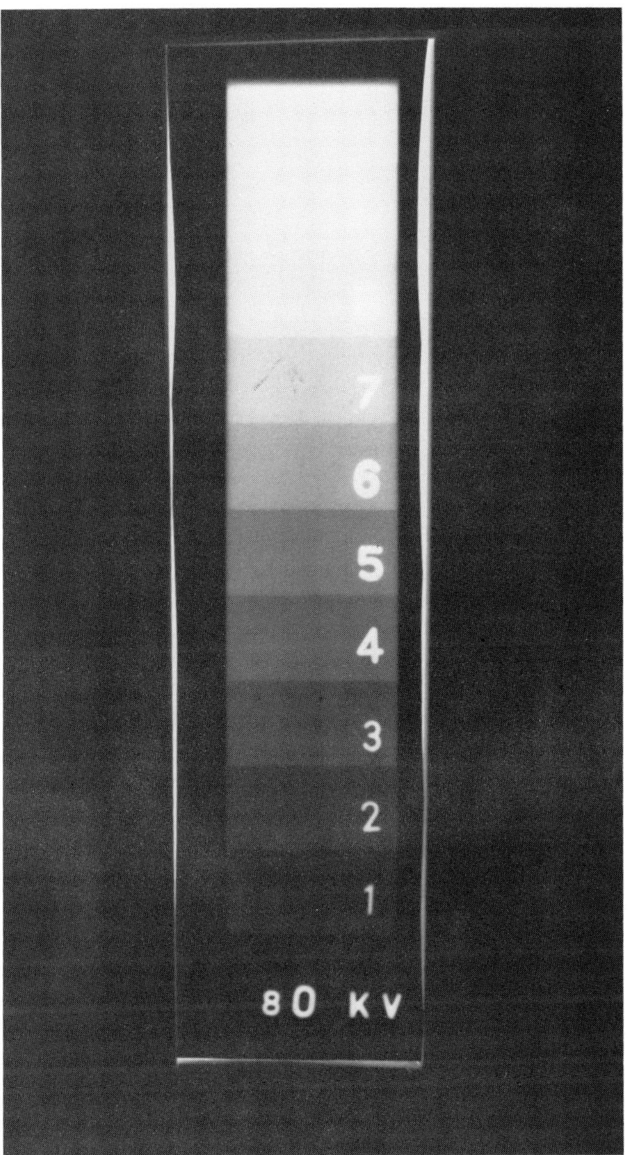

**FIGURE 10–2.** Image of a penetrometer produced using 80 kVp. The steps of the penetrometer are visible as a result of the different density levels. Because each step attenuates the beam differently owing to increased thickness, contrast is visible.

## CONTRAST AND SILVER DEPOSITS

Another way to describe contrast is the distribution of metallic silver that is present following the development of the latent image. Areas of greater silver deposits have more density and areas with smaller silver deposits will have less density.

## CONTROLLING FACTOR OF CONTRAST

The technical factor that controls contrast is kilovoltage. The radiologists want to see complete im-

ages of tissue and not simply a silhouette or outline. Radiographers must produce radiographs that demonstrate the structural detail of the tissue.

## CONTRAST IS CONTROLLED BY KILOVOLTAGE.

In order for the radiologist to visualize the desired detail, the part must be adequately penetrated. Penetration of the part is controlled by the kilovoltage. Attenuation and the distribution of densities across the film are significantly affected by the kilovoltage selection. Therefore, the factor used to control contrast is kilovoltage. Figure 10–3 demonstrates the importance of kilovoltage.

## ATTENUATION AND PENETRATION OF THE PART ARE AFFECTED BY CHANGES IN THE kVp SELECTION.

The concept represented in Figure 10–3*A* demonstrates how a lower kilovoltage peak (kVp) selection will allow for only thin parts to be penetrated. The remaining parts completely attenuate the beam. The x-ray photons are not energetic enough to penetrate the part. The result is demonstrated by the use of a penetrometer in Figure 10–4.

The use of an optimal kVp selection is shown in Figure 10–4. As the kVp increases, the photons have sufficient energy to penetrate the multiple thicknesses but with different amounts of attenuation. The thickest part is slightly penetrated, and the adjacent layer of thickness attenuates the beam slightly less, distinguishing it from the two layers on either side. The result is the visualization of each layer with only a slight variation in density. The tissue structures to be demonstrated must be adequately penetrated in order to have sufficient contrast to make the detail visible.

Milliampereseconds (mAs) changes the quantity of photons in the beam and cannot be used as a substitute factor to alter contrast on a radiograph. Penetration is not affected by increases or decreases in the mAs. No appreciable amount of increase in beam quantity can make up for a lack of energy of the x-ray photons in the beam. In other words, do not use mAs as the technical factor to produce changes in contrast. Kilovoltage controls contrast and mAs controls density.

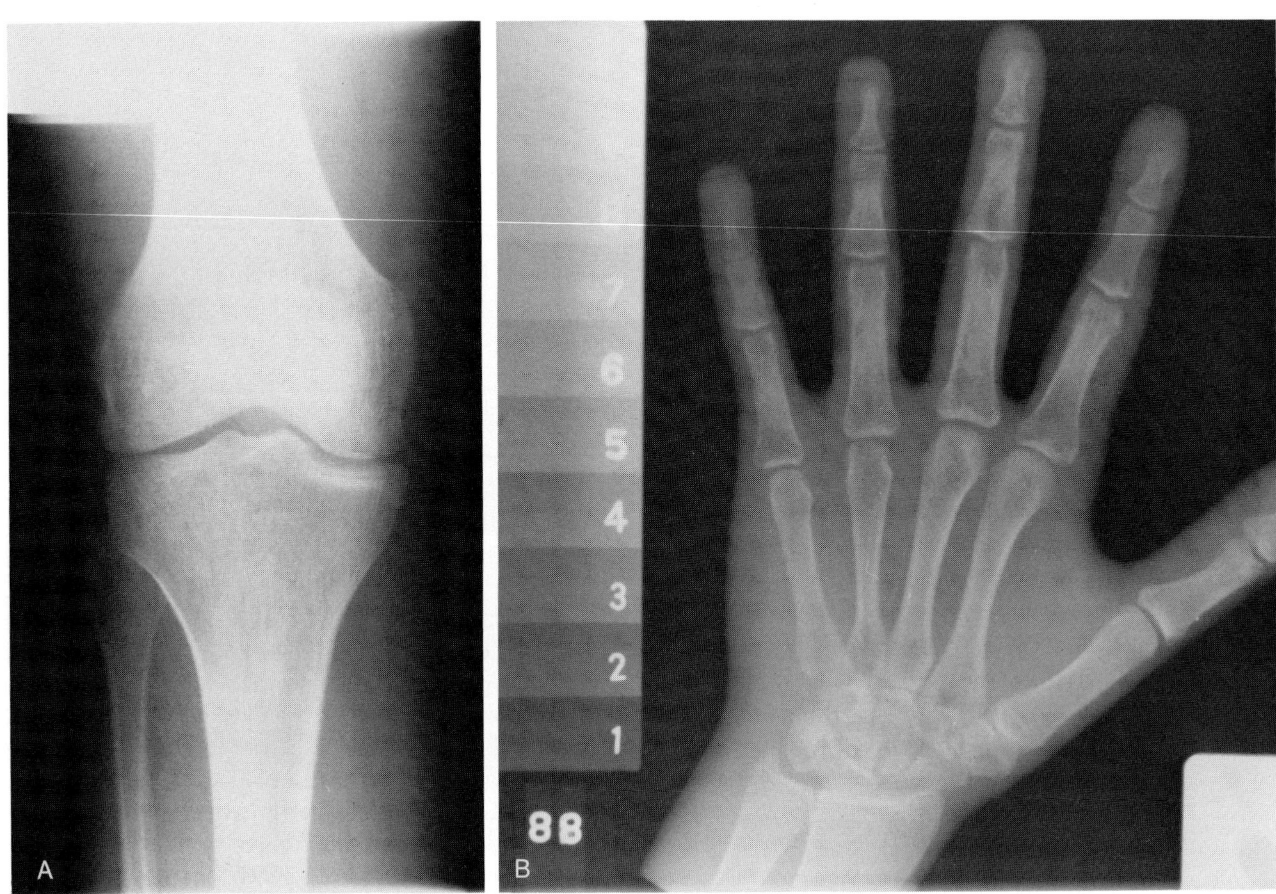

**FIGURE 10–3.** Exposures made with high and low kVp selections. *A* was produced using 45 kVp. *B* was produced using 88 kVp. *A* is an image that is mostly black and white, whereas *B* is an image with overall gray tones and many shades of gray.

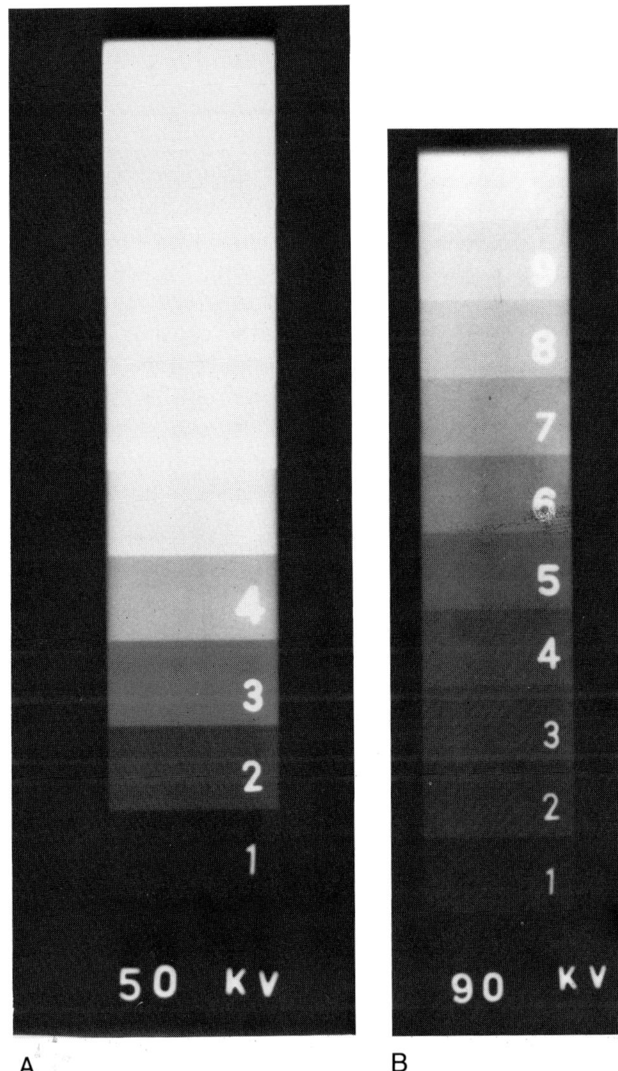



**FIGURE 10–4.** Radiographs of the penetrometer made with high and low kilovoltage selections. *A* was produced using 50 kVp. There are few shades of gray, producing a shorter scale of contrast, or high contrast. *B* was produced using 90 kVp. There are many shades of gray, described as a longer scale of contrast, or low contrast.

## TYPES OF CONTRAST

In diagnostic radiology, two types of contrast are generally recognized: subject or tissue contrast and film contrast. The ability to see skeletal structures on a radiograph is due to the presence of subject contrast.

Subject contrast is the difference in density of adjacent structures. Subject contrast is present with bone and its surrounding soft tissue. When one images the kidneys, ureters, bladder, and gastrointestinal (GI) tract, little or no subject contrast is present. The density differences are not great enough to allow for borders to be visible. If these structures are to be visualized, an external agent called contrast medium must be utilized. For example, contrast media are injected into the venous system in order to visualize the drainage system of the kidneys (Fig. 10–5).

---

## SUBJECT CONTRAST IS THE DIFFERENCE IN DENSITY OF ADJACENT STRUCTURES.

---

The contrast medium has a higher atomic number and will increase attenuation of the beam, resulting in increased subject contrast. Figure 10–5A shows a plain radiograph of the abdomen, whereas Figure 10–5B demonstrates how the presence of contrast medium will produce an image of the urinary system.

---

## CONTRAST MEDIA CAN BE USED TO INCREASE SUBJECT CONTRAST.

---

Subject contrast is controlled by the quality of the x-ray beam. The energy of the photons must be great enough to penetrate the anatomic parts. This depends on the structure, thickness, and characteristics of the tissue composition. Tissue with greater water content requires more energy to penetrate the part than tissue composed mainly of fat or air. Bone requires greater energy to penetrate than any soft tissue structure in the body. Therefore, when the combination of these tissue types is present in the area to be exposed by the primary beam, subject

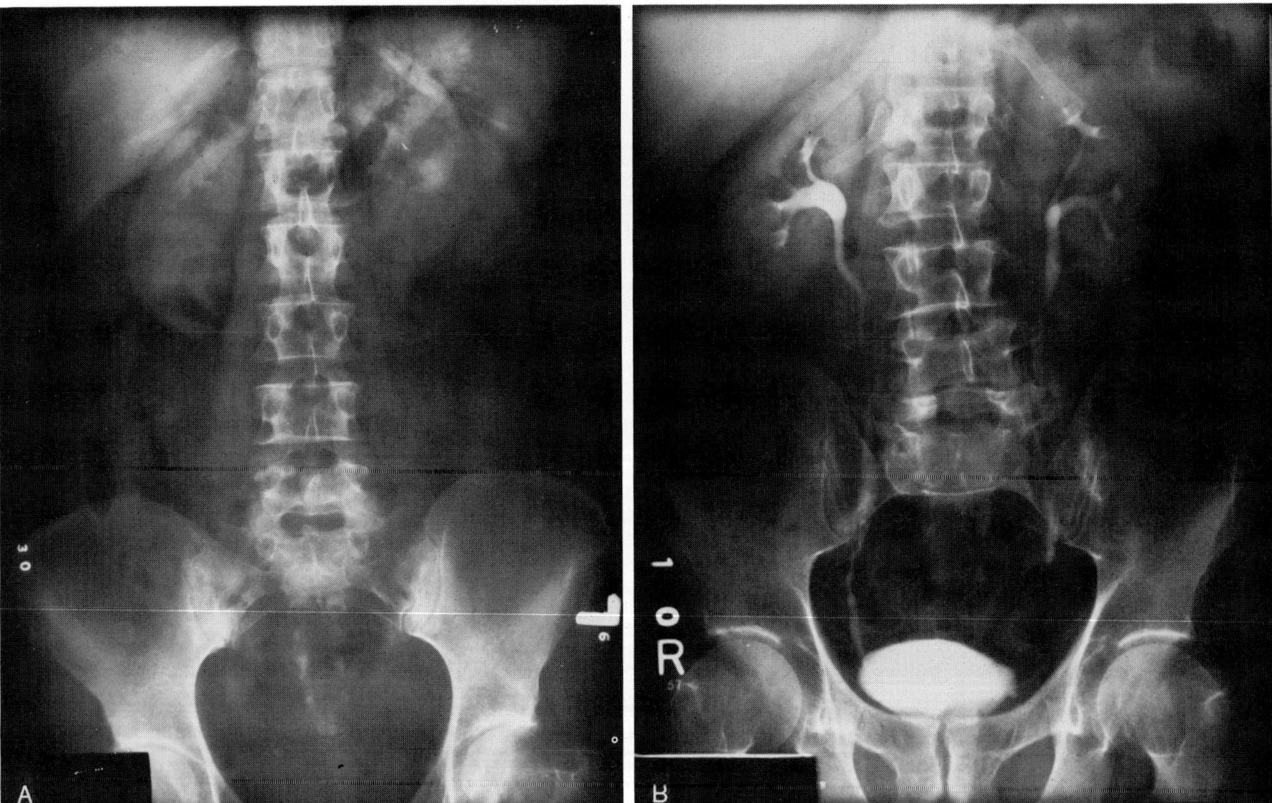

**FIGURE 10–5.** Contrast of the anatomic part produced by the use of contrast medium. *A* shows an abdominal radiograph produced without contrast medium. The kidneys are present owing to their tissue density. Other parts of the urinary system are visualized in *B* after contrast medium has been injected into the venous system of the patient. Contrast medium enhances the subject contrast to show the drainage system, ureters, and bladder.

contrast will be evident. Gas (air) shadows can be seen in the GI tract, and bone with surrounding tissue can be visualized, as demonstrated in Figure 10–6.

Pathology is also a factor in subject contrast. Disease processes often change the tissue structures and composition by making them more or less dense. These changes can be visualized by subject contrast if the tissue changes are sufficient.

## FILM CONTRAST

Film contrast refers to those qualities of x-ray film that result in the recording of high contrast or low contrast. The qualities are inherent in the preparation of the emulsion. Fog and scatter affect film contrast. Fog and scatter are undesirable density that produces gray tones on the film, which decrease contrast.

---

FILM CONTRAST IS INHERENT IN THE PREPARATION OF THE FILM EMULSION.

---

## CHARACTERISTICS OF CONTRAST

In order for a radiographer to consistently produce radiographs with acceptable contrast, he or she must be familiar with the use of kilovoltage and the characteristics exhibited on a radiograph. The language of contrast becomes a critical factor.

Contrast is described as either long scale, short scale, or moderate scale. Scale refers to the number of different densities present on the radiograph. If a radiograph was cut up into tiny little squares (each representing a density level) and the squares lined up in a graduated column with the lightest

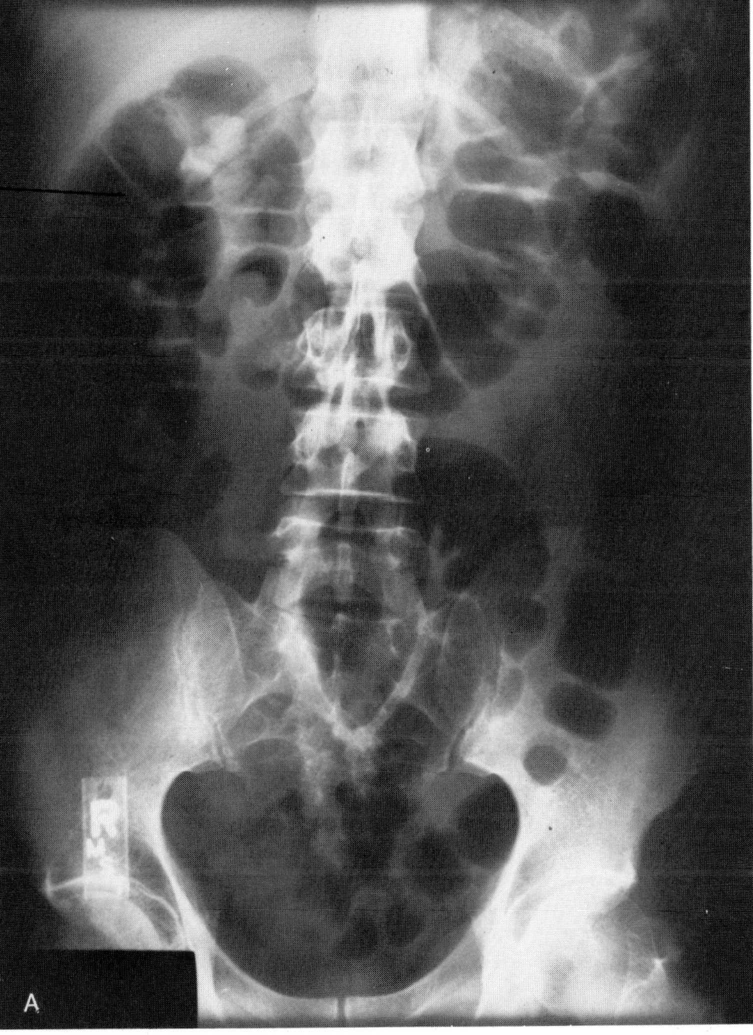


**FIGURE 10–6.** Subject contrast is demonstrated in *A* with gas in the large intestine.

*Illustration continued on following page*

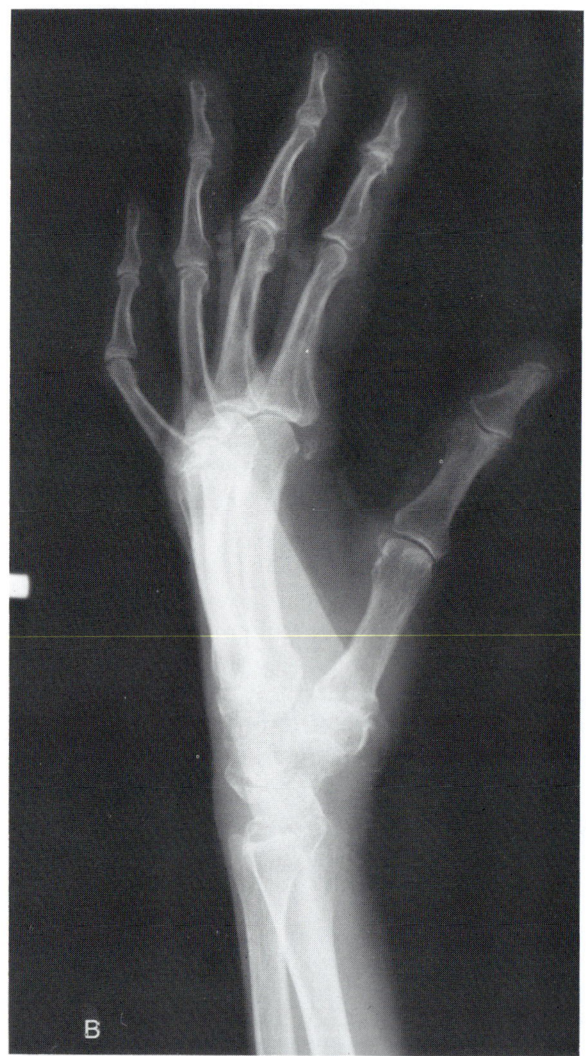

**FIGURE 10–6** *Continued* Skeletal and soft tissue can be seen in *B*.

square at the top and the darkest square at the bottom, this would represent a scale of contrast (Fig. 10–7).

---

CONTRAST SCALE REFERS TO THE NUMBER OF DIFFERENT DENSITY READINGS PRESENT ON THE RADIOGRAPH.

---

Long scale of contrast would be represented by a *long* column, with many squares representing each density level. The change from one square to the next would be gradual (Fig. 10–8).

---

LONG SCALE OF CONTRAST IS REPRESENTED BY MANY DIFFERENT DENSITY LEVELS ON THE RADIOGRAPH.

---

Short scale of contrast would be represented by a column with fewer squares (Fig. 10–8*B*). Fewer density levels would be shown from the lightest to darkest square. The change in density from one square to the next would be more pronounced.

---

SHORT SCALE OF CONTRAST IS REPRESENTED BY ONLY A FEW DENSITY LEVELS ON THE RADIOGRAPH.

---

## Long Scale of Contrast

Long scale of contrast means the difference in recorded density of adjacent structures is very small and many density levels are present. There are many different shades of gray between the lightest and darkest density values. Radiographs with a very long scale appear gray (Fig. 10–8*A*).

The advantage of a long scale of contrast is the visualization of more structural detail. Most tissue densities have been penetrated and structural detail is visible. Long scale is a result of higher kilovoltage. The higher the kilovoltage, the more gray tones are present on the radiograph. Part of the grayness is a result of increased scatter radiation produced by the increase in kilovoltage. The gray appearance produced by long scale reduces the overall contrast, and, in many cases, it is unwanted and undesirable.

---

LONG SCALE OF CONTRAST HAS MANY SHADES OF GRAY AND IS THE RESULT OF HIGH kVp.

---

Terms to describe long scale can be confusing. For example, long scale means low contrast, low degree of contrast, decreased or not enough contrast. Low contrast and low degree of contrast refer to very small density difference from one square to the next on the scale. "Not enough contrast" is a term used by many who believe a long scale has too many gray tones and not enough subject contrast (Fig. 10–8).

Increased exposure latitude is present with long-scale (high-kVp) techniques. Increased exposure latitude means that the margin of error is greater for acceptable exposure using high kilovoltage selections and results in a long scale of contrast.

Figure 10–9 presents the elements of long scale of contrast.

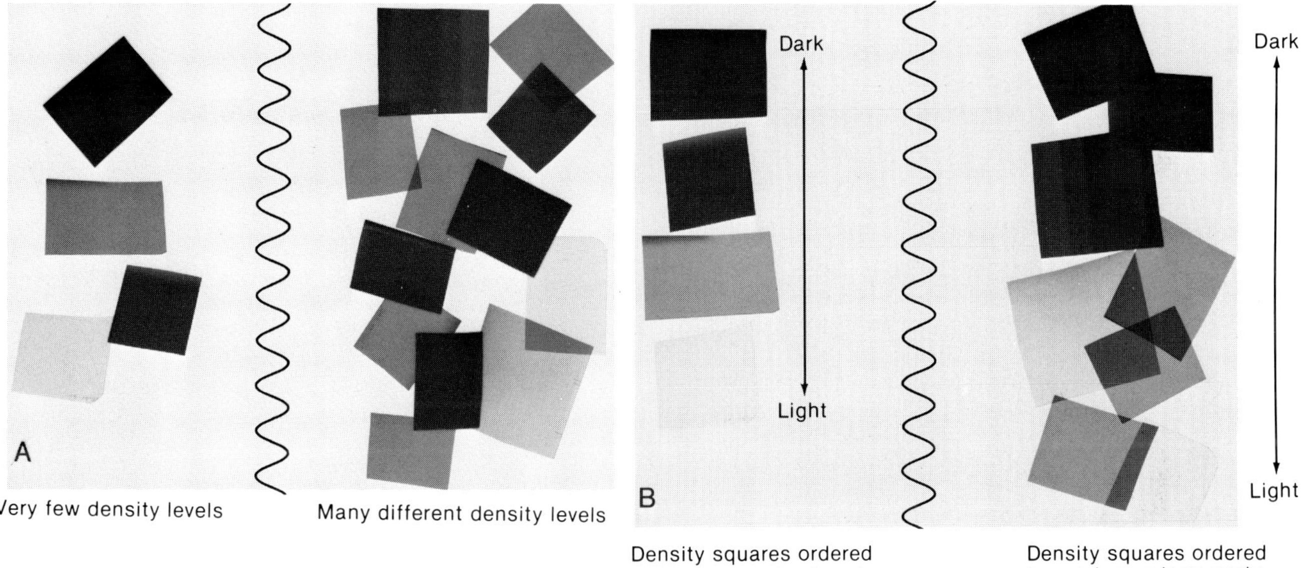



**FIGURE 10–7.** Radiographic contrast is demonstrated by the presence of squares of density. To produce contrast scale, the small squares are lined up with the darkest squares at the top and the lightest ones at the bottom. The result is contrast scale. In *A*, the left group has only a few shades of density and the group on the right has many different density squares. In *B*, the squares on the left have been ordered with the dark squares at the top and the light squares at the bottom. The result shows a short scale of contrast. The group on the right has also been reorganized with the darkest squares at the top and the lightest squares at the bottom. There are more squares representing shades of gray, producing a longer scale of contrast.

## Short Scale of Contrast

The opposite of long scale is short scale of contrast. Short scale of contrast is present when the density differences in adjacent structures are abrupt or pronounced. Short scale of contrast is produced by the use of low kVp selections.

The column of density levels shown in Figure 10–8*B* will be short, with few shades of gray tones between the lightest and darkest areas. The borders of the structures are evident, and, to many, radiographs exhibiting a short scale of contrast are better for viewing. The most positive characteristic for short scale is the enhanced contrast shown with skeletal studies (Fig. 10–10).

> SHORT SCALE OF CONTRAST HAS A SMALL NUMBER OF GRAY TONES AND IS THE RESULT OF LOW kVp.

A shorter scale of contrast is more ideal to examine bone structures, as shown in Figure 10–10. Radiographs appear black and white, with very little gray tones.

The disadvantages of a scale of contrast that is too short are important. Exposure factors selected to produce a short scale of contrast use a low

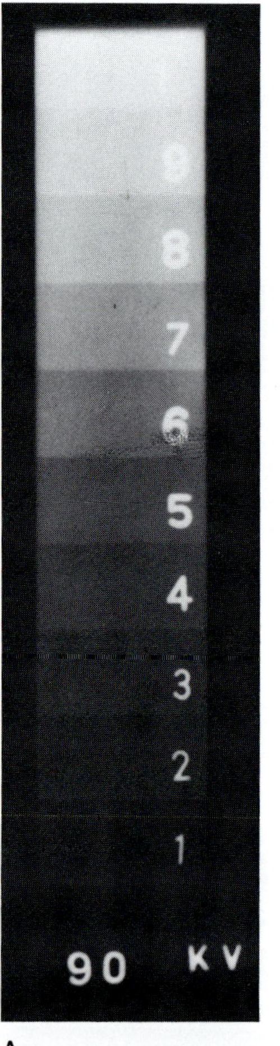


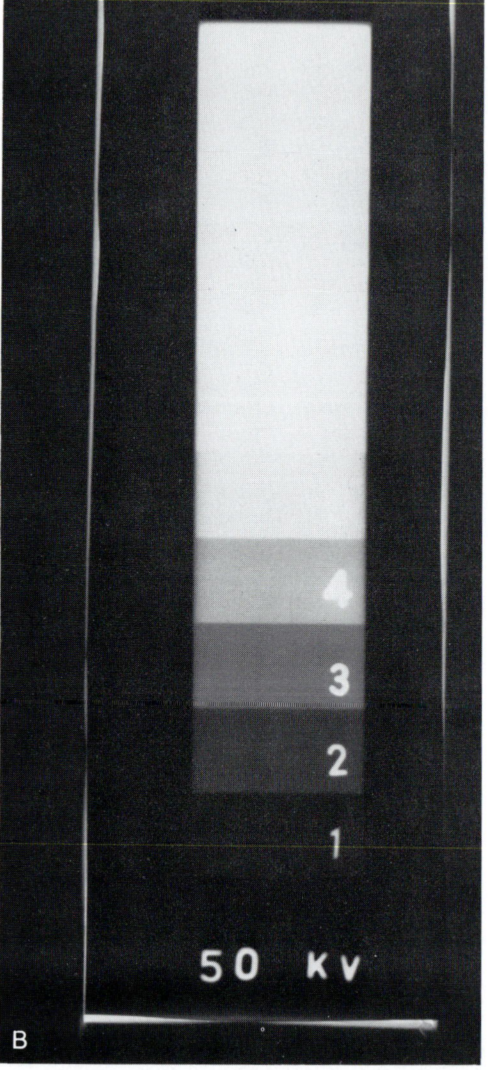


**FIGURE 10–8.** Long scale versus short scale. *A,* Long scale of contrast has many shades of gray between the lightest and darkest density values. *B,* Short scale of contrast has fewer density levels between the lightest and darkest squares. The change from one step to the next is more pronounced.

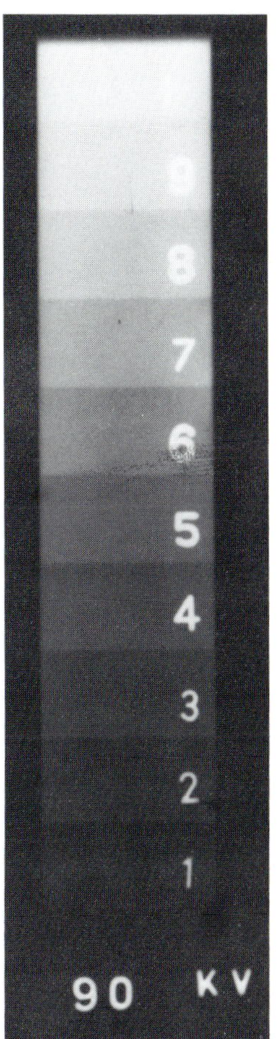



**FIGURE 10–9.** The elements of the long scale of contrast.

kilovoltage selection. Radiographs of the spine, skull, and other more dense anatomic structures may produce images with the thickest areas underpenetrated. Lower kilovoltage selections needed to produce a short scale of contrast may be inadequate for penetrating thicker body parts. Close examination reveals a silhouette without visualization of structural detail (Fig. 10–11).

The areas where inadequate penetration by the x-ray photons exists are clear (white) because no exposure reached the film, resulting in an absence of black metallic silver deposits. There is no image recorded on the film without adequate penetration of the part. Frequently, radiographs with a short scale of contrast exhibit significant clear areas where penetration did not occur. A scale of contrast that is too short may have limited diagnostic value although it looks pleasing to the human eye.

Another point to remember with short scale of contrast is that because lower kVp selections are used, the amount of radiation absorbed by the patient increases.

The terms associated with short scale of contrast

are higher contrast, high degree of contrast, and more contrast (Fig. 10–12).

High contrast or high degree of contrast refers to the abrupt and pronounced borders that are present. There is no gradual change with small difference in density; the changes in adjacent densities are abrupt. The phrase "more contrast" refers to the appearance of mostly black and white or clear areas. If a densitometer was used to measure each density level present, the number of readings would be less than with a long scale of contrast. The lower kVp exposures for short scale have less exposure latitude. The margin of error is small for producing a good radiograph.

Radiographic contrast is an extremely complex factor as radiographers attempt to consistently achieve high-quality radiographs. The selection of factors is extremely important. Kilovoltage is the factor that controls contrast. High kVp produces long-scale and low kVp produces short-scale contrast. To review the facts associated with kVp, radiographers must understand that high kVp produces more scatter; however, the amount of scatter radiation absorbed by the patient is less.

## KILOVOLTAGE CONTROLS CONTRAST.

With low kVp, less scatter is produced and the radiograph does not have many gray tones; however, the amount of radiation absorbed by the patient is increased.

To compromise with the scale of contrast, radiographers must try to produce radiographs with a moderate scale. A moderate scale of contrast is "in between" a long and short scale, as demonstrated in Figure 10–13. The kVp selection is made to achieve optimal penetration of the part. This is called optimal kVp selection. The kVp selection is neither very low nor very high. Optimal kVp will assure that the finished radiograph demonstrates structural detail without the excessive gray tones of long scale (Fig. 10–14).

## FACTORS THAT AFFECT RADIOGRAPHIC CONTRAST

### Film-Screen Systems

Film-screen systems must be selected with the desired characteristic of contrast in mind. In general, the use of screens will increase contrast. The

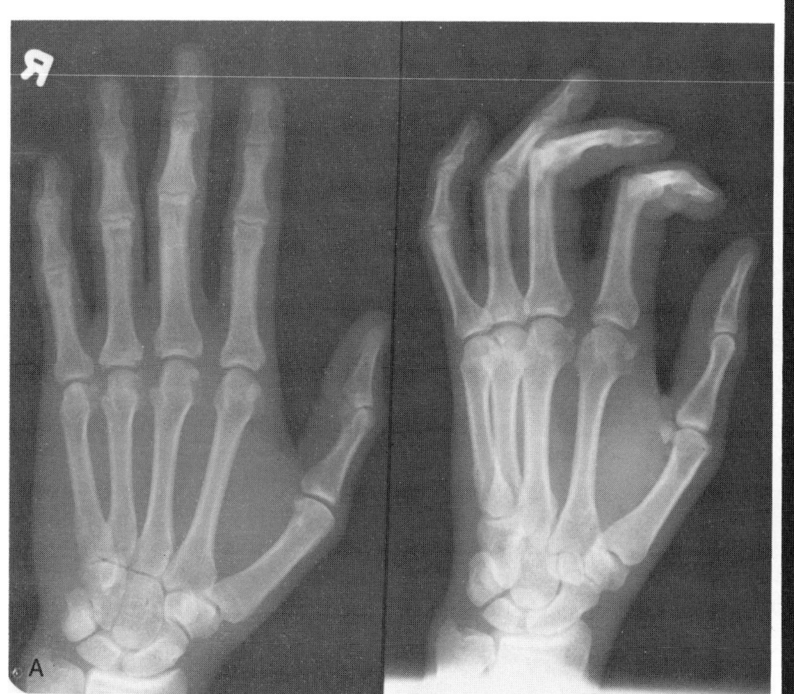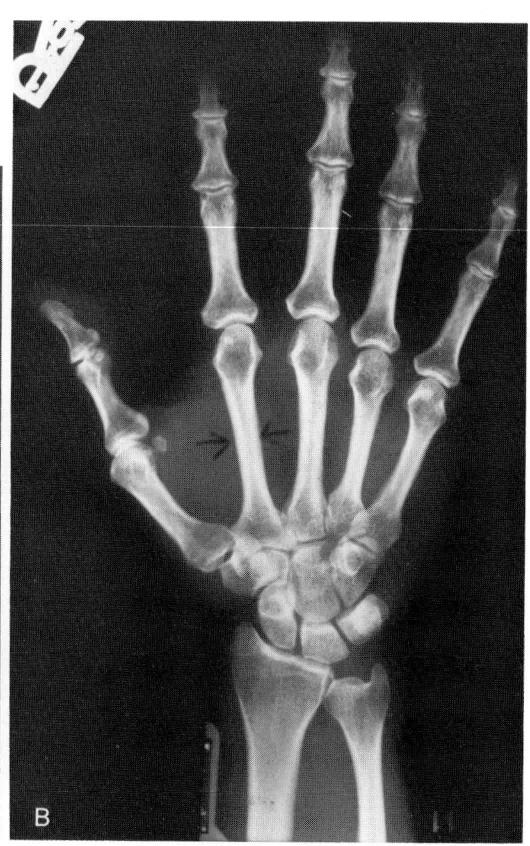

**FIGURE 10–10.** Radiographs of extremities representing long scale and short scale of contrast. *A,* Radiograph representing long scale of contrast. The image has an overall gray appearance with very little contrast between the soft tissue and skeleton. *B,* Radiograph with short scale of contrast. It has more of a black and white appearance, and there is a pronounced difference between the skeleton and soft tissue.

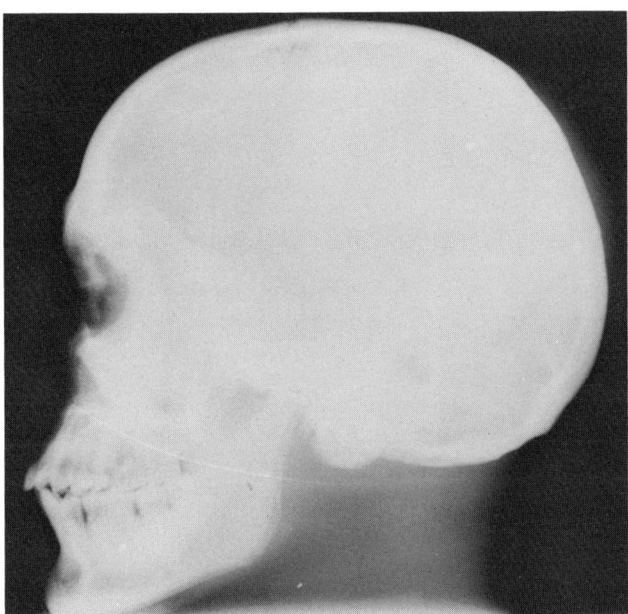

**FIGURE 10–11.** Radiograph of the skull demonstrating underpenetration of the part.

The objectives in the selection of a film-screen system should be: acceptable speed, good contrast (moderate scale), and the ability to adequately visualize the structural details of the anatomic areas of interest.

## Processing

The proper time-temperature relationship and chemical mixtures are necessary to build proper contrast during the processing cycle. Chemical fog will tend to prevent good contrast. Fog may result if temperatures are too high. If the temperatures are too low, the density will not be sufficient to build adequate contrast on the film. Underdevelopment prevents the film from building adequate contrast.

faster the screen, the greater the contrast or the shorter the scale. This is most evident in the use of calcium tungstate screens with regular-speed x-ray film. In general, slow screens produce the longest scale or lower contrast, and high-speed screens produce the shortest scale, with more contrast. Images with moderate scale of contrast tend to provide more diagnostic information; therefore, the selection of the film-screen system is very important.

IN GENERAL, AS INTENSIFYING SCREENS INCREASE IN SPEED, CONTRAST INCREASES.

The use of rare earth phosphors has produced new technology in the film-screen selection process. Studies have shown that rare earth phosphors work best at approximately 70 to 80 kVp. This kVp range provides optimal kVp for a moderate contrast scale. In addition, the speed of rare earth provides the advantage of a slightly shorter scale of contrast.

RARE EARTH SCREENS PRODUCE RADIOGRAPHS WITH A SLIGHT INCREASE IN CONTRAST OVER CALCIUM TUNGSTATE SCREENS.

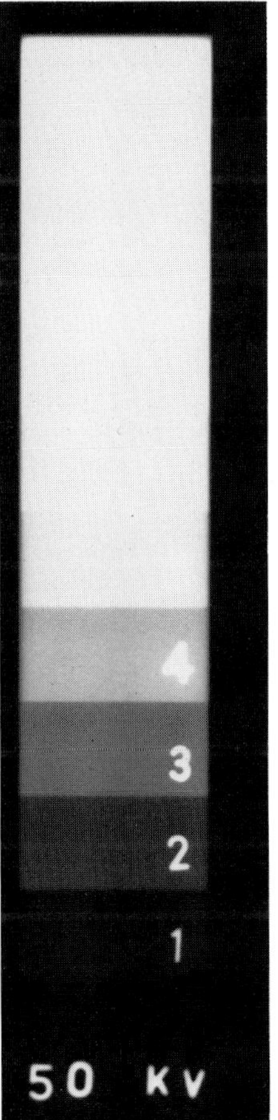


**FIGURE 10–12.** The elements of the short scale of contrast.

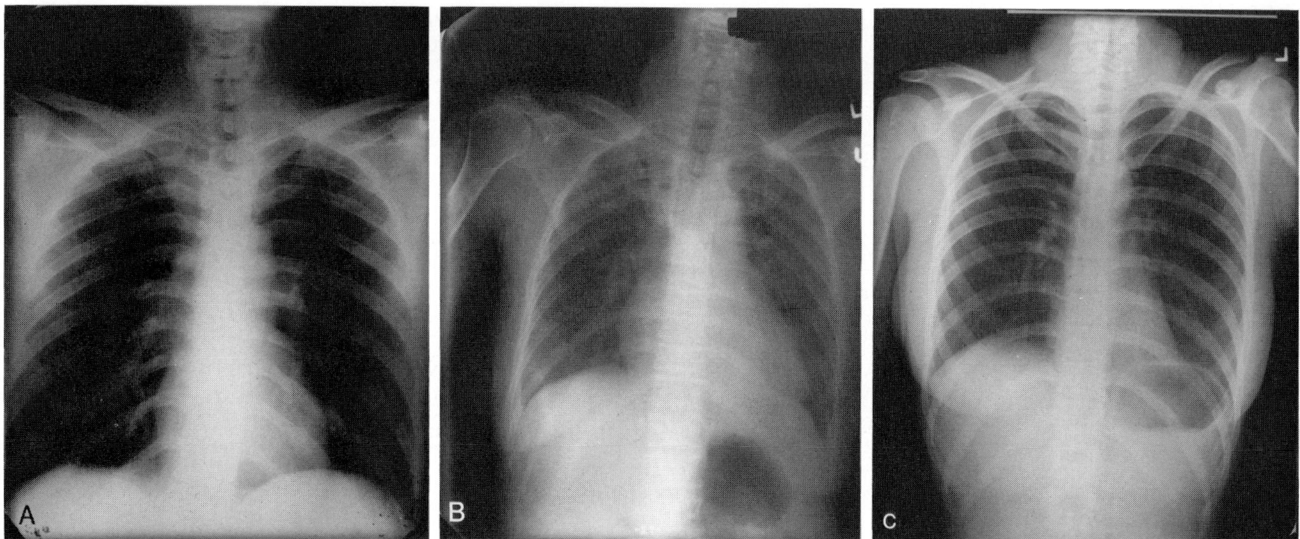

**FIGURE 10–13.** Radiographs of the chest exhibiting different scales of contrast. *A,* A short scale of contrast. *B,* A very long scale with many gray tones. *C,* A more moderate scale of contrast.

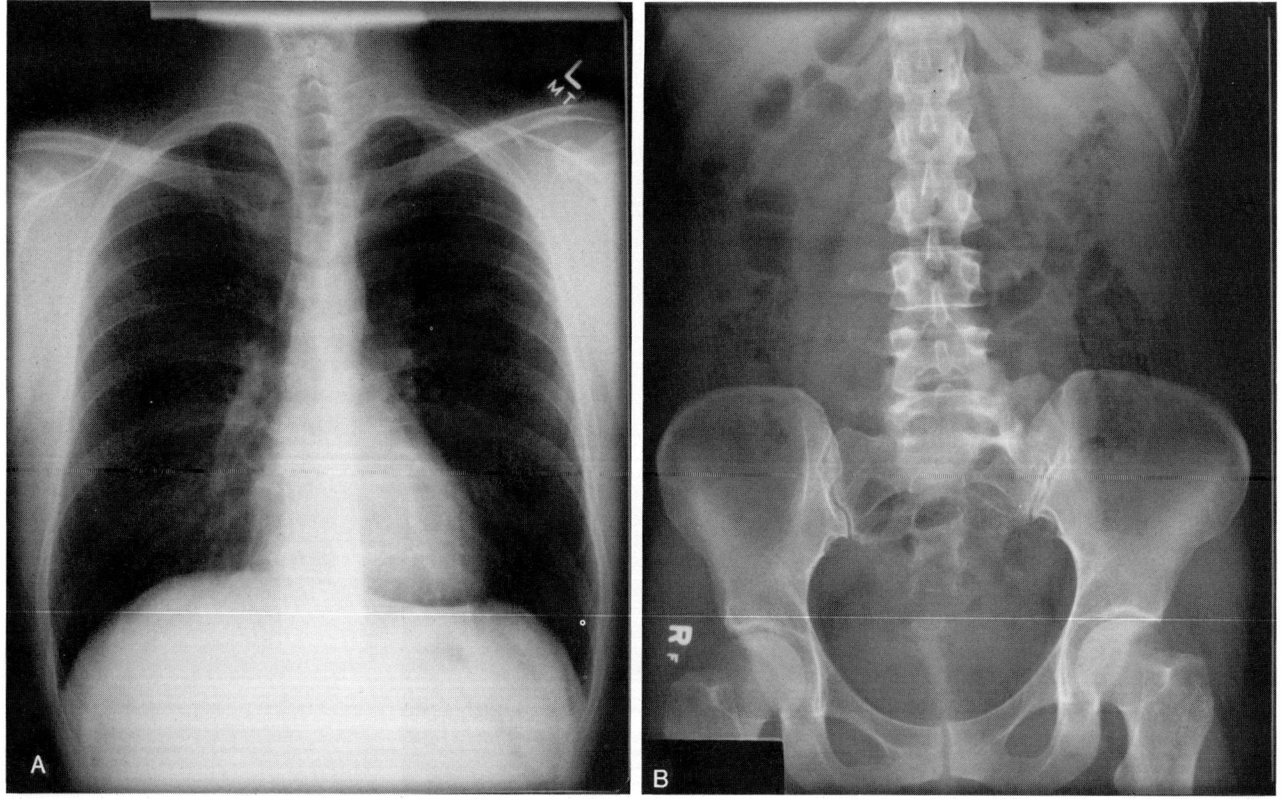

**FIGURE 10–14.** High-quality radiographs with slightly different contrast scale. *A,* Chest radiograph representing a moderate scale of contrast. *B,* A radiograph of the abdomen representing a longer scale of contrast that enhances the many different tissue densities that are present.

PROCESSING MUST BE OPTIMAL TO
PRODUCE ADEQUATE CONTRAST.

## Beam Restriction

The use of beam restriction is very important in the recording of good contrast. As the beam becomes more restricted to the actual size of the part, less scatter radiation is produced, which in turn reduces fog, resulting in greater contrast on the film. Scatter hinders the production of radiographs with good contrast. The use of beam restriction will increase contrast and produce radiographs with a shorter scale of contrast.

BEAM RESTRICTION PRODUCES AN INCREASE
IN CONTRAST.

## Grids

Grids are devices located between the patient and the film. When a grid is in place, it absorbs scattered x-rays that travel in many directions to prevent hitting the film. Scatter rays that travel nearly parallel with the remnant primary x-ray photons exiting the body will not be absorbed by the grid. The use of grids will require an increase in exposure factors; however, there will be an increase in the contrast, and the result will be a radiograph with a shorter scale of contrast.

**TABLE 10–1.** FACTORS THAT AFFECT CONTRAST

| Controlling Factor | Influencing Factor |
| --- | --- |
| Kilovoltage (kVp) | Tissue composition |
| | Contrast media |
| | Pathology |
| | Fog |
| | Scatter radiation |
| | Film-screen systems |
| | Processing |
| | Beam restriction |
| | Grid |

THE USE OF GRIDS PRODUCES AN INCREASE
IN CONTRAST.

## Pathology and Composition of the Part

The composition of the anatomic part of interest is important in understanding the characteristics of contrast as recorded on the film. Disease processes that increase water content will result in radiographs exhibiting longer scale. The same is true for fat content. Obese patients with increased fat content will exhibit radiographs with longer scale. On the other hand, disease processes that cause tissue destruction such as osteoporosis will generally exhibit a short scale of contrast. The same is true for tissue filled with air or gas shadows—the recorded contrast is greater. Contrast on a radiograph can be enhanced by the use of compression. Abdominal tissue can be compressed by exposing the patient using the posterior-anterior projection instead of the anterior-posterior projection.

Table 10–1 reviews contrast and the factors that control and influence contrast.

# C H A P T E R  11

# Radiographic Definition and Distortion

● ● ● ● ● ● ●

## CHAPTER OBJECTIVES

1. Define the term "maximum definition."
2. Define umbra and penumbra.
3. Describe the relationship of penumbra and unsharpness.
4. Explain the umbrella concept for image definition.
5. List the factors associated with image definition.
6. Define or describe:

   Recorded detail    Visibility of detail
   Distortion

7. List the geometric factors associated with recorded detail.
8. Explain how each of the geometric factors (OFD, FFD, and FSS) affects image unsharpness.
9. Describe how motion interferes with image distortion.
10. List examples for reducing unsharpness with the geometric factors and motion.
11. Define quantum mottle.
12. Describe the conditions that produce mottle.
13. Explain the effects on image resolution by the thickness of the phosphor layer and the conversion efficiency of the phosphor.
14. Describe the bar test used to evaluate the resolving power of the imaging system.
15. Explain how screen-film contact affects image definition.
16. Define image distortion.
17. Differentiate between foreshortening and elongation.
18. Identify the factors that cause size and shape distortion.
19. Define the term "visibility of detail."
20. Define magnification factor and write the formula.
21. Differentiate between overexposure and underexposure, and list the causes.
22. Describe how fog and scatter affect visibility of detail.
23. Explain how kVp and mAs can affect visibility of detail.

## KEY WORDS AND TERMS

Definition
Sharpness of the image
Maximum definition
Umbra
Penumbra
Unsharpness
Visibility of detail
Focal spot size (FSS)
Focal-film distance (FFD)
Object-film distance (OFD)
Geometric factor
Voluntary motion
Involuntary motion
Blurring of image
Restraints
Immobilization of part
Compression bands
Sand bags

Screen mottle
Quantum mottle
Screen "noise"
Phosphor layer
Phosphor conversion efficiency
Image resolution
Bar-test pattern
Line pair/mm
Screen-film contact
Distortion
Size distortion
Magnification
Shape distortion
Elongation
Foreshortening
Magnification factor
Overexposure
Underexposure

## RECOMMENDATIONS FOR GENERAL DISCUSSION QUESTIONS

1. Discuss each factor related to definition (umbrella).
2. Describe the difference in recorded detail and visibility of detail.
3. What are the requirements to achieve good recorded detail?
4. What are the requirements for assuring the best visibility of detail?
5. What should be included in a procedure guide for producing well-defined radiographs?
6. What steps should be taken to eliminate or reduce distortion of the image?

## DEFINITION

Radiographic definition describes the clarity and sharpness of the image. The term "definition" means to make definite, clear, and refers to the sharpness of outlines and the detail or sharpness of minute markings.

### DEFINITION DESCRIBES THE CLARITY AND SHARPNESS OF THE IMAGE.

Maximum definition in radiography describes an image that outlines objects extremely well. The lines and markings of the actual anatomic part are the best possible. Maximum definition implies that a radiograph shows minimum magnification and distortion and has clarity that enhances the visibility of the anatomic markings.

There are inherent limitations in radiography that prevent the production of a perfect radiograph. For example, the anatomic part of interest is inside the body and therefore cannot be placed next to the film. This causes the part to be recorded larger than its actual size. In addition, there is no specific point source for the production of x-rays. Photons that originate from different points on the target area cause some unsharpness as they traverse the borders of objects. This results in slight blurring of the object.

In radiography, the true object recorded on the film is called the *umbra* and the small or thin area of blurring around the umbra is called the *penumbra* (Fig. 11–1).

### UMBRA IS THE TRUE OBJECT RECORDED ON THE FILM. PENUMBRA IS THE THIN BLURRED AREA AROUND THE UMBRA.

Penumbra is also known as *unsharpness.* Penumbra places a limitation on radiographic definition. Figure 11–2*A* shows unsharpness around the edge of the image with a wide beam, whereas Figure 11–2*B* shows less unsharpness with a narrow beam. Radiographers cannot completely eliminate penumbra or unsharpness; however, it can be minimized so that image quality is not compromised.

### PENUMBRA IS UNSHARPNESS.

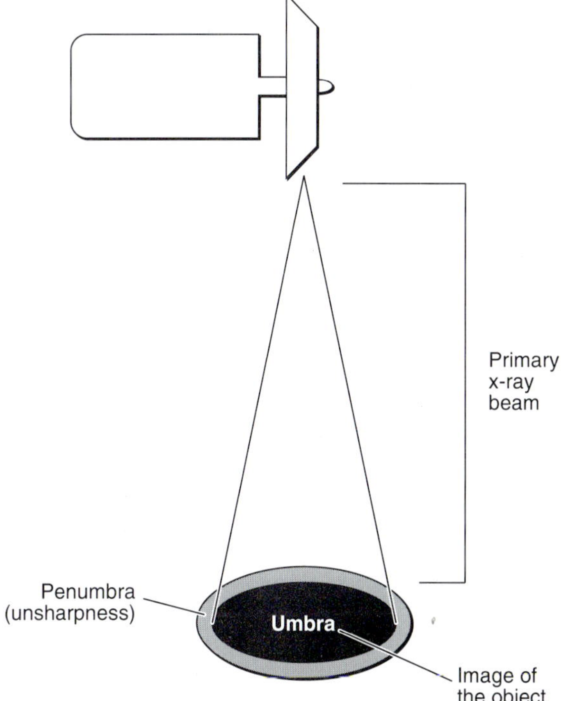


**FIGURE 11–1.** The true image of the object recorded on the film is the umbra. The blurring around the edge of the umbra is the penumbra or unsharpness.

Factors must be combined in such a way that an image with the best possible sharpness and detail is produced. Good definition is present with minute lines and details visible, and it enables the radiologist to evaluate for abnormalities. Figure 11–3 shows a radiograph with good definition.

In radiography, definition is an all-encompassing term that includes all of the visible characteristics of a radiograph (Fig. 11–4).

As indicated in the diagram in Figure 11–4, definition is a comprehensive term. It includes all factors used to produce a radiograph that will directly affect the image detail and sharpness, as well as all factors that affect the visibility of detail.

Those characteristics associated with definition are recorded detail, distortion, and visibility of detail. Radiographers use these factors to produce and evaluate radiographs.

### THE CHARACTERISTICS OF DEFINITION ARE RECORDED DETAIL, DISTORTION, AND VISIBILITY OF DETAIL.

### Recorded Detail

Recorded detail is the actual or visible detail of the part of interest recorded on the film. Recording

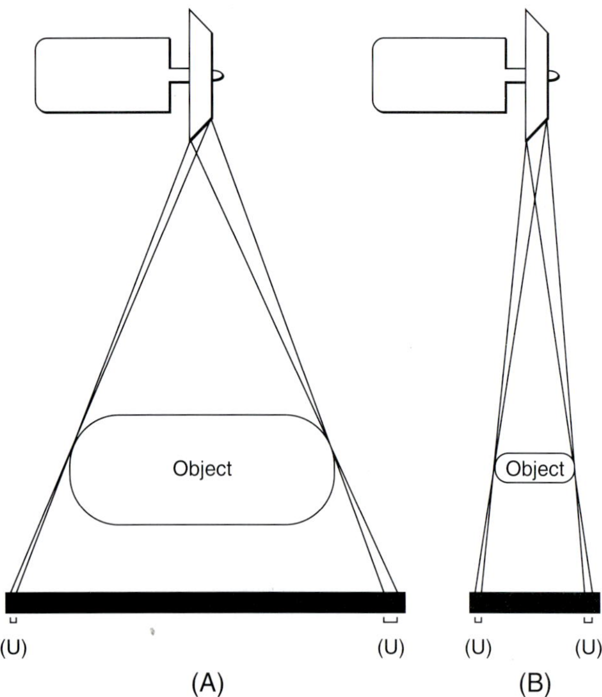



**FIGURE 11–2.** A wide-angle primary beam (*A*) will result in more unsharpness (U) or penumbra than a narrow-angle beam (*B*).

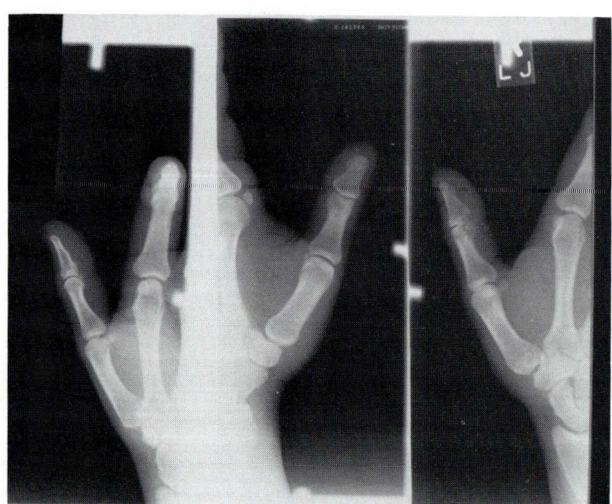

**FIGURE 11–3.** Radiograph that exhibits good definition. The skeletal markings are visible with good differentiation between bone and soft tissue. The borders of the bones and soft tissue are very distinct. Recorded detail is adequate; there is minimal distortion, and visibility of detail is very good.

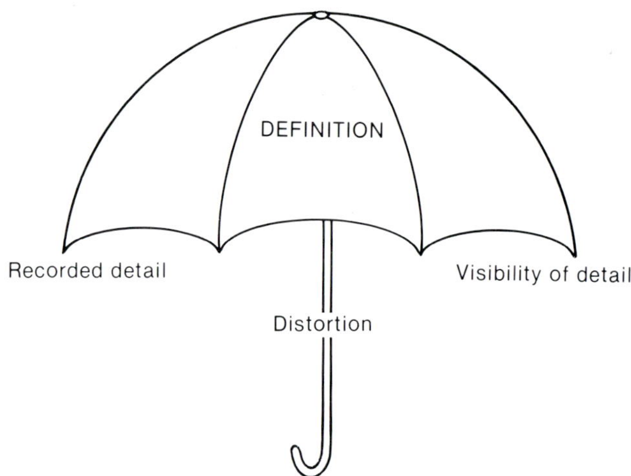



**FIGURE 11–4.** Radiographic definition is a comprehensive term that includes all factors that are used to produce a radiograph. All factors are related to recorded detail, distortion, and visibility of detail.

the image detail is dependent on the focal spot size (FSS), the distance between the focal spot and the x-ray film (focal-film distance [FFD]), the distance between the part of interest and the film (object-to-film distance [OFD]), absence of object movement, and the type of recording system used to produce the image. FSS, OFD, and FFD are significant factors that control unsharpness by their geometric nature in the production of x-rays. FSS, OFD, and FFD are called the "geometric factors."

**THE GEOMETRIC FACTORS IN RECORDING DETAIL ARE FFD, OFD, AND FSS.**

## Focal Spot Size

Figure 11–5 is an enhanced diagram that demonstrates how the use of a large focal spot will increase unsharpness on the image.

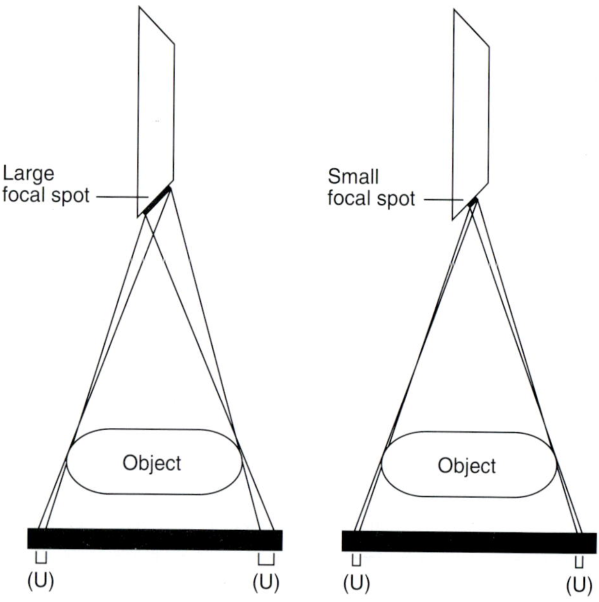



**FIGURE 11–5.** The use of a large focal spot will result in increased blurring (unsharpness [U]) around the object. The unsharpness is caused by x-rays that originate from different points on the focal spot striking the edge of the object.

The illustration demonstrates how the use of a large FSS results in increased image unsharpness. The unsharpness is caused by x-rays originating from different points on the focal spot. As they travel tangentially across the edge of the anatomic part of interest, the outer edge of the object receives x-ray photons from all areas of the focal spot to help record the image on the film. The effect produces a fuzzy, unsharp border around the area of the object. The human eye reads this as unsharpness. As unsharpness increases, the outlines of the objects become more difficult to identify. Increased unsharpness on a radiograph interferes with the radiologist's ability to evaluate the structures.

## THE SMALLER THE FOCAL SPOT SIZE, THE GREATER THE IMAGE SHARPNESS.

At the time of the selection of the exposure factors, care must be taken to select the smallest possible focal spot that is practical. This will result in the best possible image sharpness. Caution must be exercised. The radiographer should consult rating charts to determine if the selection of the FSS and technical factors are compatible with that specific x-ray tube.

## Focal-Film Distance

Distance between the focal spot and the x-ray film will affect sharpness. Figure 11–6 demonstrates how changes in the FFD will affect unsharpness. The illustration shows that unsharpness increases as the FFD is decreased.

The illustration demonstrates the concept that x-rays originate from the entire surface of the focal spot and not from a single point source. Photons that originate from these different points pass tangentially across the edge of the object and record information in a slightly different area. The result is unsharpness. As the FFD decreases, the unsharpness will increase.

## THE LONGER THE FFD, THE GREATER THE SHARPNESS OF THE IMAGE.

Radiographers must utilize the longest FFD that is practical to minimize unsharpness. In most radiology departments, examinations are performed

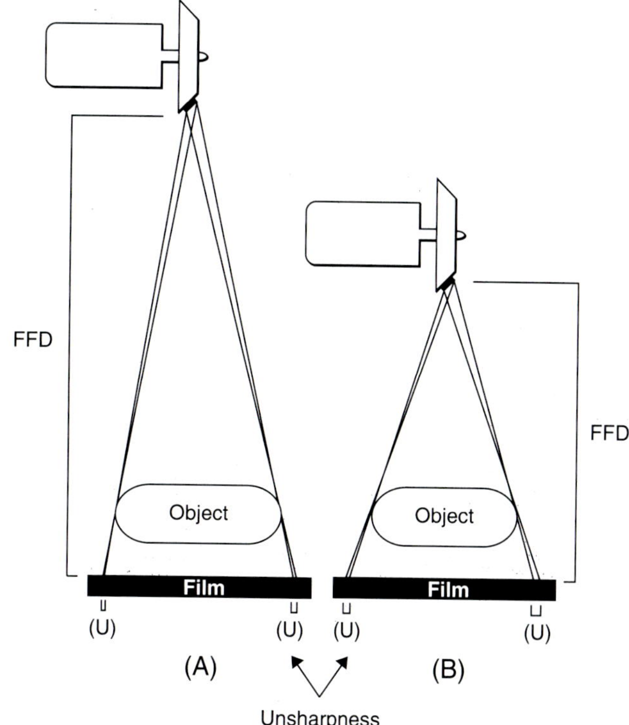


**FIGURE 11–6.** As the focal-film distance (FFD) increases, unsharpness of the image will decrease.

with a standard FFD. It is important to follow the standard guide and to refrain from making arbitrary changes in the FFD.

## Object-Film Distance

One of the first principles to be learned when positioning a body part to be imaged is to place the anatomic part of interest as near the film as possible. This principle is very important in radiography. The primary reason for placing the part as near the film as possible is to produce maximum recorded detail. The OFD is a factor in size distortion. As the OFD increases, so does the image unsharpness and size distortion (magnification).

## THE SHORTER THE OFD, THE GREATER THE IMAGE SHARPNESS.

The distance from the part of interest and the film is the third geometric factor for evaluating recorded detail. Figure 11–7 illustrates how changes in the OFD will contribute to unsharpness.

As the distance between the object and the film increases, so will the unsharpness. The concept is

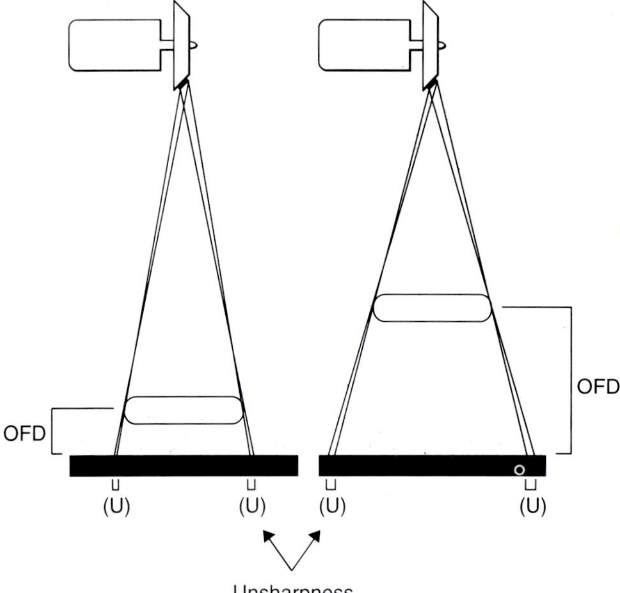



**FIGURE 11–7.** An increase in the object-film distance (OFD) will increase unsharpness.

the same as described for FFD and OFD. The photons originate from different points on the target and result in a slight difference in recording the image on the film.

It is important always to place the part as near the film as possible. Inasmuch as the part cannot be placed directly next to the film, the geometry of the illustrations indicates some unsharpness will always be present.

Geometric unsharpness as produced by the FFD, FSS, and OFD can be minimized by a long FFD, small FSS, and a short OFD.

## Motion

The biggest enemy in the production of a good radiograph is motion. No matter how well the job is done with the selection of the technical and geometric factors, if the part moves during the exposure, detail can not be accurately recorded. The result is a blurred image that is useless to the radiographer and radiologist. The examination must be repeated. Motion must be eliminated in general radiography (Fig. 11–8).

To better understand how to eliminate motion, one must first understand the characteristics of motion. Motion that is voluntary is easiest for radiographers to control. Movement of the extremities, body movement, and breathing are considered to be voluntary. This means that instructions must be given by the radiographer and understood by the

patient so that movement does not occur at the time of the exposure.

## MOTION OF THE PART MUST BE ELIMINATED DURING THE EXPOSURE.

Patients are often anxious and apprehensive at the time a radiograph is produced, and movement may occur even if the patient understood the instructions. Minimum restraints that will provide security to the patient, such as sand bags across an extremity, can help reduce the possibility of motion.

Involuntary motion is present in the gastrointestinal tract, cardiovascular system, and with patients who may be incoherent or unconscious and cannot hold their breath for the short time period needed to make a radiographic exposure. Involuntary motion presents a real challenge to the radiographer. Suggestions for controlling involuntary motion at the time of the exposure would be to use the shortest possible exposure time as well as immobilization through the use of compression bands, sand bags, etc. Special pediatric restraints are available for radiography of small children and babies.

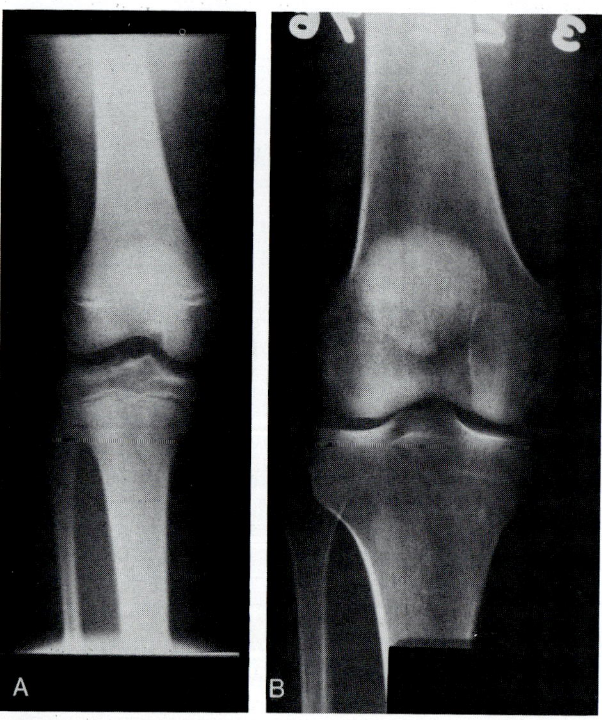



**FIGURE 11–8.** Motion can be a major problem in producing radiographs with good definition. *A,* A radiograph with the part in motion at the time of the exposure. Overall blurring of the image has prevented the recording of good image detail. *B,* A radiograph with improved image detail in the absence of motion of the part.

## Recording System (Film-Screen Combinations)

The imaging system composed of the screen-film combination will also control and influence the recording of detail. Film graininess, screen structure, and screen mottle or quantum mottle (noise) must be considered in the evaluation of screen-film effectiveness in recording detail.

Film graininess is another factor; however, it is not a major factor in diagnostic radiology. Film graininess refers to the inherent uneven distribution of silver crystals in the film emulsion. Film graininess would be a factor if radiographs are enlarged for viewing.

Screen structural defects may be present in the manufacturing process, producing imperfections in the phosphor layer. Neither of these factors is of great significance in general radiography.

Screen mottle or quantum mottle (noise) is the fluctuation in the number of photons absorbed by the screen phosphors. The x-ray beam is made up of different energies. The multiple energies in the primary beam, along with the fluctuation in the photon absorption by the screen, result in non-uniform light exposures to the film. Mottle looks like a "snowy" television screen and prevents the recording of good detail.

Quantum mottle is more evident in high-speed systems. An exception would be with screens where the layer of phosphors has been increased in thickness to produce faster speed. In the manufacture of screens using new technology, a more efficient phosphor rather than increased thickness of the phosphor layer is used to produce speed.

The fast screens with a thicker phosphor layer will absorb more photons and require the mAs to be reduced. The increased thickness of the phosphor layer produces more light diffusion, which obscures the mottle. However, the increased diffusion of light will increase unsharpness of the image, as shown in Figure 11–9. Rare earth systems, on the other hand, are more efficient and do not produce as much light diffusion and unsharpness. The increased ef-ficiency of the rare earth phosphors does not require a thicker layer to achieve an increase in speed. Therefore, with rare earth screens, the diffusion of light that reduces image definition is not a factor in image production.

INTENSIFYING SCREENS WITH MINIMAL LIGHT DIFFUSION WILL PRODUCE BETTER RECORDED DETAIL.

Quantum mottle is easier to recognize as the film speed and screen speed increase. The milliampere-seconds (mAs) is reduced and the patient receives less radiation; however, fewer photons will be available to produce the image. With fewer photons available, a non-uniform pattern of light strikes the film, producing an increase in quantum mottle. Quantum mottle is most significant with high kilo-voltage peak (kVp) and low mAs exposure used with fast imaging systems. Quantum mottle will obscure recorded detail.

WITH FAST IMAGING SYSTEMS, MOTTLE IS A PROBLEM WITH EXPOSURES USING HIGH kVp AND LOW mAs; MOTTLE WILL OBSCURE RECORDED DETAIL.

## Image Resolution

Image resolution is the term used to evaluate a screen-film system's ability to record detail. The ability of an imaging system to provide good image resolution can be measured using a leaded bar-test pattern (Fig. 11–10). The test pattern is sectioned with bars of lines, with interspacing in a specific pattern. The test pattern is radiographed. The film is processed and viewed by the radiographer to

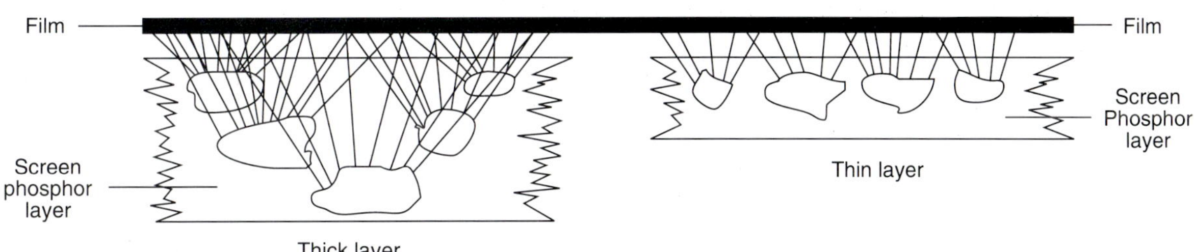


**FIGURE 11–9.** A thicker phosphor layer produces greater light diffusion. As the amount of light diffusion increases, unsharpness will decrease.

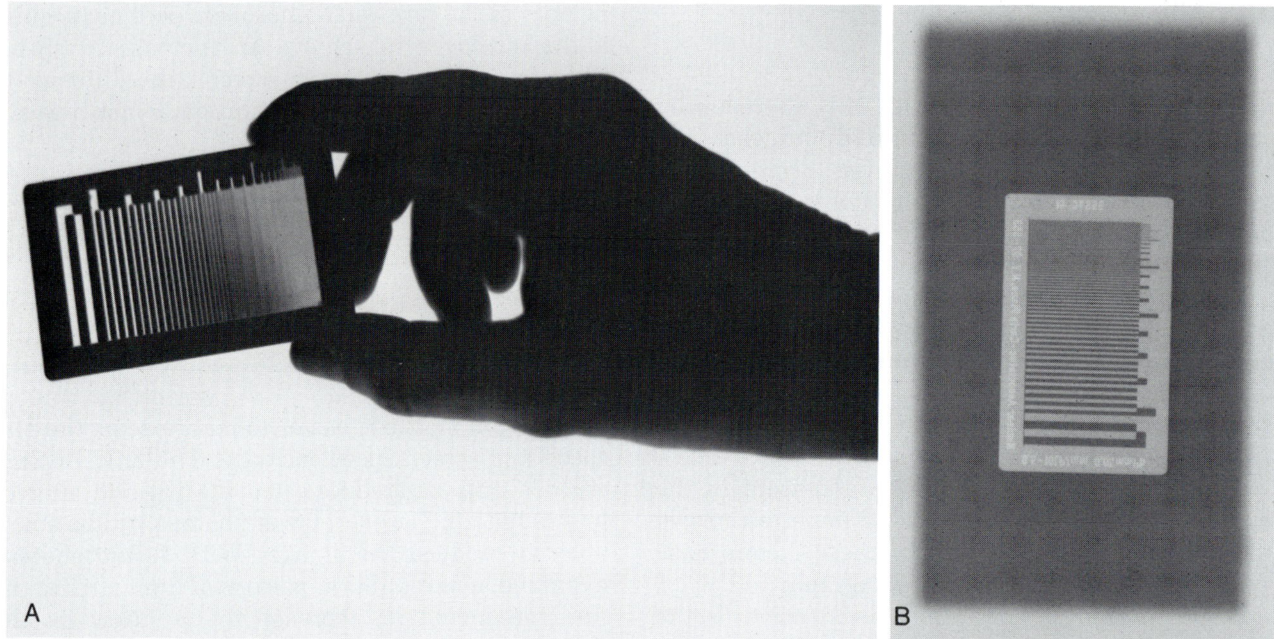

**FIGURE 11–10.** Image resolution can be tested using a leaded bar test pattern. *A,* The bar test pattern is held in front of a viewbox, and the pattern of bars is visible. *B,* A radiograph made using the test pattern.

determine the number of line pairs that can be visualized.

A line pair is one line (bar) and one interspace. For example, if eight line pairs are visible, this means that eight bars and eight interspaces are visible, and the system has a resolution value of 8 line pairs/mm. The higher the number of line pairs/mm that are visible, the greater the resolving power of the imaging system and its ability to record detail.

---

THE GREATER THE RESOLVING POWER OF THE IMAGING SYSTEM, THE GREATER THE RECORDED DETAIL.

---

How many line pairs/mm can be visualized? The answer is dependent on the observer. A particular screen-film system with the ability to produce good detail may demonstrate 8 to 10 line pairs/mm. Table 11–1 compares sample screen systems.

**TABLE 11–1.** SCREEN SPEED AND RESOLUTION

| Screen Type | Speed | Line Pairs/MM |
| --- | --- | --- |
| Calcium tungstate | Slow (50) | 15 |
| Calcium tungstate | Fast (200) | 5–7 |
| Calcium tungstate | Medium (100) | 10 |
| Rare earth | 400 | 10 |
| Rare earth | 1200 | 6–8 |

## Screen-Film Contact

Screen-film contact is the pressure exerted by the film holder as it encloses the x-ray film. The pressure should be evenly distributed across the surface of the film. Screen-film contact is essential to record detail accurately. Poor screen-film contact reduces sharpness of the image. Screen-film contact can be evaluated by the radiographer, as described in Chapter 5. A wire mesh is imaged using the film holder suspected of poor screen contact. The result would show area(s) of increased or decreased density representing poor contact and decreased sharpness (Fig. 11–11).

---

GOOD FILM-SCREEN CONTACT MUST BE PRESENT TO ACHIEVE MAXIMUM DETAIL.

---

## DISTORTION

The misrepresentation of size and/or shape of the object is called distortion. In almost every radiograph there is distortion of the part in the form of size distortion (magnification). Magnification of the part occurs because the part is never in direct contact with the film. It would be best to have a zero OFD, but it is not realistic in medical radiography. Radiographs are usually made with 2 to 10 inches between the part and the film.

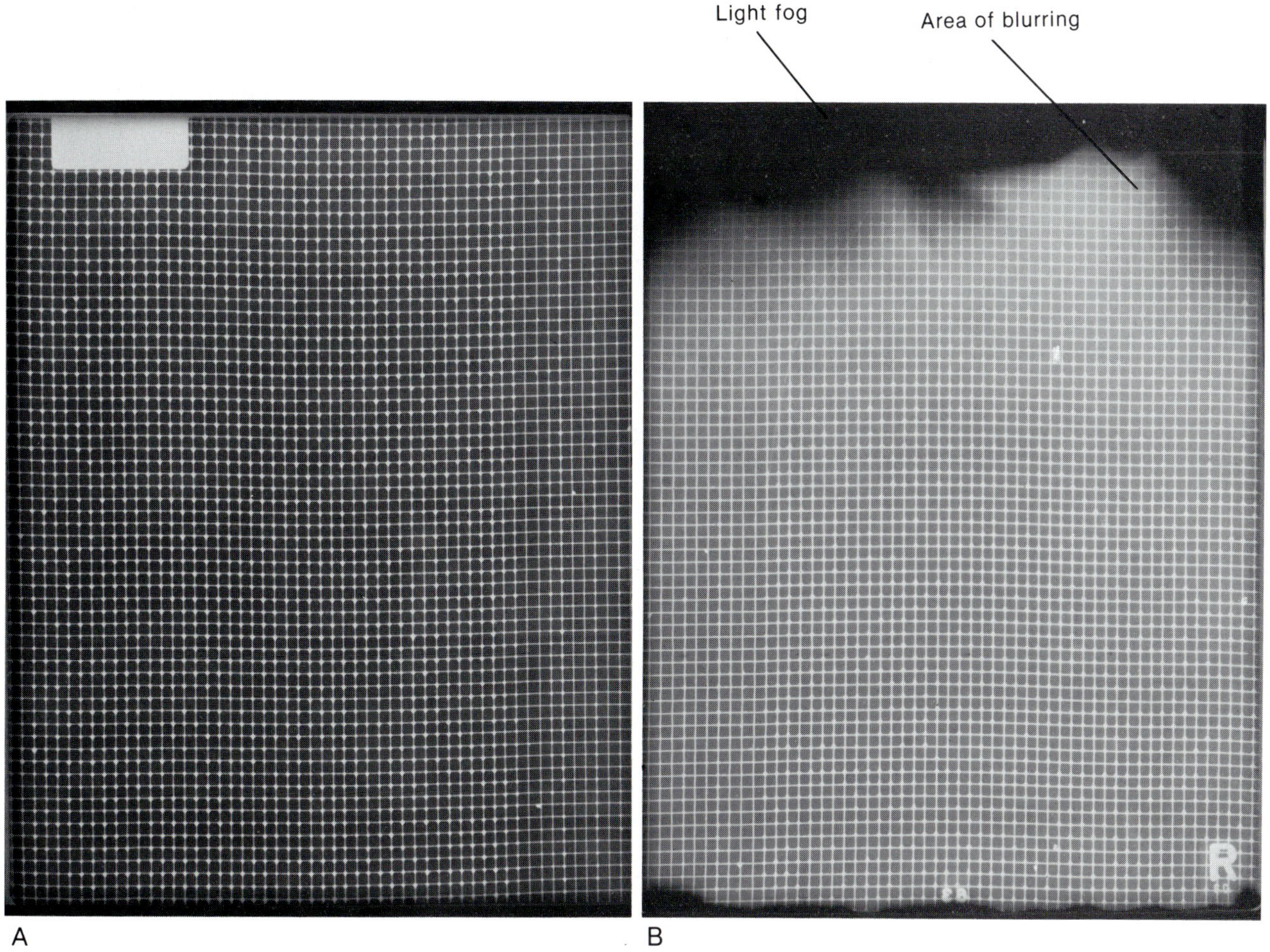

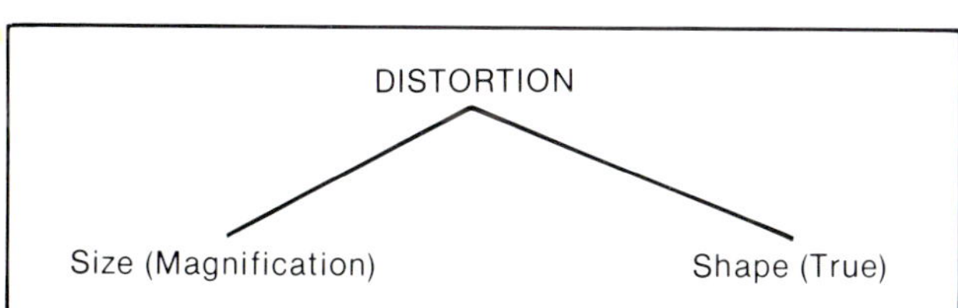


**FIGURE 11–11.** Film-screen contact is important in producing a radiograph with good definition. *A,* A radiograph representing a test for screen-film contact. Because the overall density and image detail is very good, the screen-film contact is adequate. *B,* A radiograph with poor film-screen contact, especially on the upper edge. The screens do not come together, and light entered the cassette to expose the film. The image of the wire mesh is also blurred near the fogged area.

**DISTORTION IS THE MISREPRESENTATION OF THE SIZE AND/OR SHAPE OF THE PART BEING RADIOGRAPHED.**

There are two types of distortion: size distortion (magnification) and shape distortion (true) (Fig. 11–12).

Size distortion or magnification occurs whenever

DISTORTION

Size (Magnification)          Shape (True)

**FIGURE 11–12.** The two types of distortion—size (magnification) and shape (true).

the OFD is greater than zero. The greater the OFD, the greater the magnification. The thickness of the part will affect the OFD. For a lateral projection of the lumbar spine, a slightly obese patient will produce a significantly longer OFD, whereas a thin patient would allow for a shorter OFD. Patient thickness and part thickness are factors that cannot be changed. Skill must be used to place the part as near the film as possible. Magnification distortion is demonstrated in Figure 11–13.

**MAGNIFICATION CAN BE REDUCED WITH A SHORT OFD.**

Radiologists are accustomed to viewing radiographs with specific amounts of magnification. However, when tumors or other abnormalities are present, it may be important to know the approximate

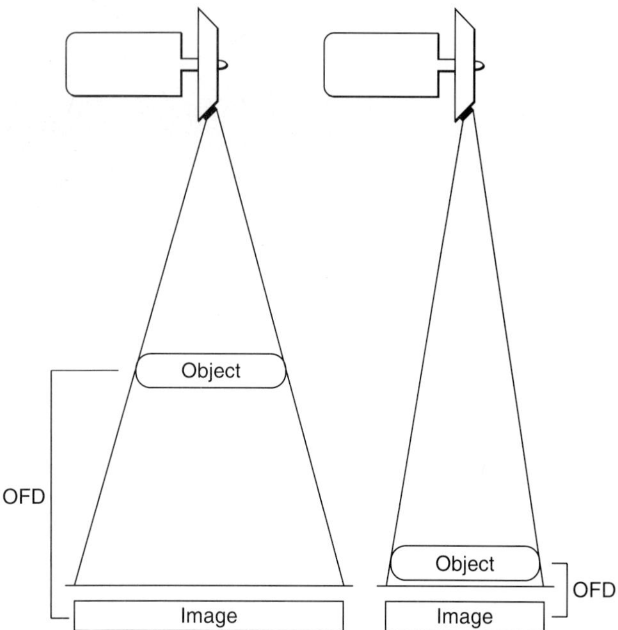


**FIGURE 11–13.** As OFD increases, the amount of magnification will increase. To reduce magnification, place the object as near the film as possible.

amount of magnification. This can be calculated using the formula to determine the magnification factor.

Magnification factor:

$$M = \frac{FFD}{FFD - OFD}$$

EXAMPLE:

What is the magnification factor for an object that is located 4″ from the film with a 40″ FFD?

$$M = \frac{40}{40 - 4}$$

$$M = \frac{40}{36}$$

$$M = 1.1$$

The example indicates that an object imaged with a 40-inch FFD and a 4-inch OFD will have a magnification factor of 1.1. The factor indicates the amount of magnification of the object. The example shown is magnified by a factor of 1.1. If the actual size of the object is 2.5 cm, the image will be 2.5 × 1.1 or 2.8 cm on the finished radiograph.

Shape distortion or true distortion is present when the image does not represent the true shape of the actual object. As indicated earlier, size distortion is almost always present; however, shape distortion is not. When the shape of the object is distorted, it is described as elongated or foreshortened. Elongation refers to an image that is "stretched" and appears longer than the actual size. The stretching of the image is produced when the x-ray tube or film holder is improperly aligned, with an excessive angle (Fig. 11–14).

---

ELONGATION AND FORESHORTENING ARE THE RESULT OF IMPROPERLY ALIGNED TUBE, FILM, AND PART.

---

Foreshortening occurs when the object appears shorter than its actual size; it results from poor alignment of the part and the film. Radiographs should be produced with a minimum of foreshortening and elongation (Table 11–2).

The four rules listed in Table 11–2 are necessary for practicing radiography. For special views of certain anatomic parts, such as small joints or articulations, tube angle or part rotation may be necessary for adequate visualization of the part. For example, in radiography of the cervical vertebrae, a 45° angle of the body part is required to demonstrate the intervertebral foramina.

## VISIBILITY OF DETAIL

A vacationer driving over the Golden Gate Bridge into San Francisco on a clear day can see the lovely city by the bay in all of its beauty. But from time to time, the vacationer may only see a thick layer of fog. The fog has obscured the view of the city. Is the city there? Yes; however, the fog has prevented visibility of the city. The analogy can be used to describe visibility of detail in radiography. Fog from scatter radiation is a detriment to the visibility of detail.

---

VISIBILITY OF DETAIL IS THE ABILITY TO SEE DETAIL RECORDED ON THE FILM

---

**TABLE 11–2.** ACTIONS TO REDUCE DISTORTION

The radiographer should:
1. use the longest acceptable FFD.
2. place the part as near the film as possible; short OFD.
3. place the object of interest as near parallel to the film as possible.
4. use a perpendicular central ray.

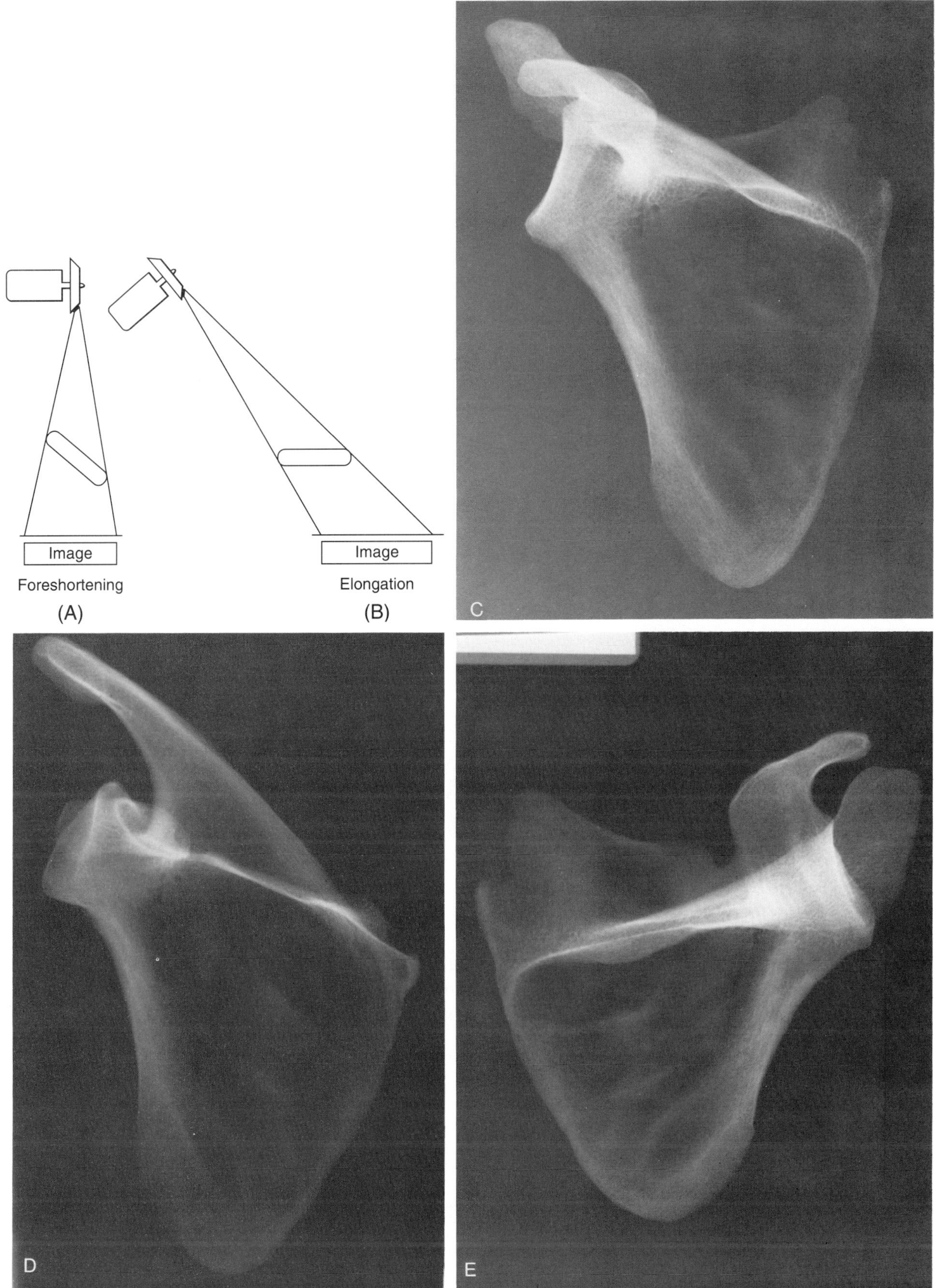


FIGURE 11–14. *A,* Foreshortening occurs when the part is improperly aligned with the tube and film. *B,* Elongation occurs when the x-ray tube is aligned with an excessive angle. The scapula is used to demonstrate image distortion. *C,* A scapula with minimum distortion. The object was placed as near parallel to the film as possible. *D,* An image of the scapula produced with an extreme tube angle. The image has been elongated. *E,* An image produced with the part angled. The result is foreshortening of the object.

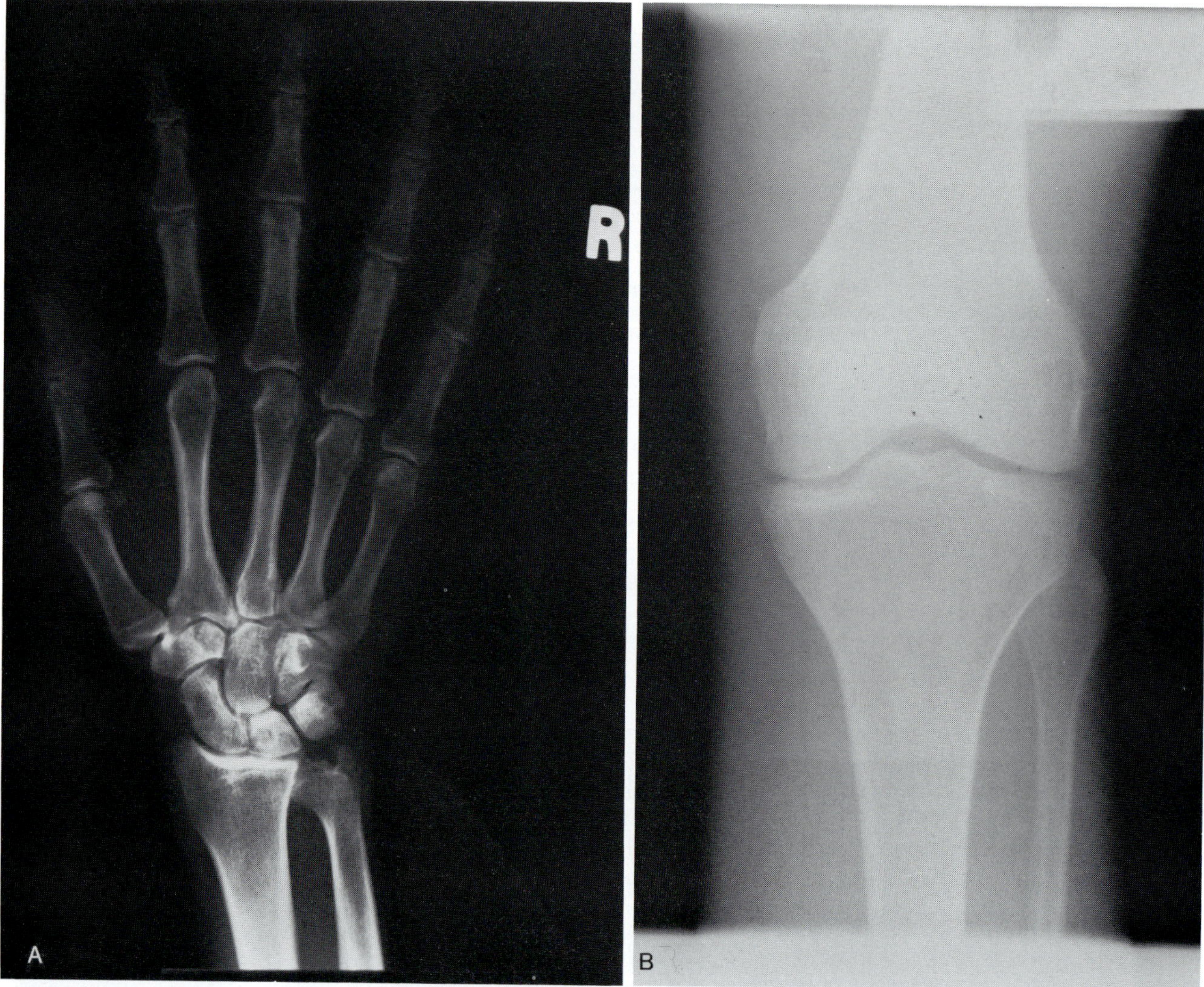


**FIGURE 11–15.** Radiographs that have been overexposed or underexposed do not have adequate visibility of detail. *A,* A radiograph with too much density to adequately visualize the parts of interest. *B,* A radiograph with too little density. There is not enough blackening on the film to produce adequate contrast and make detail visible.

## Overexposure and Underexposure

In order for visibility of the image to be at its best, proper density is critical. Density must be sufficient to exhibit good contrast of the various tissues. Too much density or too little density is a result of overexposure or underexposure (Fig. 11–15).

VISIBILITY OF DETAIL DEPENDS ON THE PRESENCE OF SUFFICIENT DENSITY AND CONTRAST.

A radiograph that is overexposed has too much density. The blackening on the film is so great that it obscures the detail of the image. This is the result of too much radiation exposing the film or possibly a result of fog from scatter or processing chemicals.

A radiograph that is underexposed is one that does not have adequate density. The amount of blackening is not great enough to exhibit contrast sufficient to see image detail.

**TABLE 11–3.** QUALITY CHARACTERISTICS AND RELATED TECHNICAL FACTORS

| Quality Characteristic | Technical Factor |
| --- | --- |
| Density | Milliampere (mA) |
|  | Time (S) |
| Contrast | Kilovoltage (kVp) |
| Definition | Distance |
|   Recorded detail |  |
|   Visibility of detail |  |
| Distortion | Distance |

Density, in the proper amounts, must be present on the radiograph in order to have contrast. Contrast is important to make detail visible. Without proper density, anatomic details will not be visible, even though they have been recorded on the film.

All factors that influence density and contrast will also affect the visibility of detail. Scatter radiation will reduce visibility of detail. The selection of accessories must be such that scattered x-rays are absorbed or reduced to prevent fog on the film. Accessories, such as collimators and grids, are important in achieving the best visibility of detail.

---

**SCATTER RADIATION MUST BE REDUCED TO PROVIDE MAXIMUM VISIBILITY OF DETAIL.**

---

Penetration of the part is essential to produce good visibility of detail. Kilovoltage must be adjusted high enough to penetrate the part but not so high as to produce increased scatter radiation.

In summary, all factors related to contrast, density, and scatter radiation are important and must be properly controlled for the best possible visibility of the detail on the radiograph. Table 11–3 summarizes the technical and quality factors. Table 11–4 provides a good overview of how technical and quality factors are inter-related.

**TABLE 11–4.** RADIOGRAPHIC QUALITY

| Quality Characteristic | Controlling Factor | Influencing Factor |
| --- | --- | --- |
| Density | mAs | kVp<br>Tissue thickness<br>Tissue density<br>Foreign bodies<br>Contrast media<br>Distance (FFD)<br>Scatter radiation<br>Anode heel effect<br>Processing<br>Equipment operation<br>Film-screen systems<br>Filters<br>Grids<br>Beam restriction<br>Fog |
| Contrast | kVp | Tissue composition<br>Contrast media<br>Pathology<br>Fog<br>Scatter radiation<br>Film-screen systems<br>Processing<br>Beam restriction<br>Grids |
| Definition | Focal spot size<br>Object-film distance<br>Screens<br>Motion | Density factors<br>Contrast factors |
| Distortion | Alignment of:<br>Part<br>Film<br>Tube | |

# CHAPTER 12

# Scatter Radiation, Filtration, and Patient Exposure

● ● ● ● ● ● ●

## CHAPTER OBJECTIVES

1. Describe the effects of filtration on the primary beam.
2. Describe how patient exposure is affected by the use of filters.
3. Describe the purpose of filtration.
4. Differentiate between "inherent" and "added" filtration.
5. Name the types of materials used to construct filters.
6. Discuss the advantages of aluminum versus copper as material for filters.
7. List the specific filter thicknesses for various kilovoltage settings.
8. Describe the purpose of compensating filters.
9. Give at least three examples for the use of compensating filters.
10. Describe how scatter affects film quality.
11. Discuss the advantages and disadvantages of kilovoltage as a key factor affecting the production of scatter and patient protection.
12. List three factors primarily related to the production of scatter radiation.

## KEY WORDS AND TERMS

Filtration

Filters

Inherent filtration

Added filtration

Aluminum equivalent

Patient protection

Compensating filter

Scatter radiation

Field size

Backscatter

Tissue thickness

## RECOMMENDATIONS FOR GENERAL DISCUSSION QUESTIONS

1. Describe the purpose of filtration in radiography, to include the type of materials used, patient radiation dose, and film quality.
2. Describe how scatter affects film quality and patient exposure, to include the three major factors in the production of scatter.

The major challenge to the radiographer is to protect the patient from excessive exposure to radiation, which may occur as a result of unsafe procedures or inaccurate exposure factors. In addition, as x-rays interact with matter (body tissue), they produce scatter radiation, which will also increase the amount of exposure to the patient. Scatter radiation also becomes a concern for the personnel employed in the radiology department. The exercise of precaution for the patient and department personnel is an absolute in the practice of radiography.

Precautions to be taken for patient protection must include the use of filters and beam restrictors. Patient exposure can be reduced by the use of sufficient filtration of the x-ray beam. Scatter radiation can be reduced by restricting the size of the beam that exposes the patient. Other factors associated with the production of scatter radiation are kilovoltage, part thickness, and tissue density.

## FILTRATION

Filtration of the primary beam is accomplished by the use of metal devices called filters placed in the path of the primary x-ray beam (Fig. 12–1). The purpose of the filter is to selectively remove the low-energy photons from the beam. These low-energy photons do not possess sufficient energy to penetrate the body parts and reach the film. Without the use of filters, these low-energy photons would be absorbed by the body in the first few millimeters of tissue. With the use of a filter, low-energy photons can be absorbed by the filter and removed before the x-ray beam strikes the patient. The amount of radiation absorbed by the patient depends on the number of low-energy photons absorbed by the filter. Therefore, the main function of a filter is to reduce the amount of low-energy radiation absorbed by the patient.

---

**FILTERS SERVE TO REDUCE THE AMOUNT OF LOW-ENERGY RADIATION ABSORBED BY THE PATIENT.**

---

Federal regulations, as defined by the National Council on Radiation Protection (NCRP), govern the use of filters with general diagnostic x-ray equipment. Guidelines refer to recommended thicknesses of total filtration to be used with selected kilovoltage ranges.

Total filtration refers to the sum of "inherent" and "added" filtration (Fig. 12–2). *Inherent filtration* is the amount of filtration provided by the x-ray tube structure, housing, and collimator (if attached). X-rays must pass through the glass envelope as they exit the tube. The glass envelope provides approximately 0.5 mm of aluminum equivalent. The window or port in the tube housing, along with an attached collimator, used for beam restriction, accounts for approximately 1.0 mm of aluminum equivalent inherent filtration.

*Added filtration* is the added material placed in the beam. Filters are placed between the tube and the beam restrictor device, as shown in Figure 12–1.

Aluminum is the most commonly used material for added filtration. Aluminum is very easy to work with and serves as an efficient tool in the removal of low-energy photons from the x-ray beam. Copper may also be used as material for the construction of filters. One disadvantage to the use of copper filters is the copper material itself. Copper produces characteristic radiation in the energy range of 8 kEv, as the x-ray beam passes through the filter. When copper filters are used, they must be used along with aluminum filters because the photons could interact with the copper, producing characteristic radiation that would actually increase the radiation dose to the patient. The aluminum filters must be placed nearest the patient when used in combination with copper filters so that the characteristic radiation from the copper filter can be absorbed by the aluminum filter before it reaches the patient. The aluminum filter may also emit characteristic radiation; however, the energy level of the radiation is so low that is absorbed in the air gap between the patient and the filter and does not contribute to the patient dose (Fig. 12–3).

Added filtration ranges from 1 to 3 mm Al equivalent in thickness. Increases in filter thickness will increase the attenuation of *all* energy photons. An increase in the thickness of the filter will increase efficiency in absorbing low-energy photons. As the thickness of the filter increases, so will attenuation of the primary beam; therefore, the quantity of radiation decreases. Increased thickness of the filter over the NCRP recommendations only serves to absorb or attenuate more of the high-energy photons and decrease the number of photons in the primary beam. Unfortunately, no materials exist that filter only low-energy photons without the attenuation of the high-energy photons. The use of filters will increase the mean energy of the beam, which is interpreted as improvement in the quality of the beam (Fig. 12–4).

Inherent and added filtration together become the

*Text continued on page 131*

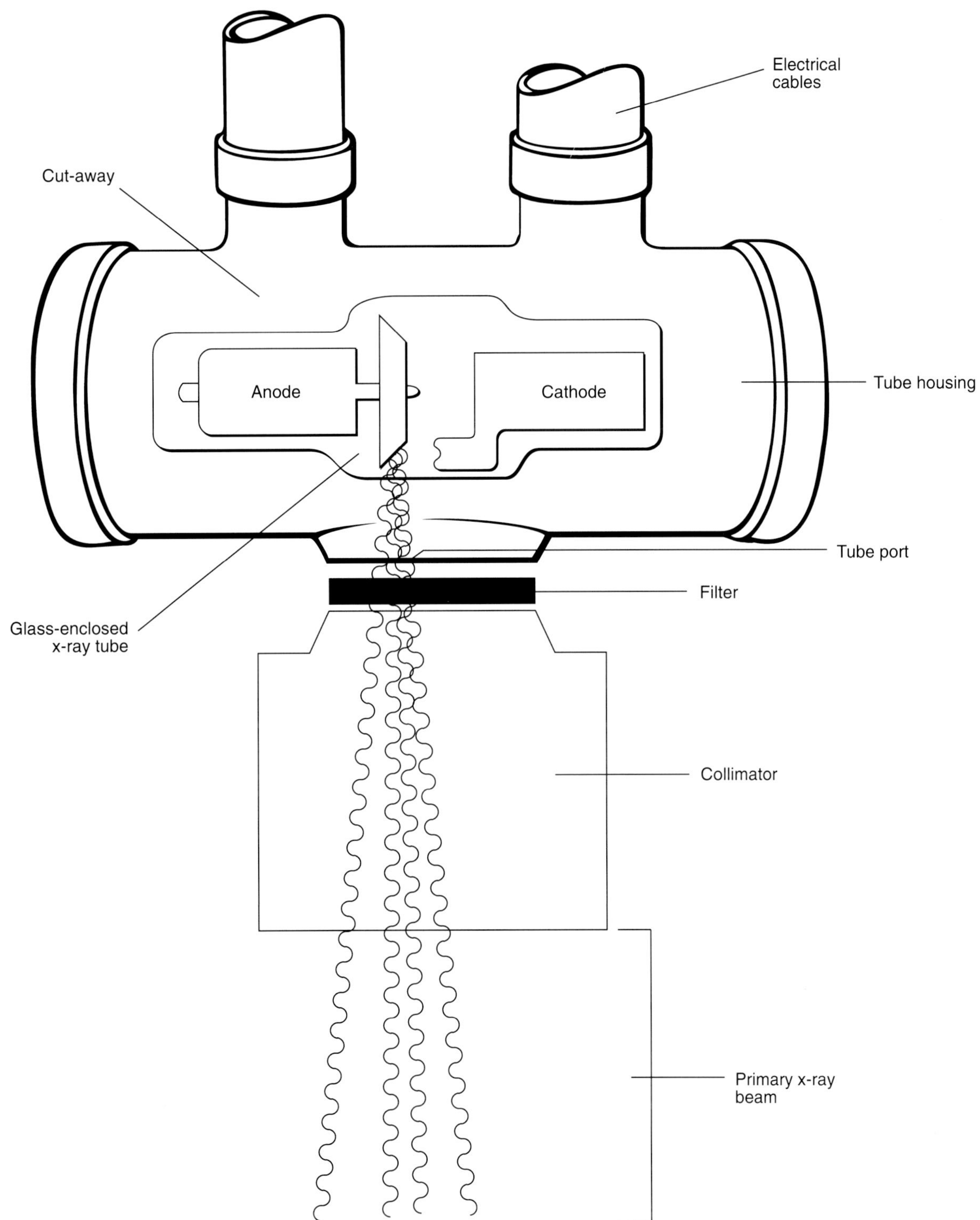



**FIGURE 12–1.** Filtration of the primary x-ray beam is accomplished by placing the filter in the path of the beam. The filter is attached to the tube port or window. Low-energy photons are absorbed by the filter. The main function of a filter is to reduce the skin dose of radiation to the patient.

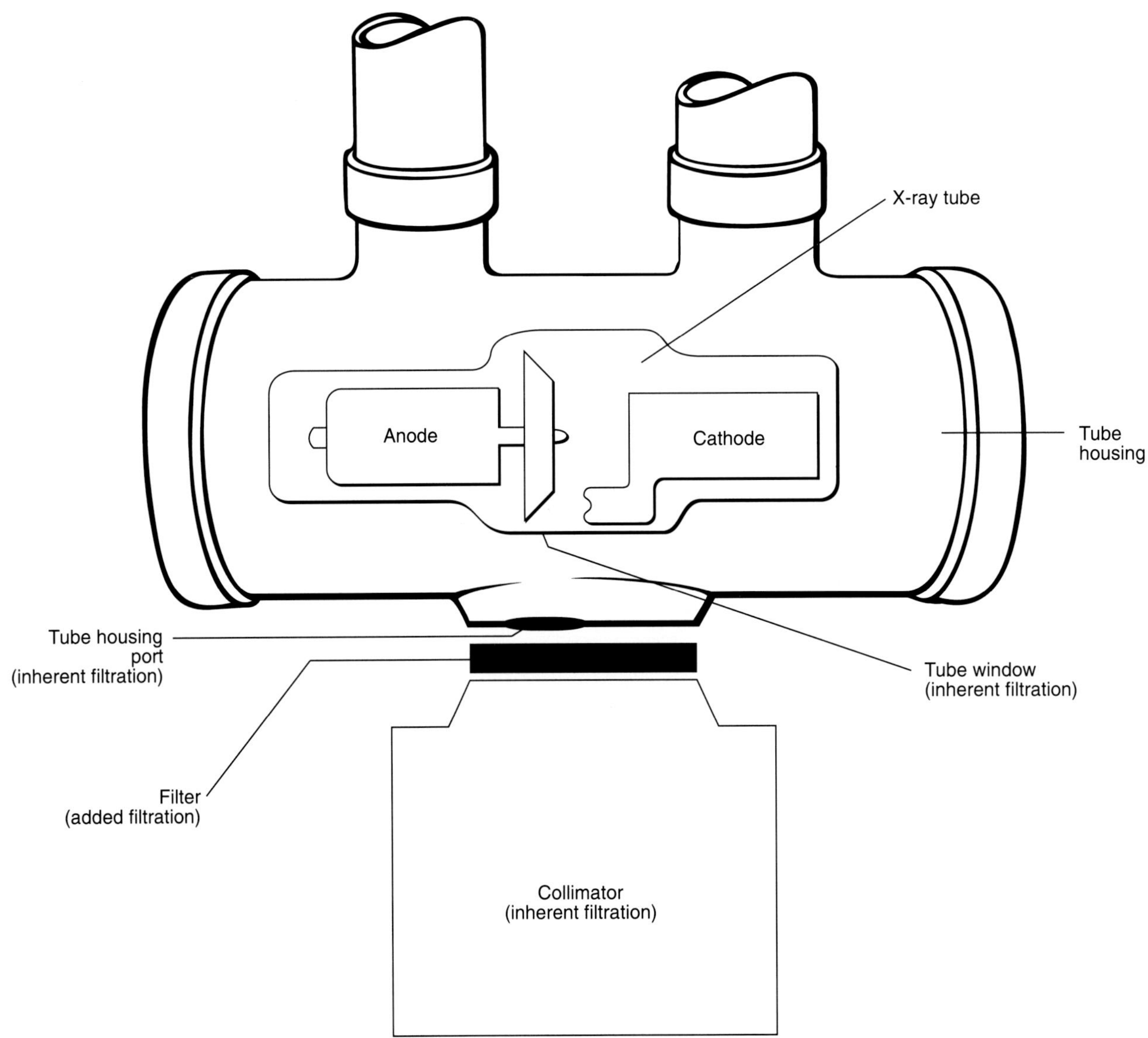


**FIGURE 12–2.** Inherent filtration of approximately 1.5 mm aluminum (Al) equivalent is provided by the tube window, tube port, and collimator. Added filtration is located between the tube and the collimator and is approximately 1 mm Al equivalent. Total inherent and added filtration is 2.5 mm Al equivalent.

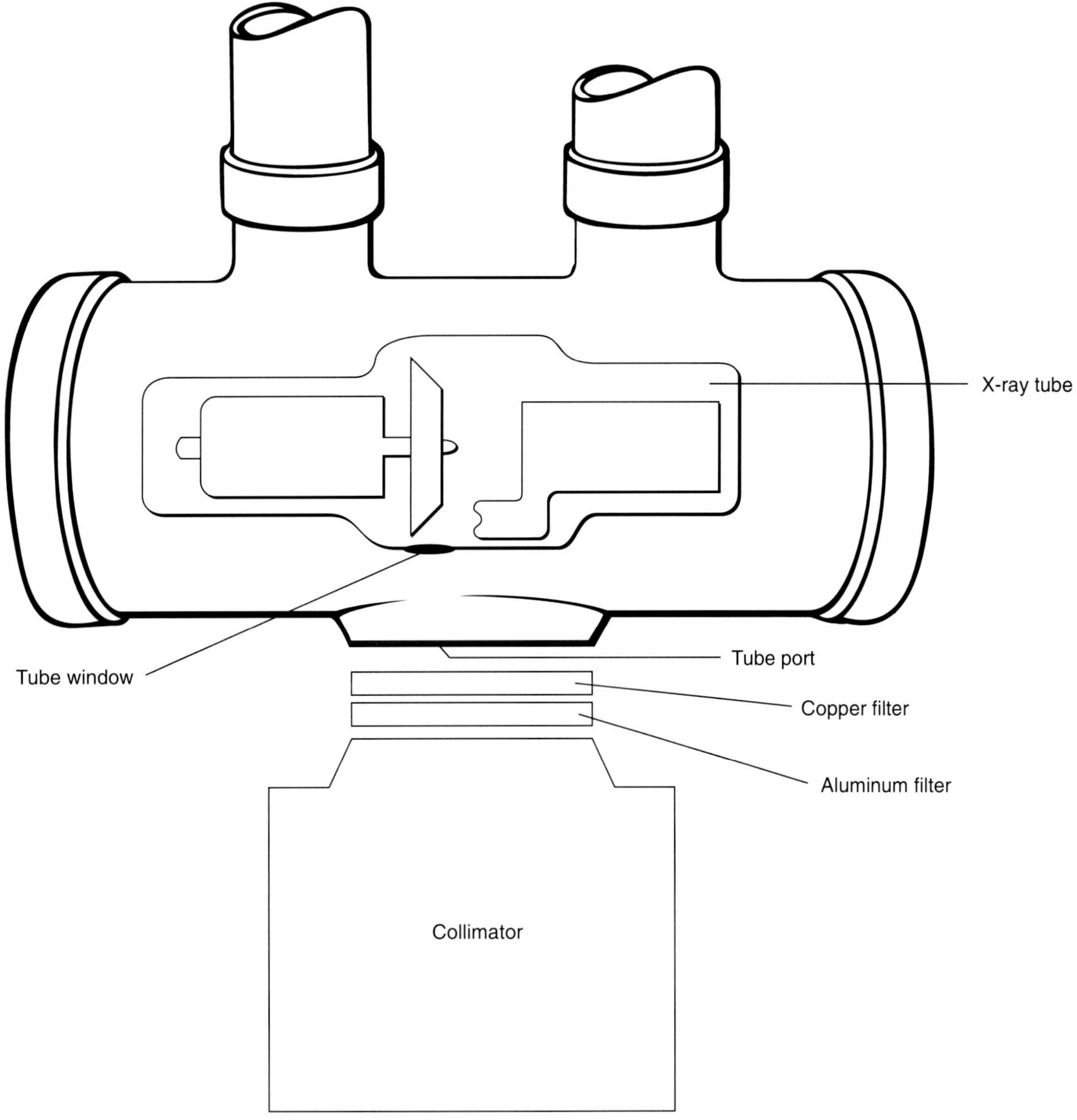


**FIGURE 12–3.** Copper filters can be used with aluminum filters. The copper filter must be placed next to the tube housing port, with the aluminum filter placed nearest the patient.

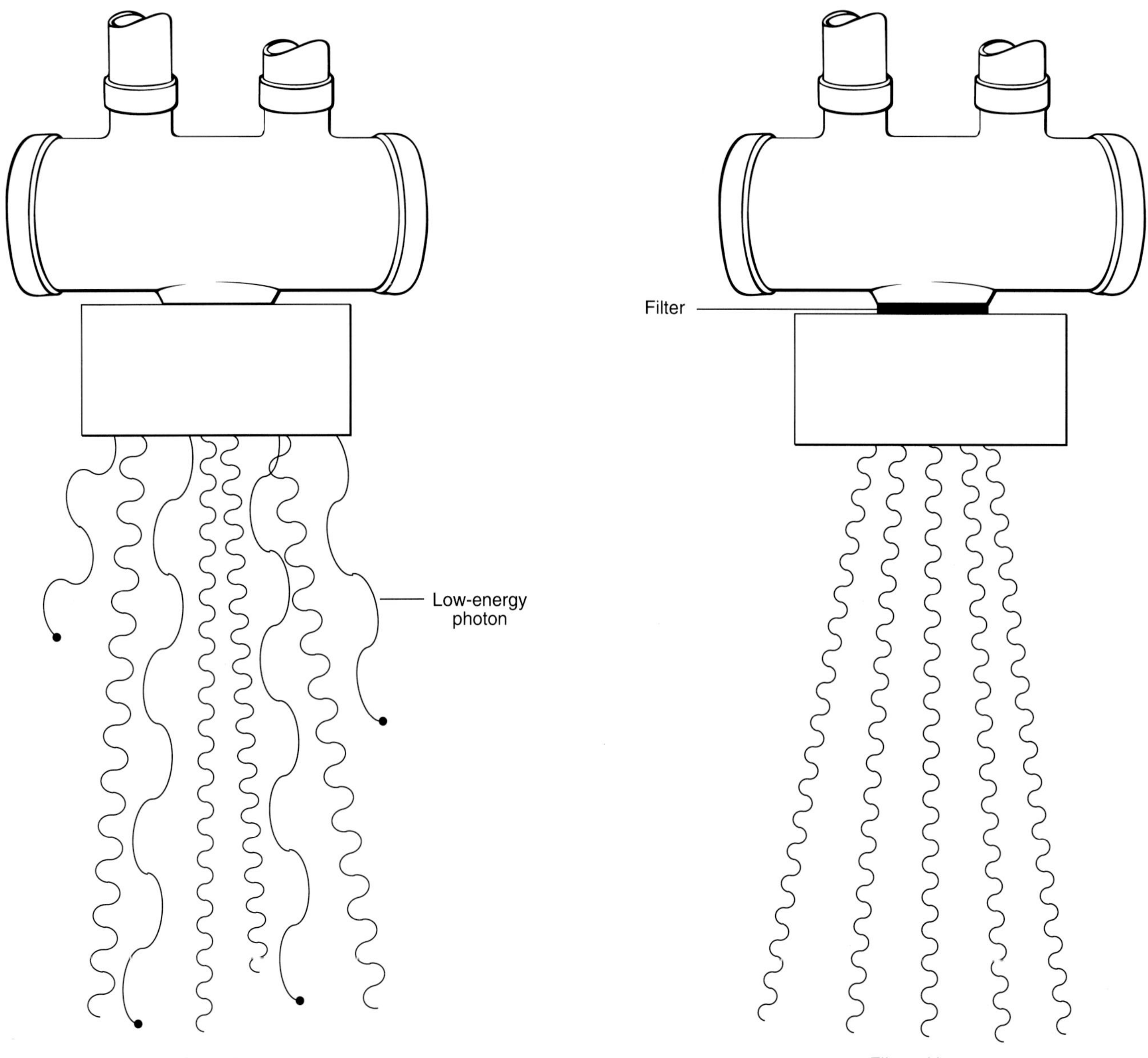


**FIGURE 12–4.** Filters remove *long*-wavelength (low-energy) radiation from the primary beam. As the amount of added filtration increases, the mean energy of the primary beam will increase.

total amount of filtration of the primary beam. The NCRP has defined the total amount of filtration required in diagnostic radiology to be:

| *Kilovoltage* | *Total Filtration (Aluminum Equivalent)* |
|---|---|
| Below 50 | 0.5 mm Al |
| 50–70 | 1.5 mm Al |
| 70 plus | 2.5 mm Al |

For most diagnostic radiographic equipment, 2.5 mm Al equivalent is sufficient to attenuate the beam in such a way as to provide the maximum reduction in the dose of radiation to the patient. Filtration of 2.5 mm Al equivalent may decrease skin dose by as much as 50%. The amount of reduction of the skin dose may vary from procedure to procedure depending on the kilovoltage selection. It must be clearly understood that filters protect the patient from excessive exposure to radiation.

---

FILTERS PROTECT THE PATIENT FROM EXCESSIVE EXPOSURE TO RADIATION.

---

## Exposure Factors

Filters attenuate all energy levels by reducing the quantity of photons in the primary beam. Using filters and increasing thickness will require a slight increase in exposure factors to maintain adequate density levels on the film.

## Mammography Units

Mammography units are designed for the very special purpose of producing high-quality detailed images of breast tissue. Breast tissue has low subject contrast, and special equipment is required to produce high-quality images. Most units operate with minimum filtration because of the extremely low energy primary beam (30 kVp range) that is required to produce maximum contrast of the tissue.

X-ray tubes for mammography units are designed for this special purpose. The glass window material is thinner to reduce the amount of inherent filtration. Inherent filtration is reduced to approximately 0.1 mm Al equivalent. Total filtration is reduced to a minimum for mammography procedures in order to maximize subject contrast.

## Compensating Filters

Filters added to accommodate variations in tissue thickness are called compensating filters. The most common type of compensating filters is the wedge (Fig. 12–5). The wedge filter would be used for examinations of the femur and thoracic spine, and angiography of the lower extremity, where the anatomic structures vary in thickness. The thickest part would be placed under the thin side of the filter. The result would be a uniform density level over the entire radiograph.

## SCATTER RADIATION

Scatter radiation degrades image quality and must be controlled by the radiographer. Figure 12–6 demonstrates two types of radiation exposing the film. Photons in the primary beam with sufficient energy will penetrate the part to become remnant radiation and emerge to strike the image receptor. Other photons may either be absorbed by the body as in a photoelectric interaction or interact with the tissue to produce Compton interactions. The latter will produce x-ray photons that emerge traveling in many directions and with a broad range of energy. This is known as scatter radiation (Fig. 12–7).

Figure 12–7A shows a radiograph with a significant amount of exposure from scatter radiation. The result is a radiograph with many gray tones. Figure 12–7B represents a radiograph with sufficient contrast and minimal exposure from scatter radiation.

Scatter radiation must be controlled in order to produce high-quality radiographs. Exposure to the image receptor by scatter radiation will cause fog on the film and reduce visibility of the detail. Scatter radiation causes increased and undesirable density (fog) on the film. In addition, scatter decreases contrast and visibility of detail, as demonstrated in Figure 12–7. Scatter also increases the patient's dose and can be a hazard to radiology department personnel. It is important to understand that scatter may account for as much as 50% of the exposure to the film for a chest radiograph and as much as 90 to 95% for a radiograph of the abdomen. Scatter contributes to the overall density but decreases film quality significantly. Most scatter offers nothing worthwhile on the finished radiograph.

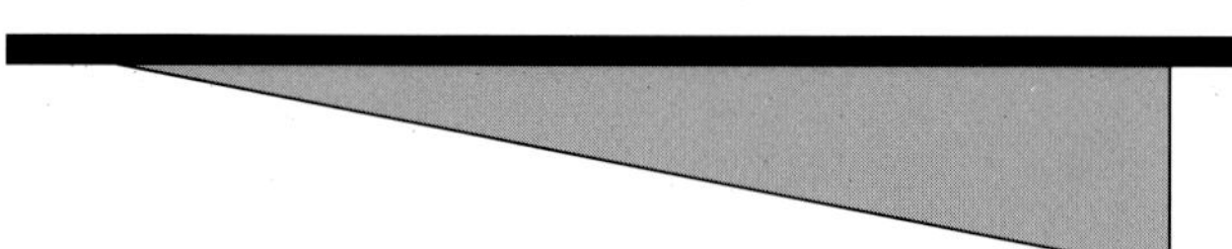

**FIGURE 12–5.** The wedge filter is used to produce a more uniform density level over the entire surface of the radiograph.

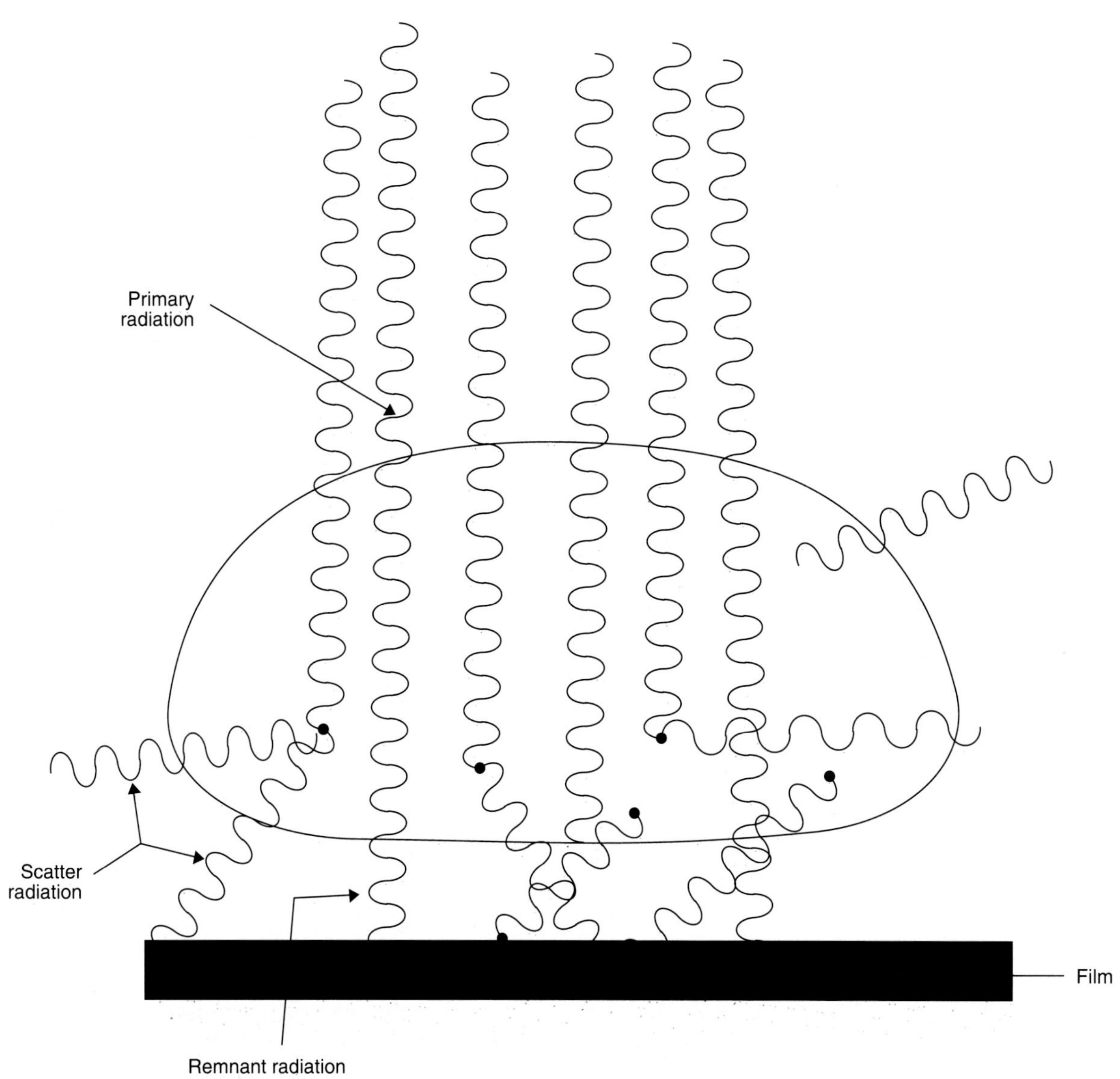


**FIGURE 12–6.** Primary radiation may penetrate the part to become remnant radiation. The film is exposed by remnant and scatter radiation.

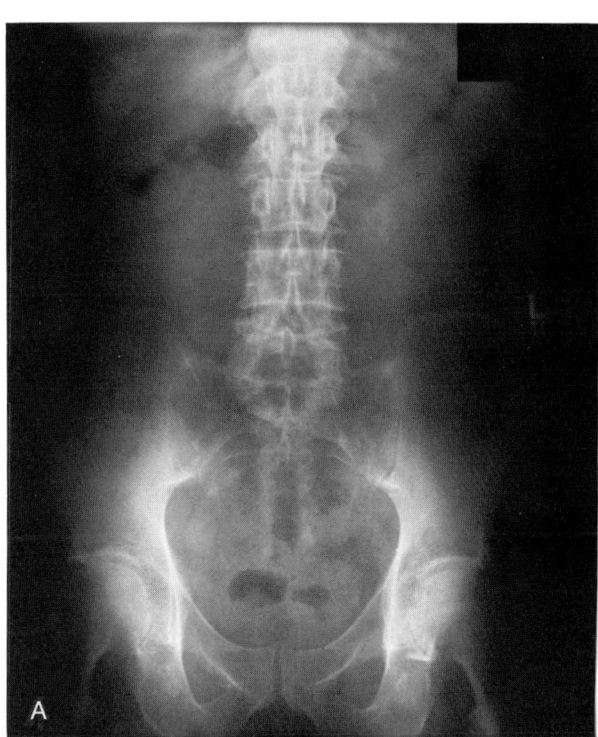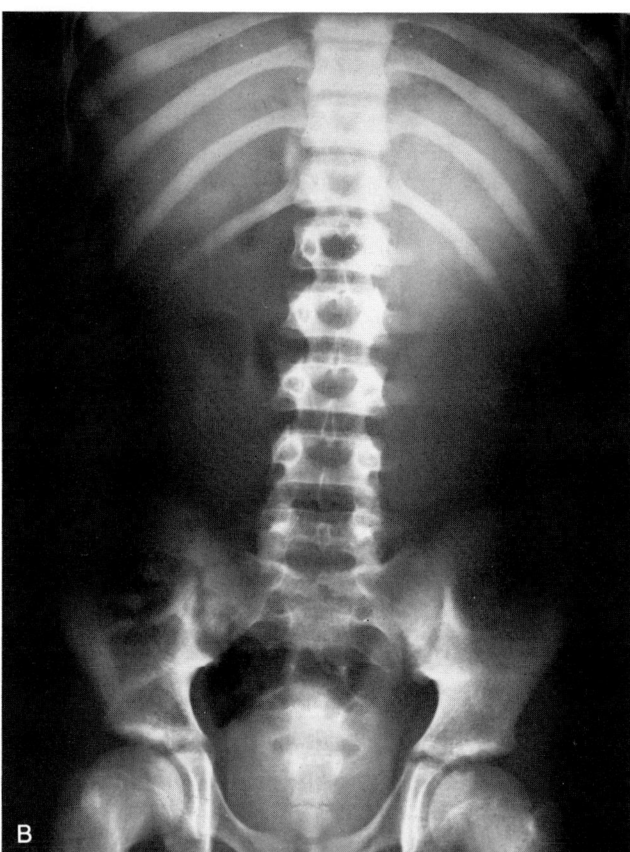

FIGURE 12–7. Scatter radiation that exposes the film reduces the visibility of detail. *A*, A radiograph with increased scatter reaching the film. *B*, A radiograph that was exposed with a minimum amount of scatter radiation. The visibility of detail is significantly improved.

## SCATTER RADIATION CONTRIBUTES TO THE OVERALL DENSITY ON THE RADIOGRAPH BUT DECREASES FILM QUALITY.

### Factors Affecting Scatter

Three primary factors are significant in determining the amount of scatter radiation reaching the film. They are kilovoltage, field size, and part thickness.

### Kilovoltage

An increase in kilovoltage will increase the effects of Compton interactions. As kilovoltage peak (kVp) is increased, the probability of any type of reaction decreases. However, with an increase in kVp, the probability increases, with any interaction that occurs, that it will be Compton interaction. This will result in an increased amount of scatter reaching the image receptor. The radiographer must make important choices. As kilovoltage is increased, scatter reaching the film will also increase.

## AS KILOVOLTAGE INCREASES, SCATTER RADIATION WILL ALSO INCREASE.

As the kilovoltage increases, the amount of scatter reaching the film will increase. However, the amount of radiation absorbed by the patient will decrease. Although the increase in kVp may cause an increase in the internal organ dose, the skin dose to the patient will be greatly reduced.

## AS THE KILOVOLTAGE INCREASES, THE AMOUNT OF RADIATION ABSORBED BY THE PATIENT WILL DECREASE.

The factor of choice, for patient protection, becomes the kilovoltage selection. Grids (described in Chapter 14) are also employed to improve the qual-

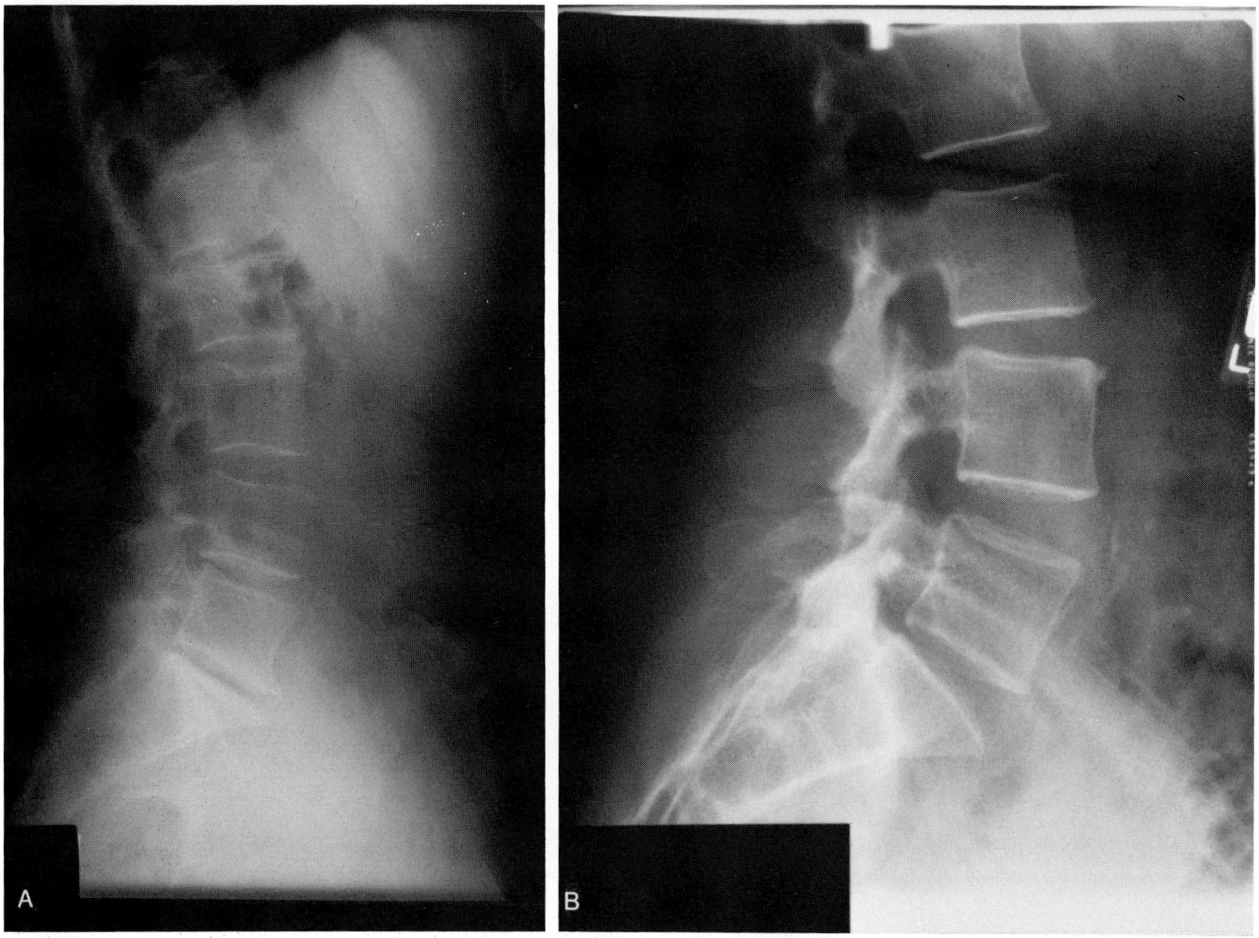

**FIGURE 12–8.** A reduction in the field size will decrease the amount of scatter exposing the film. *A,* A radiograph produced with a 14 × 17″ field size. Compare the visibility of detail with *B,* which is a smaller area of the lumbar vertebrae exposed with a 10 × 12″ field size.

ity of the film by absorbing a portion of the scatter before it reaches the film.

## Field Size and Scatter

Field size refers to the size of the area on the patient that is exposed by the primary beam. Control of the field size is probably the most important factor for controlling scatter. The larger the field size, the greater the amount of scatter, as shown in Figure 12–8. Reduction of field size decreases scat-

ter. Beam restriction is described in greater detail in Chapter 13.

Some parts of the body make it very difficult for the field size to be adjusted to expose only the part of interest. For example, a standard radiograph of the lateral lumbar spine will produce a great deal of scatter and also "backscatter" (Fig. 12–9).

Backscatter results from the primary beam striking the table-top. Scatter results from the primary beam photons interacting with the table-top and other structures on the table. Leaded rubber mask-

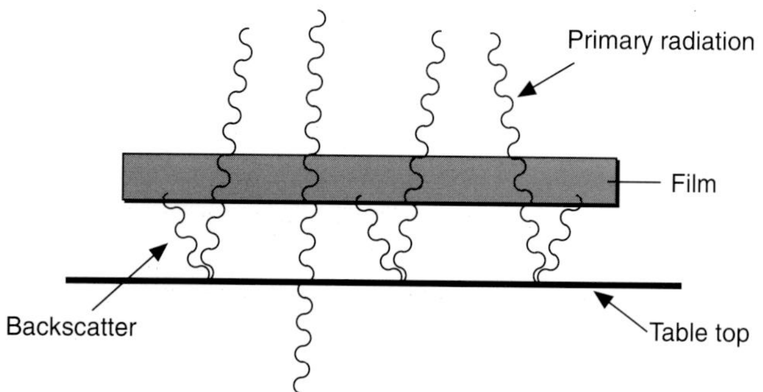


**FIGURE 12–9.** Backscatter results from x-ray photons interacting with the table top or other structures that are part of the x-ray table.

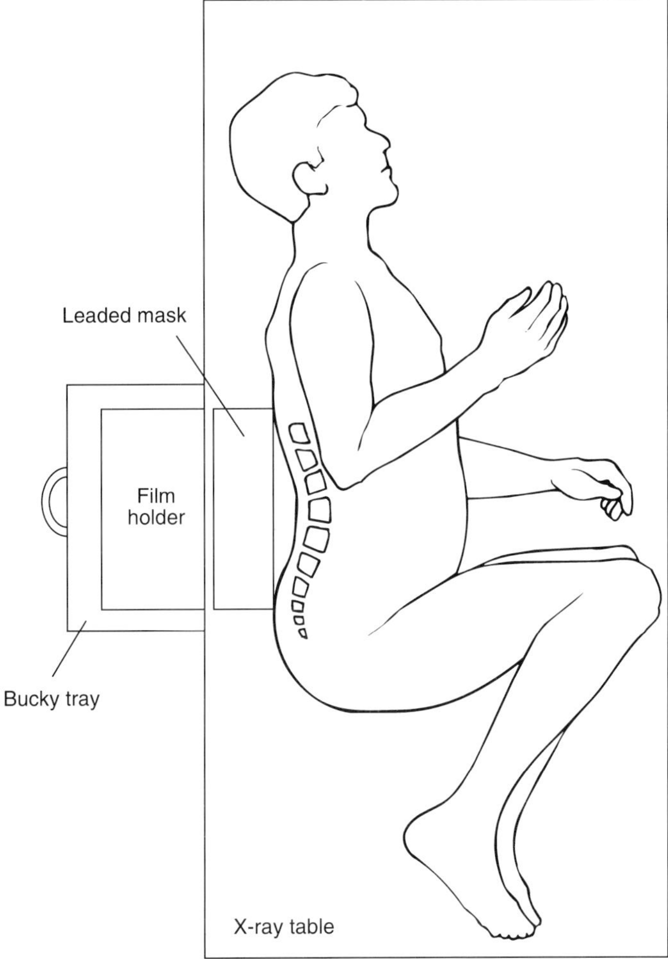



**FIGURE 12–10.** When exposing the patient for a lateral lumbar spine radiograph, significant scatter radiation is produced. Because the anatomic part of interest is more posterior, part of the primary beam will expose the film. The placing of a leaded rubber mask behind the patient will absorb primary and scatter radiation and improve the quality of the film.

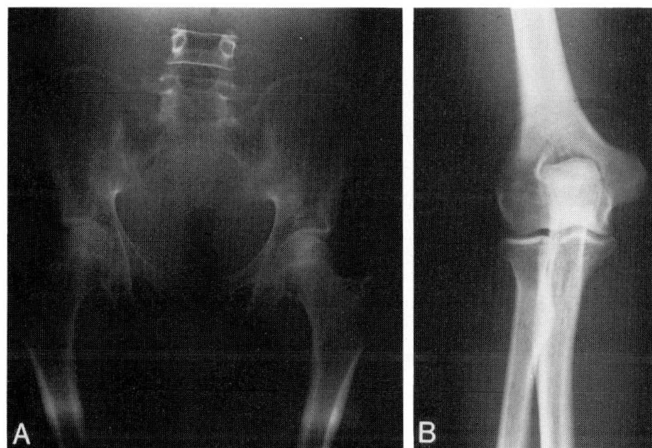



**FIGURE 12–11.** Thickness of the part to be imaged affects the production of scatter radiation. Thicker parts generally produce more scatter. *A,* A radiograph of the pelvis phantom with a gray appearance that resulted from the amount of scatter that was produced at the time of the exposure. *B,* A radiograph of a thinner anatomic part. The amount of scatter that exposed the film was minimal, producing a radiograph with improved visibility of detail.

ing will absorb photons from the primary beam that do not strike the patient and thus reduce the amount of scatter striking the patient and the film (Fig. 12–10).

## Thickness of the Part and Scatter

Thickness of the part is the third factor in the production of scatter radiation. As the part thickness and tissue density increase, scatter will increase (Fig. 12–11). Although thickness of the part is a factor that is not under the specific control of the radiographer, certain principles can be followed to reduce the effects of scatter. Compression bands can be used to reduce tissue thickness, thus reducing scatter. For an abdominal radiograph, thickness can be reduced by placing the patient in the prone position. This will decrease the amount of scatter produced.

## CHAPTER 13

# Control of Scatter Radiation: Beam Restriction

## CHAPTER OBJECTIVES

1. Discuss the rationale for beam restriction as a significant factor in protection of the patient.
2. Describe the basic principle of beam restriction.
3. Describe the degree to which scatter affects the total film density.
4. Explain how a radiographer can verify that adequate beam restriction has been accomplished.
5. List three basic types of beam restrictors.
6. Compare the effectiveness of aperture diaphragms, flared cones, cylinder cones, and collimators to determine which would be the best beam restricting device.
7. Explain the concept called "undercutting" of the photons.
8. Draw and label the collimator structure.
9. Describe the general operation of a manually operated collimator.
10. Describe the location and function of the light/mirror apparatus in the collimator.
11. List the advantages for using a collimator.
12. Differentiate between the manual and automatic collimation devices.
13. Describe the alignment test for collimators.
14. Explain the effects of beam restriction on density, contrast, and visibility of detail.
15. Identify the compensation factors used to adjust for loss of film density with a reduction in field size.
16. Calculate field size using the appropriate formula.

## KEY WORDS AND TERMS

| | |
|---|---|
| Beam restriction | "Undercutting" |
| Field size | Penumbra |
| Aperture diaphragm | Shutters |
| Flared cone | Automatic collimation |
| Cylinder cone | Positive beam limiting device (PBLD) |
| Collimator | Alignment test |

## RECOMMENDATIONS FOR GENERAL DISCUSSION QUESTIONS

1. Describe the basic principle of beam restriction, and list the advantages for patient protection and for the improvement of film quality.
2. Compare each of the following beam restriction devices with the collimator and explain why the collimator is the most effective beam restriction device: aperture diaphragm, flared cone, and cylinder cone.
3. Describe how beam restriction will directly affect image quality.

Scatter radiation is a major factor in evaluating exposure to the patient and the quality of the radiographic image. For these reasons, maximum control of scatter radiation must be exercised. Restriction of the primary x-ray beam to the size of the object to be imaged is the most effective method for the control of scatter radiation.

## BEAM RESTRICTION IS THE MOST EFFECTIVE METHOD FOR REDUCING THE AMOUNT OF SCATTER.

The amount of scatter radiation produced is directly related to the field size of the beam. The larger the field size for the primary x-ray beam, the greater the amount of scatter radiation produced. The purpose of beam restriction is to restrict the x-ray beam to irradiate the smallest area possible. In turn, the amount of exposure to the patient will be less and the quality of the image will be improved.

An important concept of scatter radiation must be understood. Although scatter radiation is undesirable, it is responsible for a significant amount of density on the radiograph. For a chest radiograph, scatter produces about 50% of the recorded density. For an abdominal radiograph, about 90 to 95% of the recorded density is attributed to scatter radiation. It is obvious that 100% elimination of all scatter would not be the goal in producing high-quality radiographs because of the enormous loss in

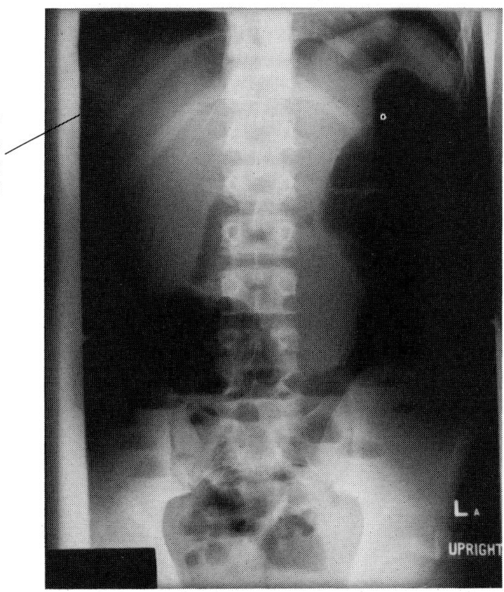



**FIGURE 13–2.** Radiograph of the abdomen illustrating borders produced by restriction of the primary beam.

density. What is important would be to control and limit the amount of scatter produced during the exposure (Fig. 13–1).

Beam restriction can be very effective in reducing the field size of the beam to the size of the part. This is accomplished by the use of effective beam restrictors that are attached to the housing of the x-ray tube. Beam restriction serves to limit the size and shape of the primary x-ray beam.

## THE PURPOSE OF BEAM RESTRICTION IS TO LIMIT THE SIZE OF THE PRIMARY X-RAY BEAM.

To determine if adequate restriction of the beam has been reached, one demonstrates an unexposed border around the edge of the finished radiograph (Fig. 13–2).

Figure 13–2 demonstrates the presence of a narrow border around the edge of an abdominal radiograph, which is the result of a beam restrictor limiting the size of the primary beam. The field size is slightly less than the film size. Figure 13–3 represents how the field size can be restricted to the actual size of the part.

### TYPES OF BEAM RESTRICTION

Beam restriction is essential in diagnostic radiology to reduce the amount of scatter. There are three basic types of beam restrictors: aperture diaphragms, cones, and collimators.

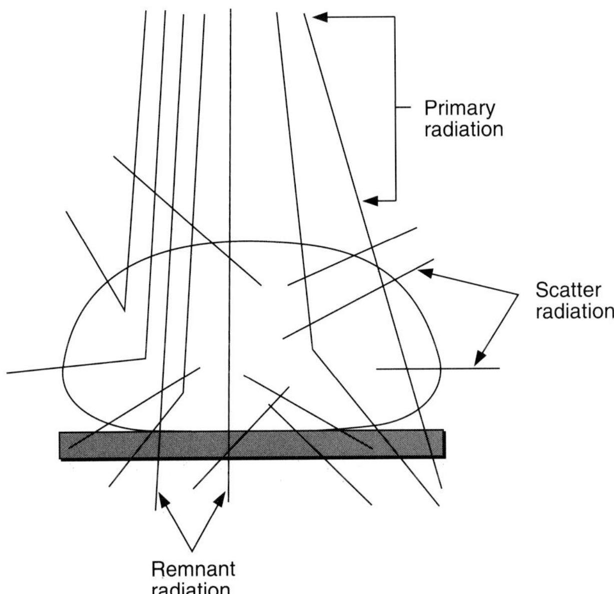



**FIGURE 13–1.** Scatter radiation contributes to the density on the radiograph. Approximately 50% of the exposure to the film for a chest radiograph is by scatter radiation.

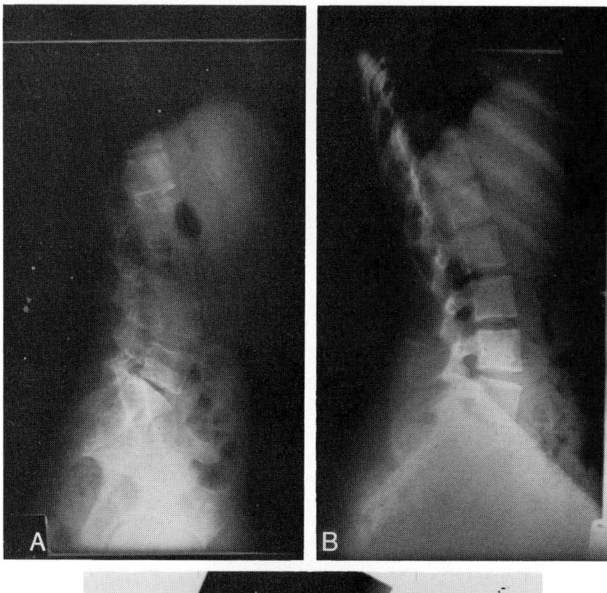

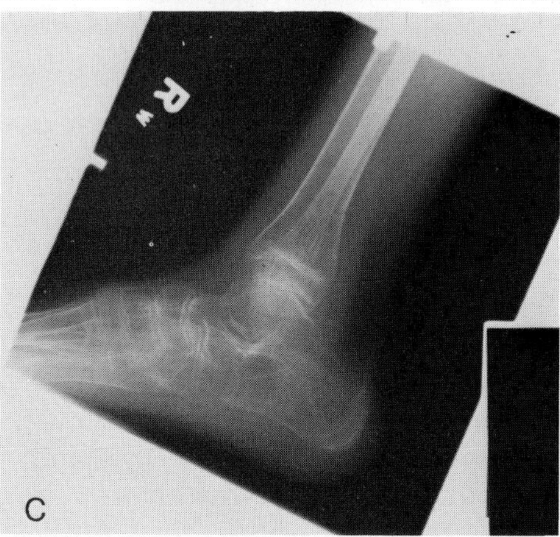

**FIGURE 13–3.** To produce the best quality radiographs, the primary beam should be restricted to the size of the part. *A* illustrates beam restriction to the size of the film. *B* illustrates beam restriction to the size of the part. Compare the visibility of detail in these radiographs. *C,* This radiograph of a smaller anatomic part demonstrates good beam restriction.

## Aperture Diaphragm

Aperture diaphragms are simple flat sheets of lead or lead-lined material with a hole in the middle. The holes may vary in size and shape according to the prescribed use. Figure 13–4 demonstrates examples of aperture openings used for beam restrictors.

Aperture diaphragms are easy to construct and simple to use. The size of the hole in the diaphragm determines the field size. There are two disadvantages associated with the use of aperture diaphragms. First, because the opening is not adjustable, only one field size can be obtained at any given focal-film distance (FFD). The second disadvantage is the increase in penumbra or unsharpness caused by the "undercutting" of the photons on the edge of the beam, as illustrated in Figure 13–5.

Undercutting occurs when x-rays that originate from different points on the target undercut or pass by the aperture diaphragm and the upper lip of a flared cone, and pass tangentially across the edge of the part. The collimator, shown in Figure 13–5*B*, eliminates most undercutting with the lower shutters, thus decreasing penumbra and increasing sharpness.

Undercutting can be significantly reduced by increasing the distance from the focal spot to the diaphragm. The closer the diaphragm to the focal spot, the greater the undercutting effect.

Overall, aperture diaphragms would be rated as poor beam restrictors; however, they are very effective when compared with exposures made with no restriction of the beam.

## Cones

Cones are heavy metal devices that are attached to the housing of the x-ray tube for the purpose of restricting the beam. They may vary from 8 to 12 inches in length, with shapes that are flared circular, rectangular, or cylindrical with added extensions (Fig. 13–6).

Flared cones are shaped to resemble the divergence of the primary beam; however, the flare is often greater than the divergence of the primary beam. This will reduce the effectiveness of the cone and is responsible for unnecessary exposure to the patient (Fig. 13–7). Penumbra is not significantly reduced. The flared cone is no more effective than the aperture diaphragm.

The cylinder cone, on the other hand, is much more effective (Fig. 13–8).

The restriction of the beam with the cylinder cone is at the end of the cylinder or "lip" furthermost from the x-ray tube. The beam is truly restricted, and the undercutting or penumbra is reduced. The most effective cylinders are the ones with adjustable extensions, as shown in Figure 13–9.

The distance from the lip to the focal spot can be increased, resulting in a significant influence on restriction of the beam.

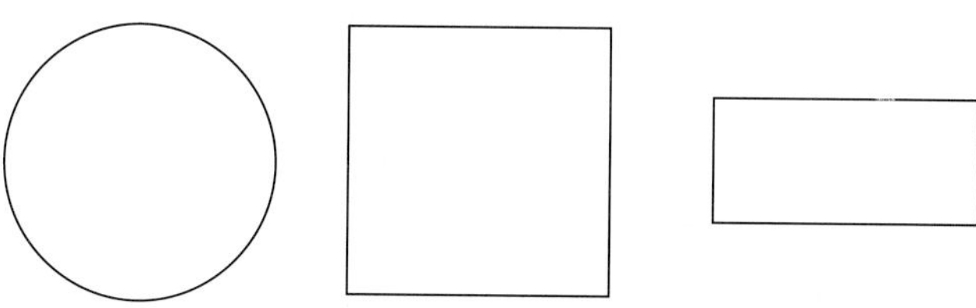

**FIGURE 13–4.** Aperture openings may vary in size and shape such as demonstrated here: circular, square, and rectangular.

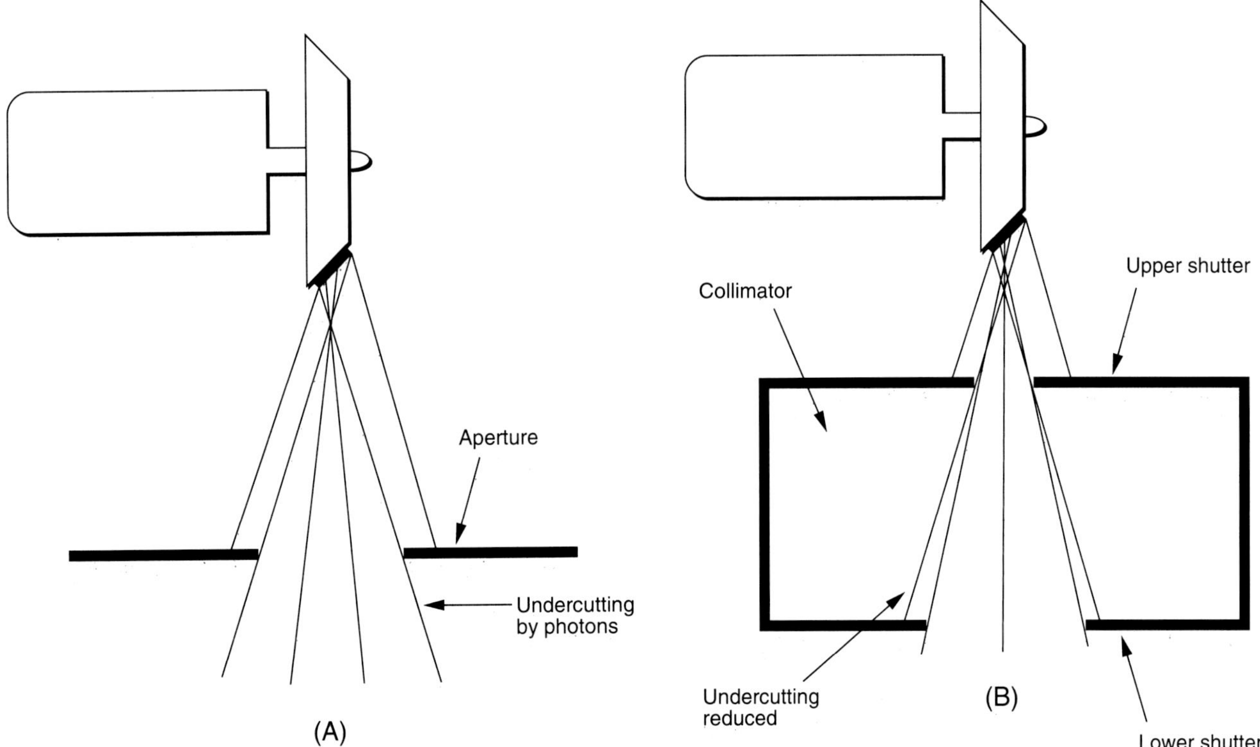



**FIGURE 13–5.** Aperture diaphragms allow undercutting of photons. As illustrated in *A*, photons from the extreme points of the focal spot undercut the diaphragm, causing unsharpness of the image. *B* illustrates how the collimator will reduce the unsharpness caused by undercutting.

The main disadvantage of the cylinder cone is the fixed size of the field; however, it can be very effective for specific examinations such as mammography or special views of the temporal bone of the skull, or joint radiography of the extremities.

## Collimators

The collimator is a box-like structure attached to the port of the x-ray tube (Fig. 13–10) for the purpose of restricting the x-ray beam. Inside the collimator are matching pairs of lead shutters resembling leaded plates. The lower shutters are mov-

able to allow for varying field sizes. The upper pair of shutters is located nearest the focal spot and is known as the port or entrance shutters. The entrance shutters are fixed to serve much like an

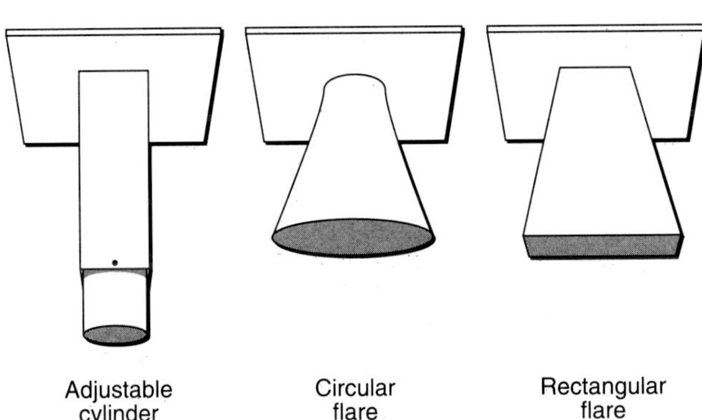



**FIGURE 13–6.** Cones are heavy metal devices that may vary in size and shape, as illustrated here.

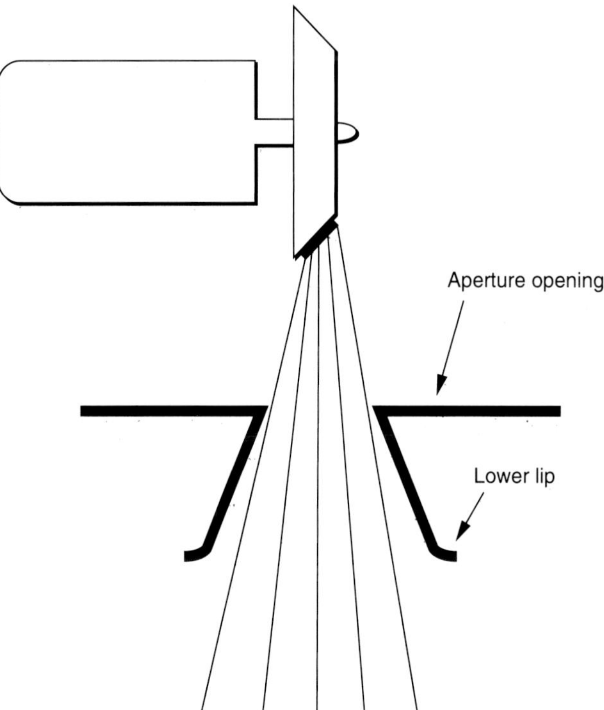



**FIGURE 13–7.** The flare of the cone is nearly parallel with the diverging photons.

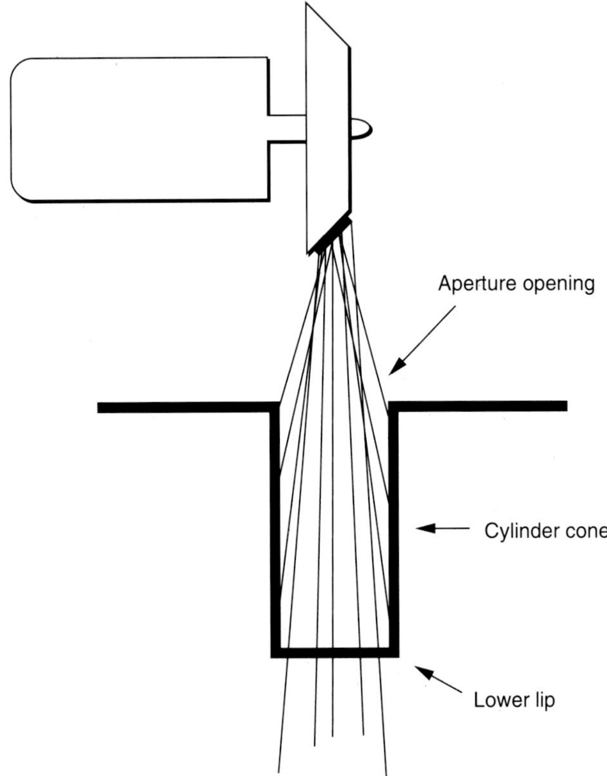



**FIGURE 13–8.** The beam is truly restricted and the undercutting by photons is reduced. Sharpness of the images will increase with use of a cylinder cone.

aperture diaphragm. The lower shutters are furthermost from the focal spot and adjust in the longitudinal and transverse directions (Fig. 13–11).

The lower shutters open and close, adjusting the border of the beam. When the shutter pairs are completely closed, they should meet in the center of the field. The two pairs of shutters are operated independently to accomplish varying field sizes. Most collimators have an external calibrated scale that can be used to select the exact size of the beam with various FFDs.

Another characteristic of the collimator is the beam centering device. Centering of the primary beam is extremely critical to prevent distortion of the image. Collimators have a light housed inside the structure that is used for centering the beam. When the light is illuminated, it is deflected by a mirror that is mounted in the middle of the collimator. The mirror is directly in the path of the x-ray beam and rests at a 45° angle. The light rays hit the mirror and are reflected through the open shutters to represent the borders of the beam (Fig. 13–12).

The shutters can be adjusted to change the field size of the beam by using the light to guide the

shutter placement. The lower portion of the collimator is usually covered with clear plastic with a crossbar in the middle. As the light passes through the crossbar, the center of the beam is marked. This is extremely helpful for accurate centering of the primary beam.

The centering device, which includes both the mirror and light, is the most vulnerable part of the collimator and may need frequent testing and adjustment. In the construction of the collimator, the placement of the bulb and mirror is very important. The distance from the focal spot to the midpoint of the mirror must be the same as the distance from the bulb to the midpoint of the mirror. This relationship is important for the light to truly represent the beam size. If the focal spot–to-mirror distance is greater than the bulb-to-mirror distance, the x-ray beam will be smaller than the light beam indicates.

The advantages of the collimator make it the best of all devices used to restrict the x-ray beam. The main advantages include its effectiveness in reducing penumbra and the variety of field sizes. The

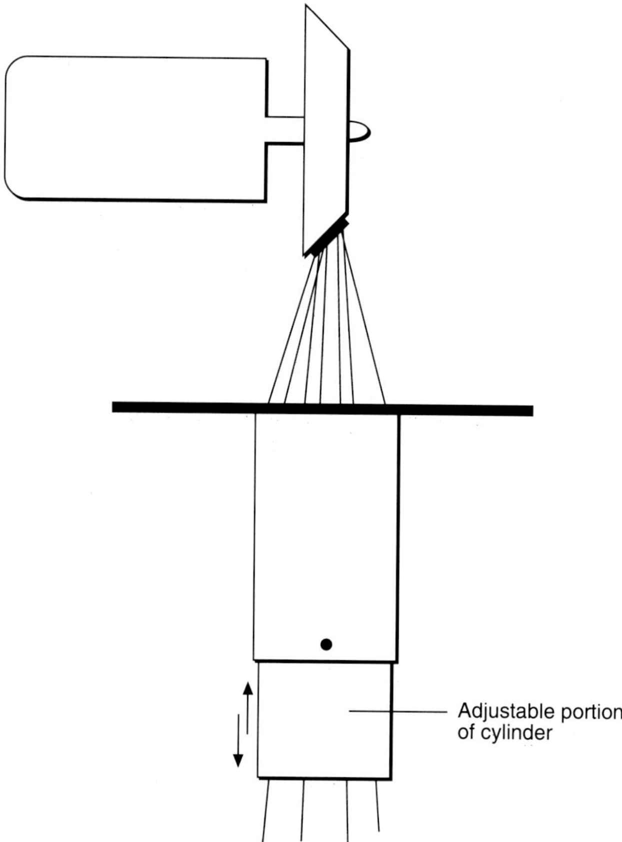



**FIGURE 13–9.** The adjustable component of a cylinder cone can be moved further from the focal spot. The greater the distance from the focal spot to the lower lip, the greater the restriction of the beam. The disadvantage is the lack of an adjustable field size.

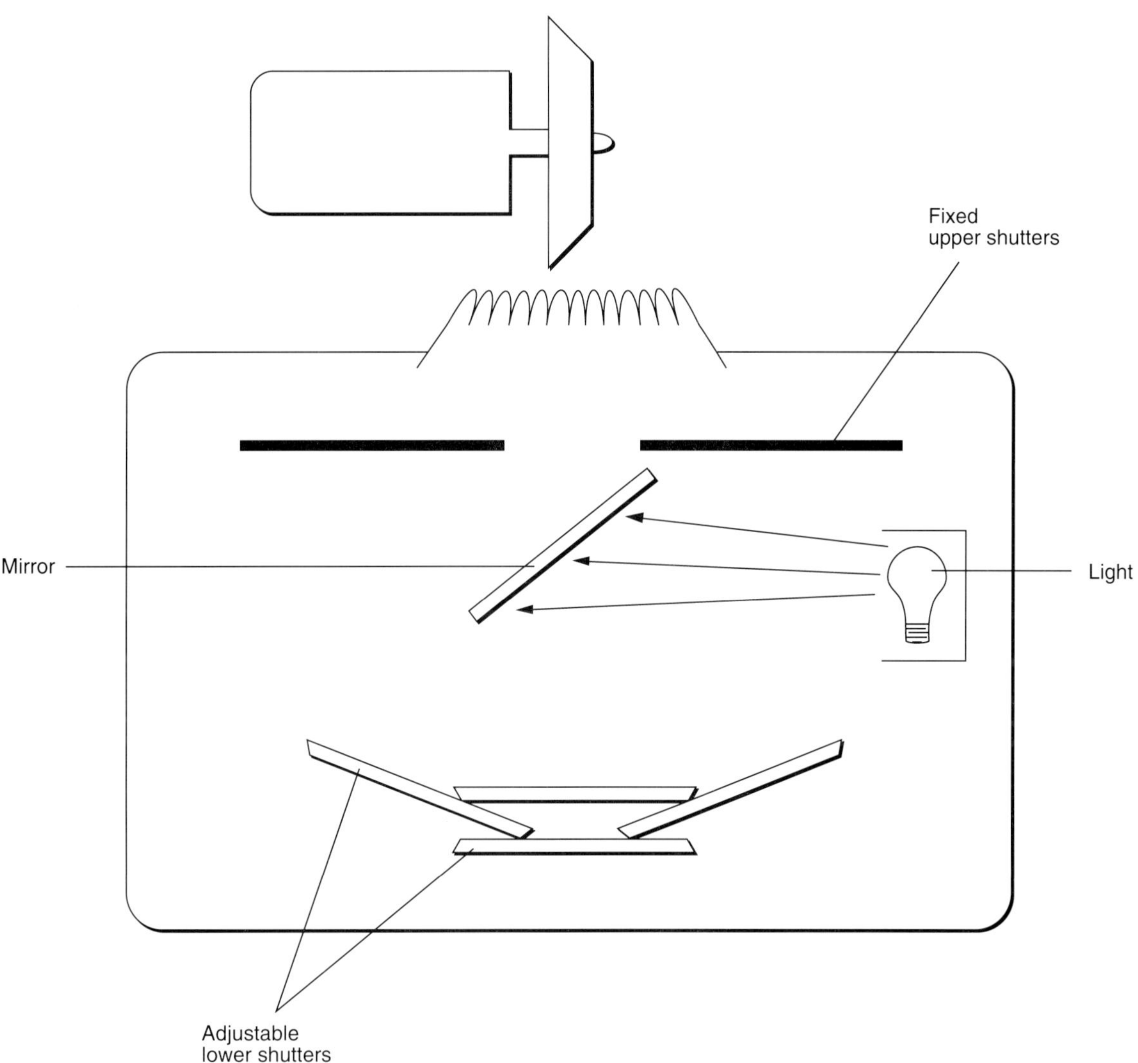


**FIGURE 13–10.** The collimator is the most effective means of restricting the primary beam. The movable lower shutters reduce undercutting and can be adjusted to fit any field size.

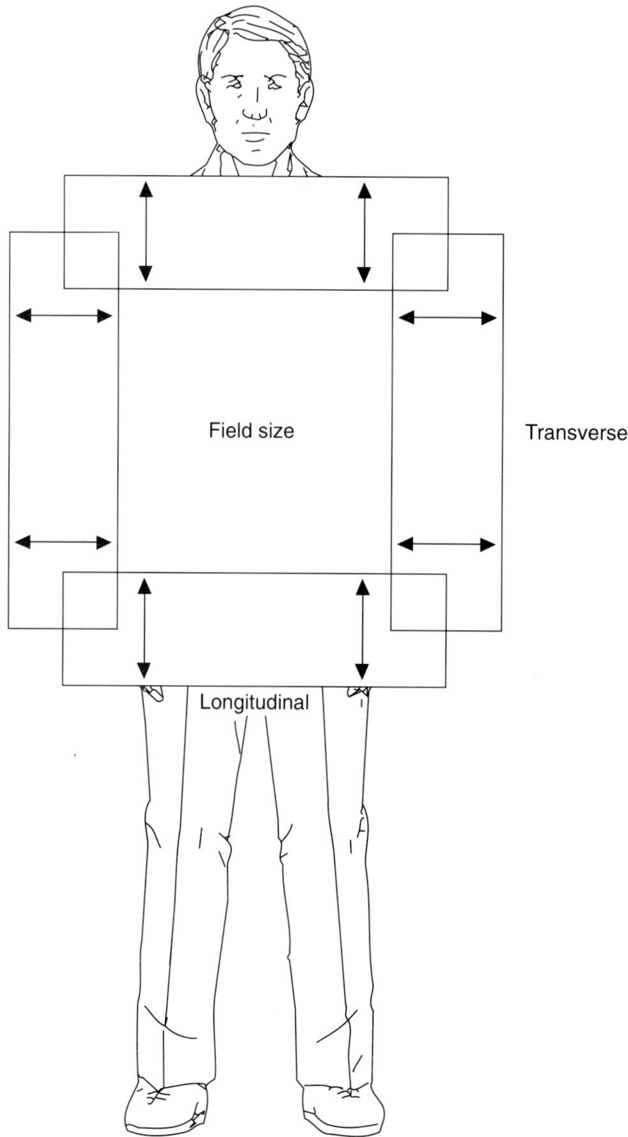


**FIGURE 13–11.** The transverse shutters adjust the side-to-side dimensions, and the longitudinal shutters adjust the head-to-toe dimensions.

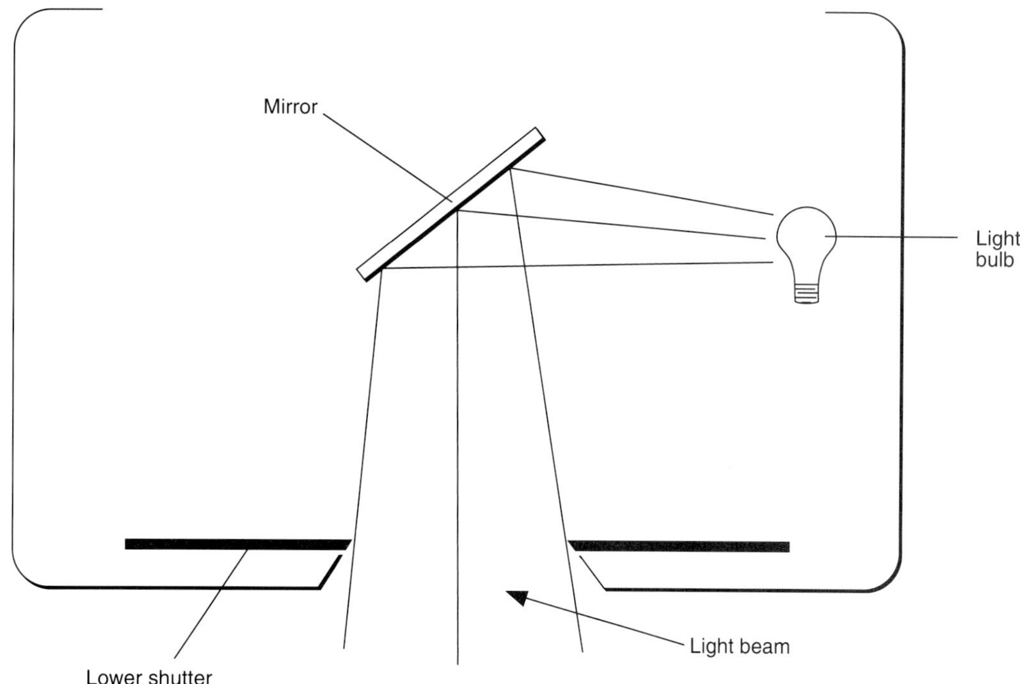


FIGURE 13–12. The light rays are reflected by the mirror to represent the primary beam. The light rays are used to adjust the longitudinal and transverse shutter to the exact field size.

beam centering apparatus allows for accuracy in placement of the beam over the centering point on the patient and with selection of the field size.

The collimator permits rectangular field sizes, which are more effective because most recording devices are rectangular in shape. Figure 13–13 demonstrates the effectiveness of rectangular or square shapes over circular field sizes. The ability to produce rectangular or square shapes provides greater and more effective beam restriction.

Collimators also add to the total inherent filtration of the x-ray beam. The collimator is the equivalent of approximately 1.0 mm aluminum, which is primarily a result of the mirror that is placed in the path of the beam.

## Automatic Collimators

The automatic collimator, also known as a *positive beam limiting device* (PBLD), works very much the same as a regular collimator. The difference with an automatic collimator is the movement of the shutters, which is accomplished with electric motors instead of manual selection. Electronic sensing devices are attached to the cassette tray. As the cassette is placed in the tray and latched, the sensors are activated to automatically adjust the shutters to the size of the film. Most automatic collimators are accurate to within 2 to 3%.

## Beam Alignment Test for Collimators

The alignment of the primary beam with the light from the collimator must remain accurate. The beam alignment test for the collimator is performed to ensure that the light beam duplicates the borders of the primary beam. The test is performed using a 14 × 17 cassette. The light beam is adjusted to leave a 2-inch unexposed border around the edge of the cassette. The corners of the light beam are marked with paper clips or other metal markers placed on the cassette. The center of the beam is also marked along with a reference point using an R or L marker. Make the exposure using approximately 2.5 milliampereseconds (mAs) and 55 kilovoltage peak (kVp). Refer to a sample test, as shown in Figure 13–14.

The test radiograph is examined to determine if the light beam, as marked by the metal objects, is identical to the primary beam. Figure 13–14 is an example of good alignment. Poor collimator beam alignments must be adjusted to prevent overexposure to the patient.

## EXPOSURE FACTORS AND FILM QUALITY—BEAM RESTRICTION

As the size of the primary beam decreases, the amount of scatter produced during the exposure will

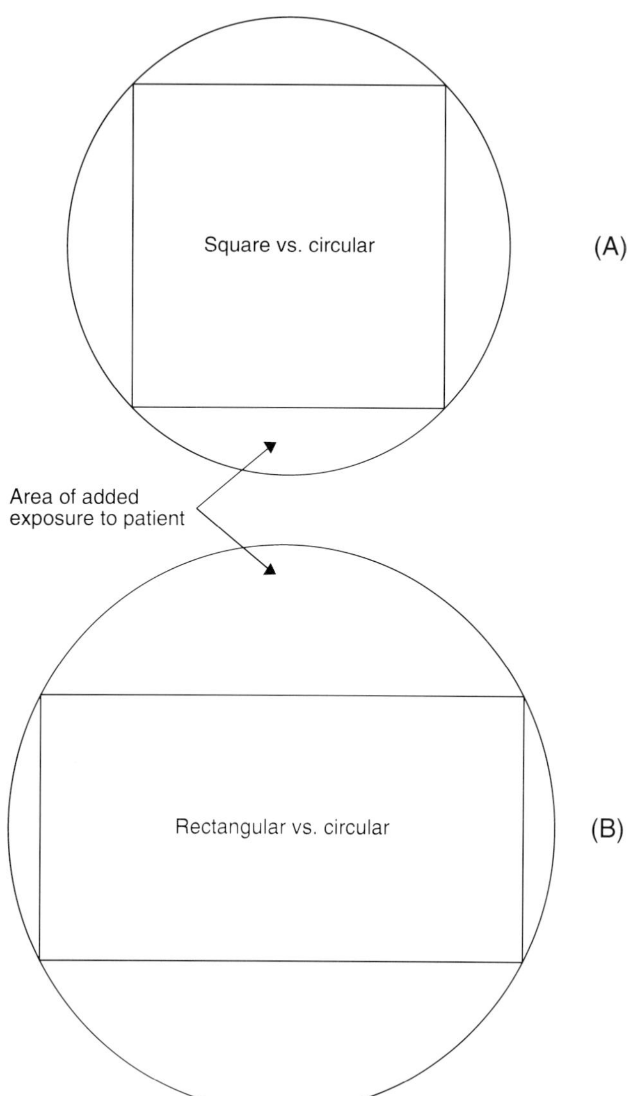


**FIGURE 13–13.** The adjustable shutters of the collimator can produce a square *(A)* or rectangular *(B)* field size that is more effective with various film sizes. As illustrated here, the use of a circular field size exposes a larger area than necessary to cover a specific film size.

also decrease. Decreasing the scatter will result in decreased density and increased contrast. Radiographs made with a small field size demonstrate fewer grays, with a more black and white appearance, which means a shorter scale of contrast.

Because beam restriction decreases the amount of scatter, increased restriction of the beam (field size becomes smaller) will result in decreased density recorded on the film, with a shorter scale of contrast.

AS THE FIELD SIZE DECREASES: SCATTER RADIATION WILL DECREASE, DENSITY WILL DECREASE, AND CONTRAST WILL INCREASE (SHORTER SCALE).

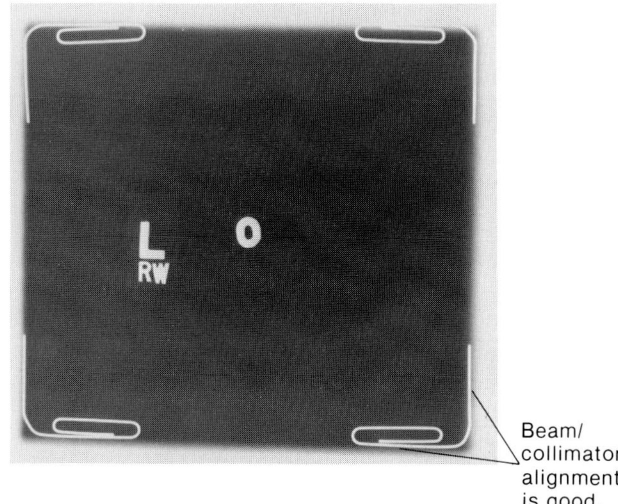


**FIGURE 13–14.** Radiograph demonstrating the procedure to test the accuracy of the collimator beam alignment. This test shows good alignment.

Increased beam restriction decreases scatter and therefore decreases density. To compensate for the decreased density, one must adjust the mAs. Table 13–1 provides a guide for changing exposure factors with a change in field size.

The increases in mAs are necessary to maintain adequate density levels when adjusting the field size.

As stated above, reducing the field size will increase contrast and provide a shorter scale of contrast. The decrease in scatter reaching the film produces a radiograph with fewer gray tones. The increase in contrast will also improve the visibility of detail. Beam restriction is extremely important in producing high-quality radiographs.

BEAM RESTRICTION IMPROVES THE VISIBILITY OF DETAIL.

## CALCULATING FIELD SIZE

When using field size adjustments, one must know the relationship between the aperture or shutter opening and the field size.

**TABLE 13–1.** ADJUSTMENTS FOR BEAM RESTRICTION

| Original Field Size (in.) | New Field Size (in.) | Increase (mAs) Needed |
|---|---|---|
| 14 × 17 | 10 × 12 | 25–35% |
| 14 × 17 | 8 × 10 | 40% |
| 14 × 17 | 5 × 7 | 60% |

For a circular opening, the diameter of the aperture will determine the diameter of the beam. If the diameter of the desired field size is known, the aperture size can be calculated by using the formula described below.

EXAMPLE:

Calculation of field size:

$$\text{Aperture opening} = \frac{\substack{\text{width or} \\ \text{diameter of} \\ \text{field}} \times \substack{\text{distance from} \\ \text{focal spot to aperture}}}{\text{focal-film distance}}$$

Calculate the aperture opening for a field size of 10″, FFD of 40″, and a 3″ distance from focal spot to aperture opening.

$$X = \frac{10 \times 3}{40} = \frac{30}{40} = \frac{3}{4}$$

The sample demonstrates that an aperture opening of ¾ inches used at a 40-inch FFD will produce a field size of 10 inches in width.

The same formula is used for a square opening. For rectangular openings, the formula must first be used to calculate width and then again to calculate length.

## CHAPTER 14

# Control of Scatter Radiation: Grids and Air Gap

## CHAPTER OBJECTIVES

1. Describe the rationale for employing grids in radiography.
2. Describe the contributions of Drs. Bucky and Potter to radiography.
3. Explain the effectiveness of grids in reducing scatter radiation exposure to the recording medium.
4. Draw examples of parallel and focused grids.
5. Differentiate between organic and inorganic interspacing.
6. List the advantages and disadvantages of moving grids.
7. Define the following as structural factors related to grids: grid ratio, grid frequency, and focal range.
8. Define the following as procedural factors related to grids: contrast improvement factor, selectivity, and Bucky factor.
9. Explain how increases and decreases in grid ratio and frequency will affect exposure factors.
10. Define grid ''cutoff'' and grid ''cleanup.''
11. List at least three conditions that will produce grid cutoff.
12. Describe how grid placement, tube alignment, and focal-film distance (FFD) will affect grid cutoff.
13. Explain how the air gap method serves as an alternative to the use of grids.
14. Compare the use of high-frequency stationary grids with that of moving grids.
15. Describe how the use of grids will affect contrast, scale of contrast, density, and visibility of detail.

## KEY WORDS AND TERMS

| | |
|---|---|
| Grid | Focal range |
| Potter-Bucky diaphragm | Grid ratio (gR) |
| Lead strips | Grid frequency (gF) |
| Slanting of strips (canting) | Contrast improvement factor (gK) |
| Interspacing | Selectivity (g$\Sigma$) |
| Linear grid | Bucky factor (bF) |
| Crossed grid | Grid cutoff |
| Parallel grid | Grid cleanup |
| Focused grid | Decenter |
| Grid cassette | Off level |
| Focus line | Air gap technique |

# RECOMMENDATIONS FOR GENERAL DISCUSSION QUESTIONS

1. Explain why grids are used in radiography when, in fact, their use requires an increase in radiation exposure to the patient.
2. Describe how parallel and focused grids are constructed to ensure effective reduction in scatter radiation exposing the film.
3. Explain the need for proper alignment of the x-ray tube, and why focal-film distance (FFD), grid placement, and alignment are essential in producing high-quality radiographs.
4. Compare the following factors and explain how they can be used to evaluate grid performance: contrast improvement factor, selectivity, and the Bucky factor.
5. Explain the concept of a grid ratio, and describe how different ratio grids affect cleanup of scatter radiation before it exposes the film.
6. Explain air gap technique and compare/contrast this method with the use of grids.

The challenge is great for the radiographer to control scatter and its effects on patient exposure and film quality. According to the type of examination, anywhere between 50 and 90% of the exposure to the film results from scatter radiation.

As described in Chapter 13, beam restrictors are extremely effective in reducing the amount of scatter produced as the x-rays interact with the patient. Patient exposure is also reduced, and the film quality is significantly improved.

The radiographic grid is an accessory used solely for the purpose of improving the quality of the radiograph. Grids are designed to absorb scatter radiation before it reaches the recording medium. Figure 14–1 shows the placement of the grid to be between the patient and the recording device.

---

## A GRID IS USED IN RADIOGRAPHY FOR IMPROVING IMAGE QUALITY.

---

The first grid was designed by Gustav Bucky in 1913. Dr. Bucky's design was improved in 1920 by the work of Hollis Potter, M.D. Dr. Potter made a device that moved the grid during the exposure. The original work done by Drs. Bucky and Potter is still the basis for the design and application of grids in radiography today.

The use of a grid complements the effects of beam restrictors. Together, the two accessories provide the most effective means available for a radiographer to produce the best possible radiographs while maintaining patient exposure at a minimum.

The grid is placed between the patient and the image receptor. As the primary x-ray beam strikes the body part and interacts, scatter radiation is produced, which travels in all directions (Fig. 14–2).

As the scatter radiation strikes the grid from an angle, it is absorbed by the grid. The grid serves to reduce the number of scatter rays striking the film. Figure 14–3 demonstrates the effectiveness of grids.

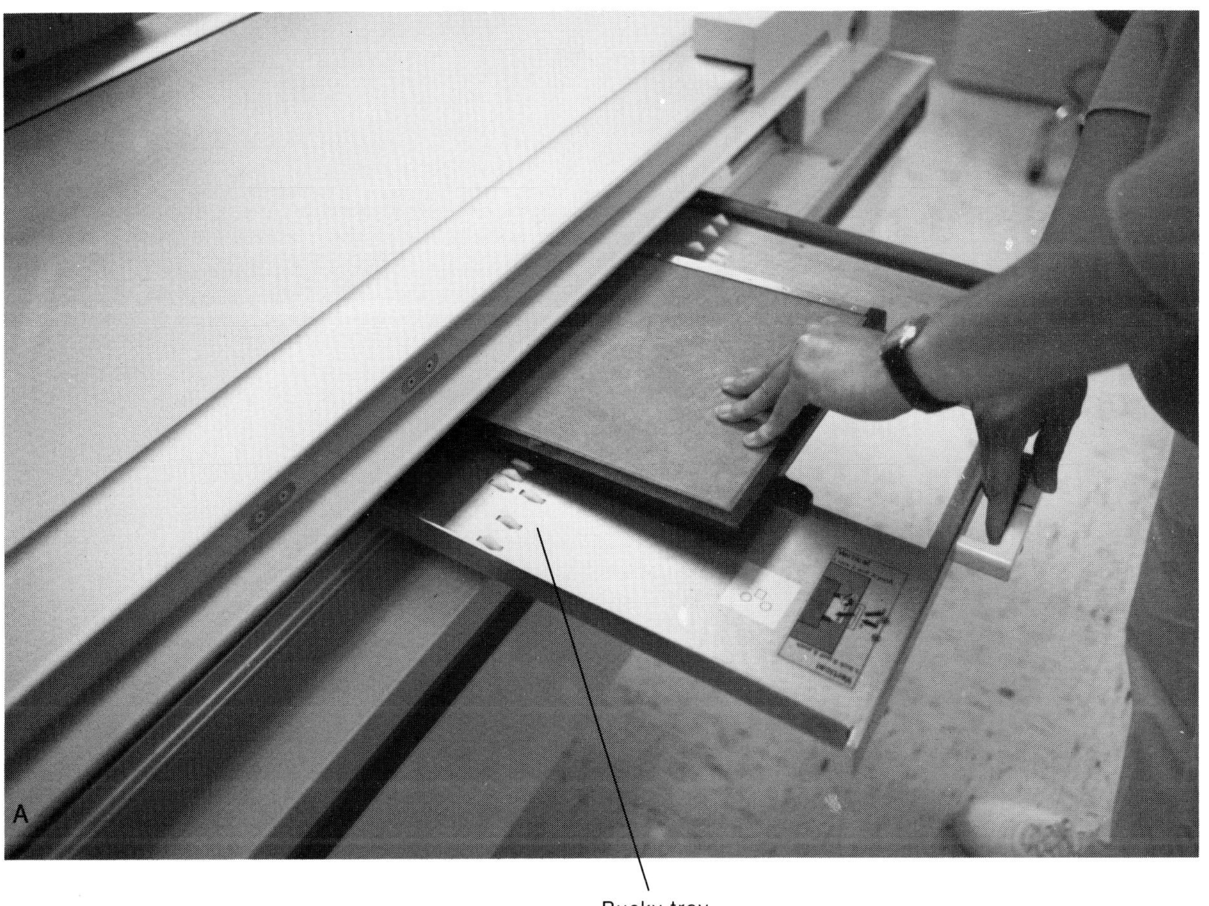


**FIGURE 14–1.** *A,* The grid is located under the table top and above the film. The device that holds the grid is called the Potter-Bucky diaphragm. The film holder is placed in the Bucky tray and moved so that the film is centered to the table top and to the midpoint of the grid.

*Illustration continued on following page*

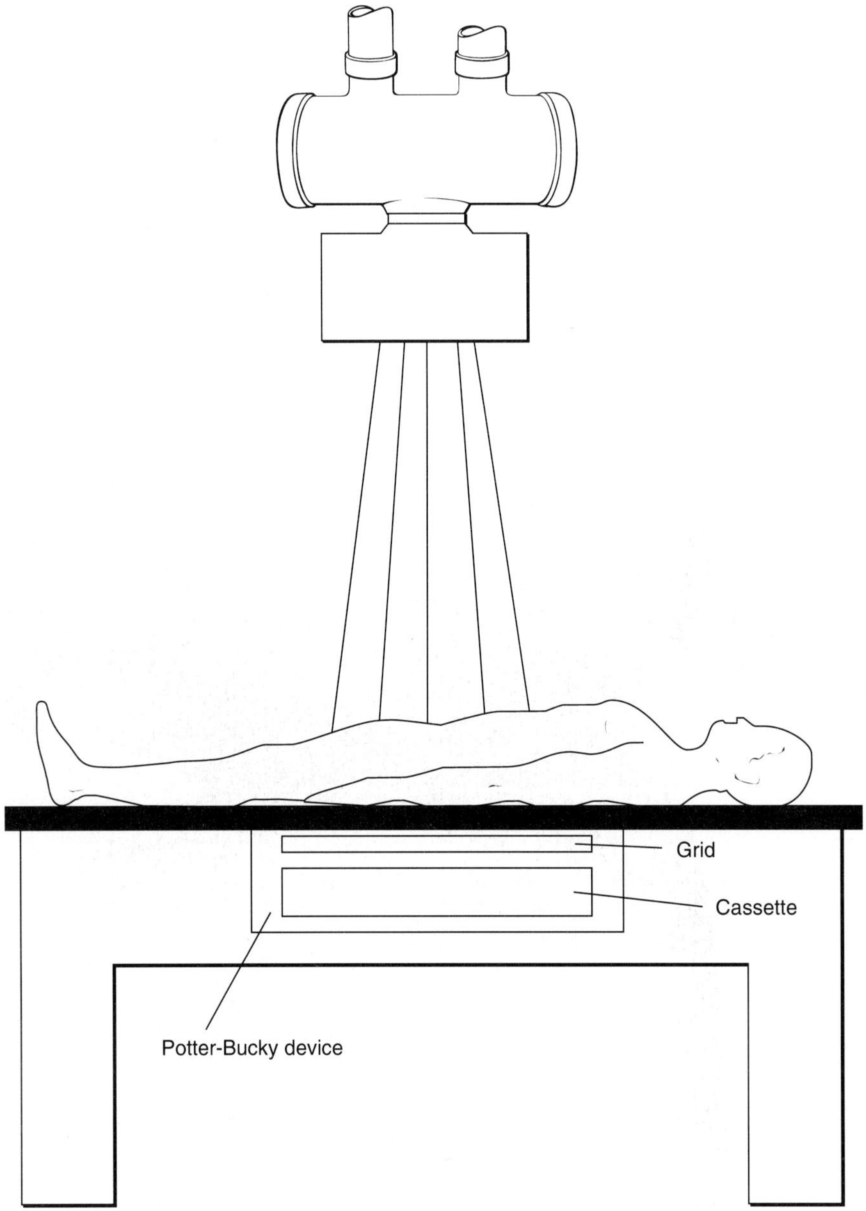


**FIGURE 14–1** *Continued B,* The Potter-Bucky device is located directly under the table top. The grid is placed between the patient and the film to reduce the amount of scatter radiation reaching the film.

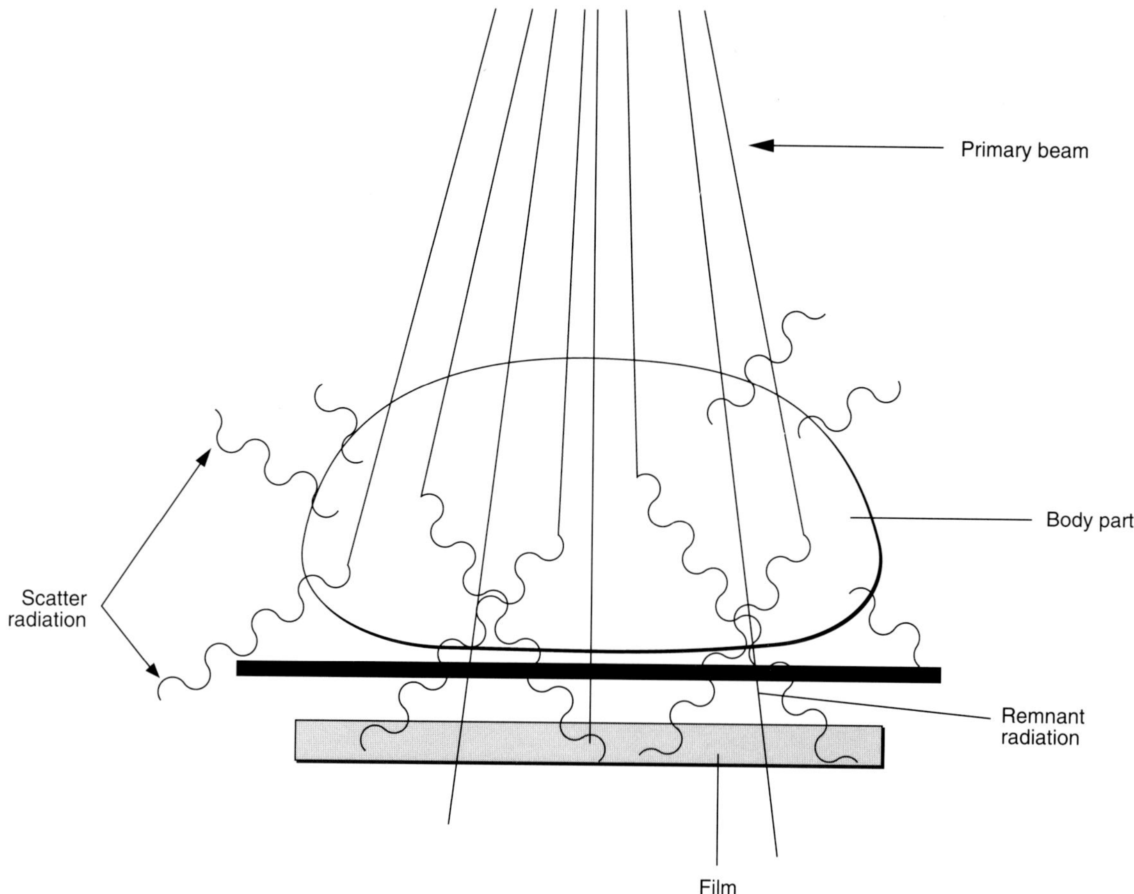



**FIGURE 14–2.** Scatter radiation is produced as the primary beam strikes the patient. The scatter radiation travels in many directions, with a significant amount striking the x-ray film and causing a decrease in visibility of detail.

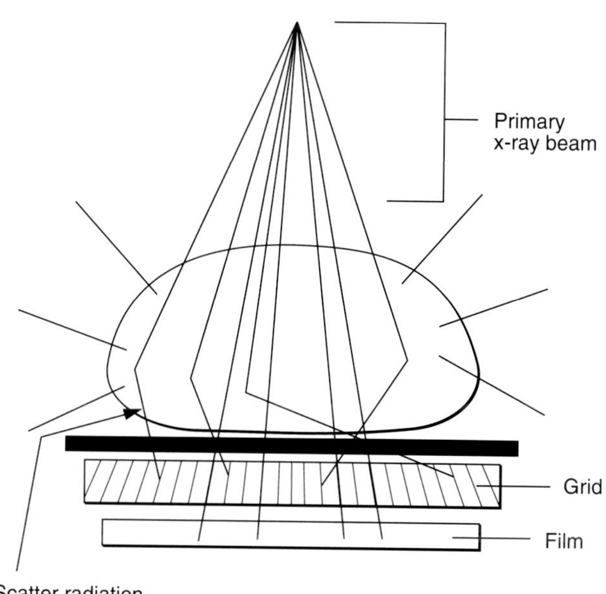



**FIGURE 14–3.** A grid placed between the patient and the film will absorb scatter radiation. The primary x-rays will travel near parallel to the lead strips to strike the film.

## THE USE OF A GRID WILL REDUCE THE AMOUNT OF SCATTER EXPOSING THE FILM.

The lead strips absorb scatter rays that travel at an angle of more than 5% from the remnant radiation. The increase in absorption of scatter will decrease the amount of exposure to the film.

The use of a grid during an exposure requires an increase in exposure factors to maintain adequate density on the finished radiograph. As the exposure factors (milliampereseconds [mAs]) increase, so does the amount of exposure to the patient. This becomes the major disadvantage for using grids during the exposure. Remember, grids are used solely for the purpose of improving film quality.

## THE USE OF A GRID WILL REQUIRE AN INCREASE IN EXPOSURE FACTORS TO MAINTAIN ADEQUATE DENSITY.

## CONSTRUCTION AND TYPES OF GRIDS

Grids are carefully constructed wafer-like devices made to be placed in grid holders located underneath the top of the x-ray table and above the tray that holds the film. Figure 14–4 shows a cross-section of a grid. Very thin lead strips measuring about 0.05 mm in thickness are placed vertically or slanted (also called canting) with interspacing material of approximately 0.33 mm. These measurements will vary with different grid designs. The strips resemble a heavy lead foil.

Lead strips with uniform quality are easily produced by manufacturers. The high atomic number of lead and its ability to absorb x-radiation makes lead the best possible choice in grid construction.

The interspacing between the lead strips is made of radiolucent organic or inorganic materials. The organic material used could be fiber, paper, cardboard, or plastic. The properties of organic materials allow for more remnant rays to pass through the grid with little or no attenuation. However, organic materials are more likely to absorb moisture, resulting in warping of the grid. The most common type of organic interspacing materials used in the production of grids is a combination of plastic and fiber.

---

GRIDS ARE CONSTRUCTED WITH LEAD STRIPS PLACED VERTICALLY OR SLANTED WITH A RADIOLUCENT INTERSPACING.

---

The inorganic material most often used in the construction of interspacing is aluminum. Aluminum has an advantage over organic materials because it will not absorb moisture, thus preventing warping. It is more durable and makes a very stable interspacing material. The major disadvantage of aluminum interspacing is the absorption of remnant rays. Aluminum interspacing increases the attenuation of the remnant x-rays and may require an increase in exposure factors. This translates into an

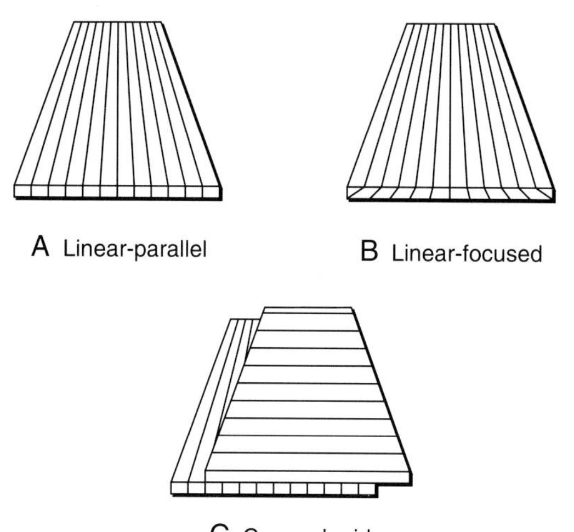



FIGURE 14–5. Grids are constructed with different designs for the alignment of the lead strips. *A,* Linear-parallel grids are constructed with the lead strips aligned parallel to each other and with the long axis of the grid. *B,* Linear-focused grids are constructed with the lead strips slanted to lie parallel with the diverging x-ray beam. *C,* Crossed grid is produced by placing two linear grids on top of each other with the lead strips aligned perpendicular to each other.

increase in exposure to the patient. As an interspacing for grids, aluminum will absorb more scatter radiation than organic materials. Radiographic contrast will increase and visibility of detail will also increase with the use of grids using aluminum interspacing.

### Types

Grids are constructed to meet the varying needs of the radiographer. Different types are available to accommodate a wide variety of radiographic procedures. The types include linear-parallel, linear-focused, crossed-parallel, cross-focused, and grid cassettes (Fig. 14–5).

The terms "linear" and "crossed" refer to the orientation of the lead strips in the grid. "Parallel" and "focused" refer to the relationship of one strip to another in cross-section.

Linear grids are constructed with grid lines aligned with the long axis of the grid. The relationship can also be described as the lead strips of the grid being aligned with the long axis of the x-ray table (Fig. 14–6).

Linear-parallel grids have lead strips that lie parallel to each other. The strips are aligned with the long axis of the grid; when used in a table examination, the strips are also aligned with the long axis of the table (Fig. 14–7).

The lead strips are aligned in the same way for a focused grid except that the strips are tilted or slanted so that they lie as near parallel to the

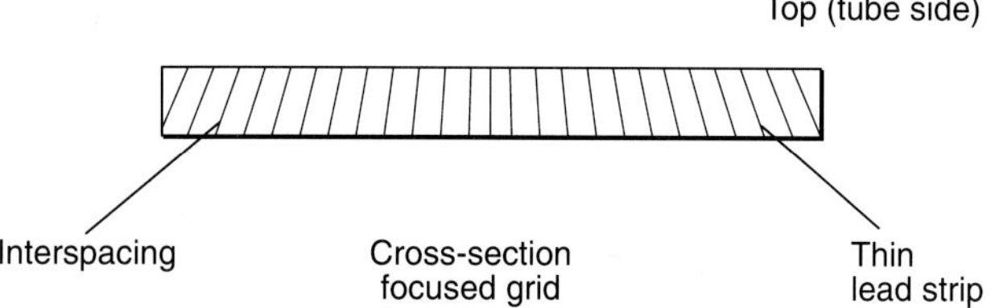



FIGURE 14–4. Cross-section of a grid. The lead strips are very thin and placed vertically and/or slanted with interspacings.

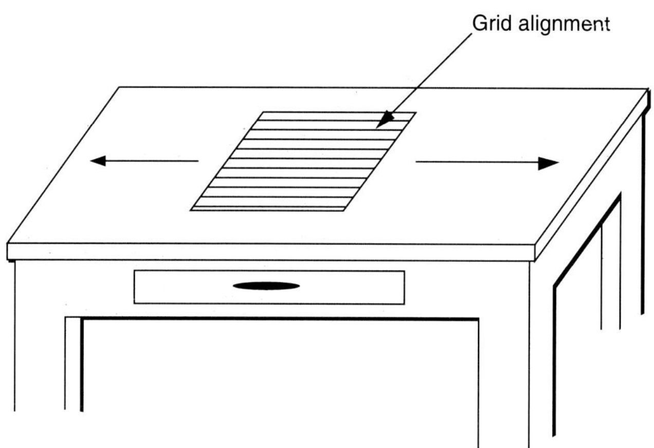



**FIGURE 14–6.** Placement of the grid is generally with the lead strips aligned with the long axis of the x-ray table.

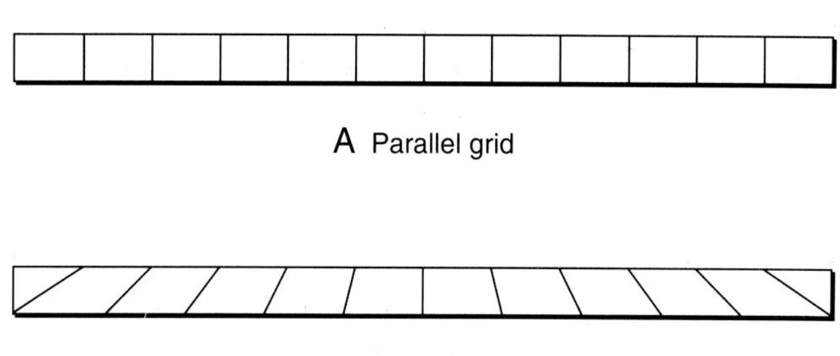



**FIGURE 14–7.** *A,* Parallel grids describe the relationship of the lead strips. The strips are vertical and parallel to each other. *B,* Focused refers to the slanting (canting) of the strips to match the diverging x-ray beam.

diverging remnant radiation as possible (Fig. 14–8).

---

# FOCUSED GRIDS HAVE GRID LINES THAT ARE SLANTED SO THAT THEY LIE ALMOST PARALLEL WITH THE DIVERGING REMNANT RADIATION.

---

The tilting of the lead strips produces a focused grid. If the strips were to be extended, they would meet at some point (Fig. 14–9). The result would be the "focus line"—a line where all grid strips would meet in a plane. The focus line identifies the distance at which the focal spot of the x-ray tube should be placed from the grid in order to reduce cutoff.

Crossed grids are generally produced by placing two linear grids on top of each other but with the lead strips aligned perpendicular to each other (Fig. 14–10). Crossed grids may be parallel or focused grids.

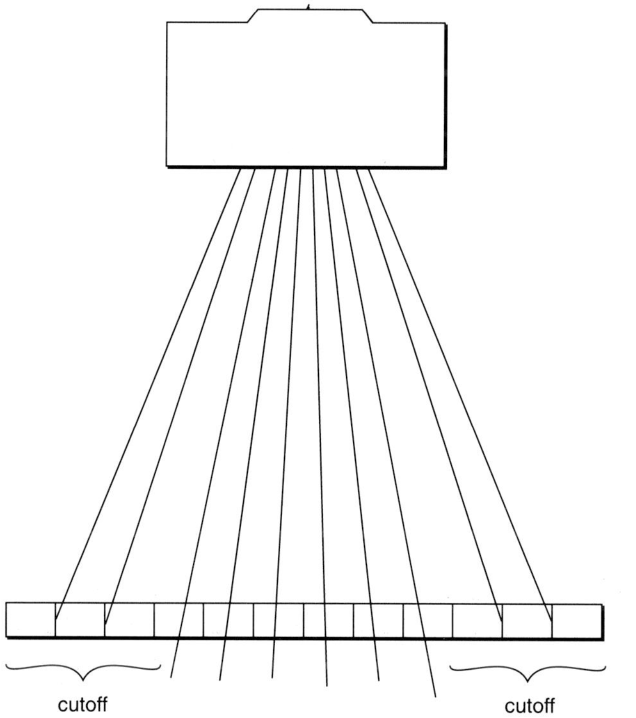



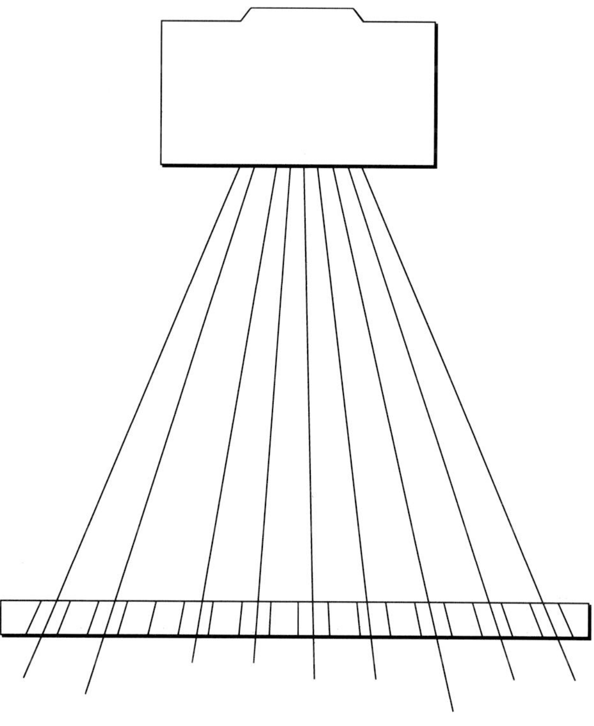



**FIGURE 14–8.** The slanting (or canting) of the lead strips allows for maximum exposure to the film by the remnant radiation. The lateral edges of a parallel grid (*A*) will absorb remnant radiation, producing grid "cutoff."

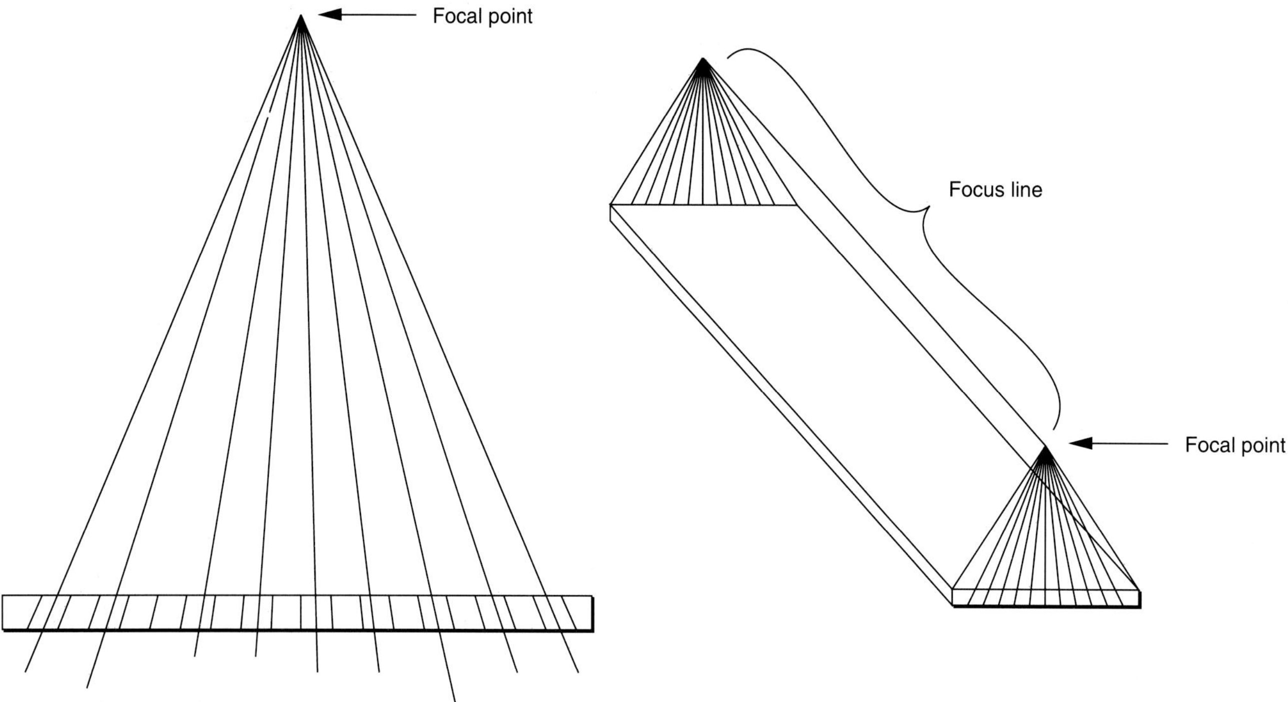


**FIGURE 14–9.** The focus line is the convergent line produced by the imaginary extension of the slanted lead strips to a point where they converge. The focus line represents the points where the x-ray tube can be placed to use a focused grid and eliminate grid cutoff.

Grid cassettes are regular cassettes or film holders constructed with a grid built into the front of the cassette. Grid cassettes may have a grid that is either parallel or focused, linear or crossed. The types of radiographic procedure to be performed will determine the type of grid cassette to be selected. Most general diagnostic procedures are best done with moving or fine-line stationary grids. Crossed grids are useful in special procedures and must be used with a perpendicular x-ray beam.

## MOVING VERSUS STATIONARY GRIDS

Dr. Potter's upgrade of the grid in 1920 produced a grid that moved during the exposure in order to

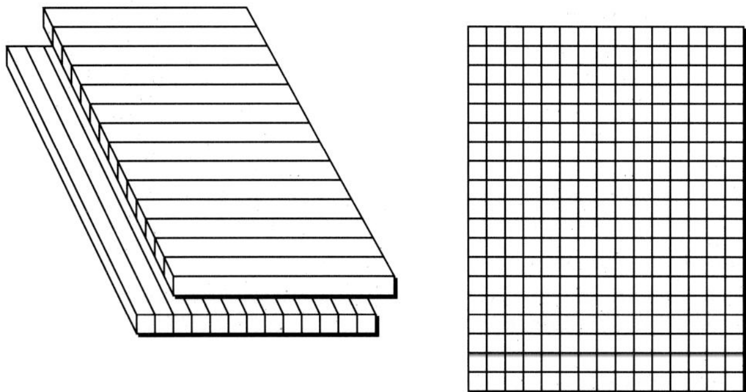

**FIGURE 14–10.** Crossed grids are produced by placing one grid on top of another with the lead strips aligned perpendicular to each other. The grids may be parallel or focused.

eliminate or blur the grid lines resulting from the image of the lead strips. For many years, radiologists have preferred moving grids because the shadow of the lead strips interfered with film quality. The apparatus that moves the grid is called the Potter-Bucky diaphragm. Different movement devices are used, producing reciprocating (back and forth) and oscillating (circular) movements.

Movement of the grid during the exposure is very successful in eliminating grid lines from the radiograph; however, the addition of an electronic device creates a disadvantage. Radiographers must contend with electrical failures, faulty or "jerky" movements, and vibration of the cassette causing motion during the exposure. Faulty movement or failure of the grid to move during the exposure causes grid lines to be visible on the radiograph. These disadvantages or malfunctions have sent manufacturers back to their labs to refine and develop grids and movement devices that attempt to overcome these problems.

MOVEMENT OF THE GRID DURING THE EXPOSURE ELIMINATES THE GRID LINES ON THE RADIOGRAPH.

Inasmuch as focused grids are the grid of choice in most procedures, the moving grid absorbs more of the remnant rays as a result of the constant decentering of the grid during the exposure. The use of a moving grid requires a slight increase in exposure factors to maintain consistent density levels on the radiograph.

Many radiology departments now prefer the use of a stationary grid with increased numbers of lead strips per inch because it will overcome many of the problems with moving grids. Most newer radiographic units use stationary linear-focused grids with 150 or more lead strips per inch.

## GRID CHARACTERISTICS

To successfully use a grid, the radiographer must understand the characteristics of the particular grid selected to use during the procedure. It is not a general practice to change grids between procedures. Grids are usually placed in the grid device and left in place. Many radiology departments assign certain procedures to specific radiographic rooms because of the requirements for that procedure along with other technical requirements such as body part, kVp, and the type of grid. This assures the best quality radiograph will be produced.

Grids are used to improve contrast and visibility of detail. The type of grid selected is determined by the following characteristics: grid ratio, grid frequency, focal range, contrast improvement factor, selectivity, and Bucky factor.

---

GRIDS ARE USED TO IMPROVE CONTRAST AND VISIBILITY OF DETAIL.

---

Grid ratio, frequency, and focal range are intrinsic or structural factors associated with the construction of grids. The contrast improvement factor, selectivity, and Bucky factor are applied to determine the effectiveness of a particular grid, and are known as extrinsic or procedural factors.

---

GRID RATIO, FREQUENCY, AND FOCAL RANGE ARE INTRINSIC STRUCTURAL FACTORS FOR GRIDS.

---

Structural factors do not vary no matter what the conditions of use may be; however, procedural factors will change as changes occur in how grids are used. For example, a change in kilovoltage would affect the procedural factors but not the structural ones.

The contrast improvement factor and selectivity may be used to compare the effectiveness of one grid with another. The Bucky factor indicates the amount of exposure increase that grids require when compared with a non-grid exposure technique.

---

CONTRAST IMPROVEMENT FACTOR, SELECTIVITY, AND BUCKY FACTOR ARE CHARACTERISTICS RELATED TO USE OF GRIDS.

---

### Grid Ratio

The ratio of the height of the lead strip to the width of the interspacing material (distance between the lead strips) is the grid ratio (gR).

---

GRID RATIO IS THE RATIO OF THE HEIGHT OF THE LEAD STRIP TO THE WIDTH OF THE INTERSPACING.

---

$$gR = \frac{\text{Height of strip}}{\text{Width of interspacing}}$$

EXAMPLE:

Height of strip          = 2.4 mm
Width of interspacing  = 0.30 mm

$$gR = \frac{2.4 \text{ mm}}{0.30 \text{ mm}} = 8$$

Grid ratio is always expressed with the ratio written over one:

$$gR = \frac{8}{1} \text{ or } 8{:}1$$

The bottom number is always one. The ratio is a way to express the grid's ability to absorb scatter. "Cleanup" is the term used to describe the grid's ability to remove scatter before it strikes the recording device. In general, higher ratio grids provide more cleanup of scatter than lower ratio grids do (Fig. 14–11).

Ratios in diagnostic radiology range from 5:1 to 16:1. The most common ratio used would be either 8:1 or 12:1. Kilovoltage selections determine the

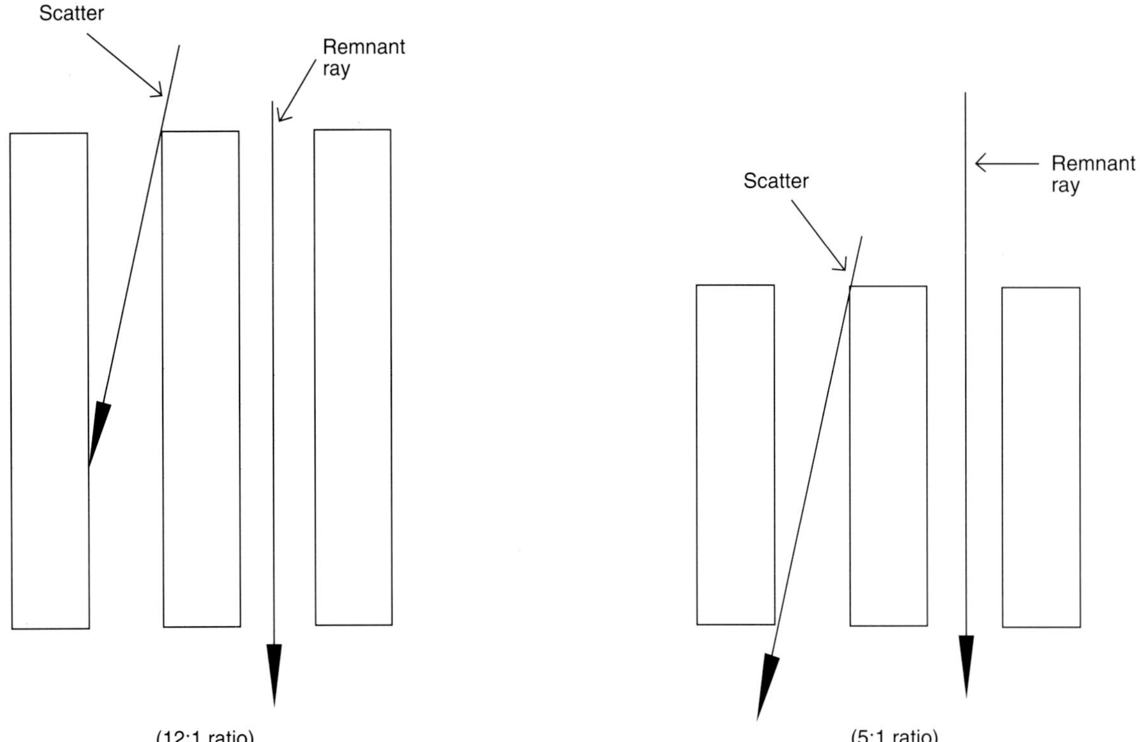



**FIGURE 14–11.** The effect of grid ratio. Scatter radiation traveling at the same angle may be affected differently with an increase in grid ratio. A scatter photon traveling at a particular angle may be able to pass through a 5:1 grid, whereas a 12:1 grid would absorb it. The 12:1 grid will provide more cleanup of scatter radiation.

grid ratio. For 90 kVp or less, an 8:1 grid is recommended. A 16:1 grid requires a significant increase in exposure factors to compensate for the loss of density. This is not desirable inasmuch as an increase in exposure factors increases the amount of radiation exposing the patient.

As the ratio increases, the amount of exposure must increase in order to maintain adequate film density. Table 14–1 provides a guide to evaluate how grid ratio (gR) may affect exposure factors.

---

THE HIGHER THE GRID RATIO, THE MORE EXPOSURE REQUIRED; THE EXPOSURE TO THE PATIENT IS GREATER.

---

**TABLE 14–1.** INCREASES IN EXPOSURE REQUIRED BY GRID USE

| Grid Ratio | Increase in mAs over Non-Grid Exposure (multiply by:) |
|---|---|
| 5:1 | 2 |
| 8:1 | 4 |
| 12:1 | 5 |
| 16:1 | 6 |

The changes recommended in Table 14–1 are estimates for grids with plastic-fiber interspacing and approximately 120 lines per inch. The factors may vary from those for grids with increased or decreased lines per inch or with aluminum interspacing. The grid most appropriate for a given procedure must be used to create a balance between high-quality radiographs and exposure to the patient.

The higher the grid ratio, the greater the improvement in contrast and visibility of detail. Again, balance is necessary to hold patient exposure to a minimum.

## Grid Frequency

The number of lead strips per inch measures the grid frequency (gF). The thickness of the lead strips becomes important. As frequency increases, the lead strips must become thinner. For example, higher frequency grids (150 to 200 lines per inch) are less likely to produce images of the lead strips because the strips are thinner and placed closer together. The range of grid frequency is from 60 lines per inch (low frequency) to as high as 200 lines per inch (high frequency). Most grids used in diagnostic radiology are stationary grids with approximately 120 lines per inch.

## GRID FREQUENCY IS THE NUMBER OF LEAD STRIPS PER INCH.

As the gF increases, the kVp range for the particular grid decreases. Thinner lead strips found in higher gF grids are more likely to allow scatter rays of higher energy to penetrate the strip. This would reduce the cleanup effectiveness of the grid.

Higher frequency grids decrease visibility of grid lines and increase contrast and visibility of detail. The one disadvantage associated with higher gF grids is the requirement to increase exposure factors (generally mAs) to maintain adequate density on the film. This results in an increase in exposure to the patient. Again the balance must be maintained to select grids with the proper ratio and grid frequency that will provide the best film quality while holding patient exposure to a minimum (Table 14–2).

## Focal Range

The design of grids limits the distance from the focal spot to the grid to a range recommended for the best performance of the grid.

## FOCAL RANGE IS THE RECOMMENDED FFD FOR THE BEST USE OF A GRID.

Focused grids must be used at the recommended focal range to prevent primary radiation absorption by the lead strips. The absorption of primary radiation as a result of poor alignment is described as grid "cutoff." Grid cutoff will occur if the lead strips are not aligned properly with the beam. Improper alignment refers to the use of the wrong FFD or off-distance FFD. (Refer to Figs. 14–8 and 14–9 for proper alignment of the FFD.) The focal line dictates the focal range for the grid.

**TABLE 14–2.** HIGH-FREQUENCY GRIDS

| Increase | Decrease |
|---|---|
| Contrast | Visibility of grid lines |
| Visibility of detail | Upper limit for kilovoltage |
| Exposure factors | |

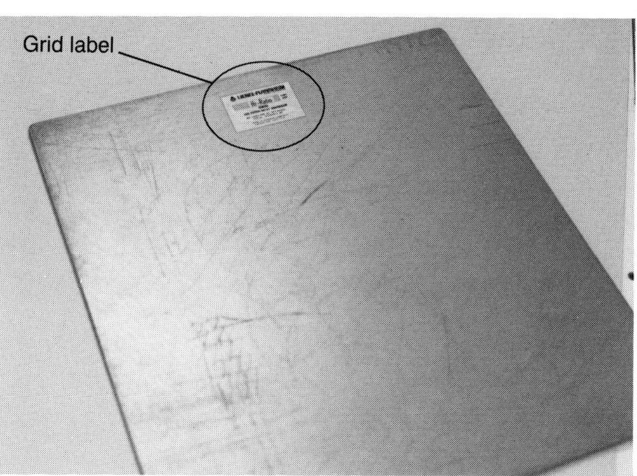


**FIGURE 14–12.** Grids are labeled to identify the tube side, focal range, and ratio.

The focal range determines the distance the focal spot may be placed from the center of the grid to prevent significant grid cutoff. Most grids are labeled with the FFD marked on the grid (Fig. 14–12).

Cross-focused grids have a focal point, and linear-focused grids have a focal line (Fig. 14–13). The focal spot of the x-ray tube must be placed at the distance marked by the focus point or focal line.

## Contrast Improvement Factor

As stated earlier in this chapter, the greater the lead content, the greater the cleanup value of a grid. Cleanup depends on the design and construction of a grid. The purpose of the grid is to increase contrast and visibility of detail by decreasing the amount of scatter reaching the film.

The contrast improvement factor (gK) is a measurement to determine the degree to which contrast is improved by using a grid.

$$gK = \frac{\text{contrast with a grid}}{\text{contrast without a grid}}$$

## THE CONTRAST IMPROVEMENT FACTOR IS A MEASUREMENT TO DETERMINE THE DEGREE TO WHICH CONTRAST IS IMPROVED WITH THE USE OF A GRID.

The gK factor measures the effectiveness of a particular grid. It is measured at 100 kVp using a phantom representing an average body part thickness of 18 to 20 cm.

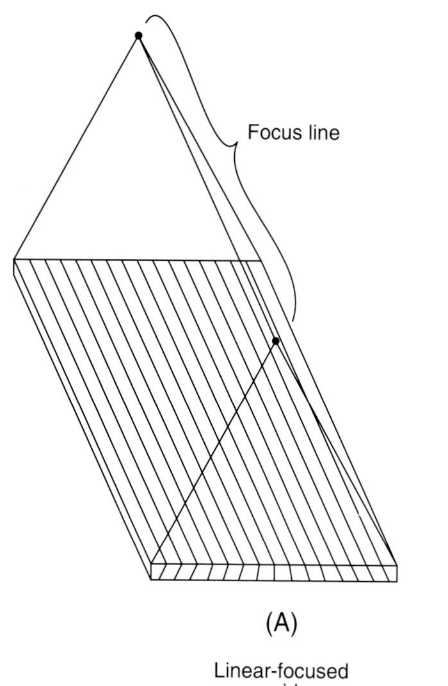


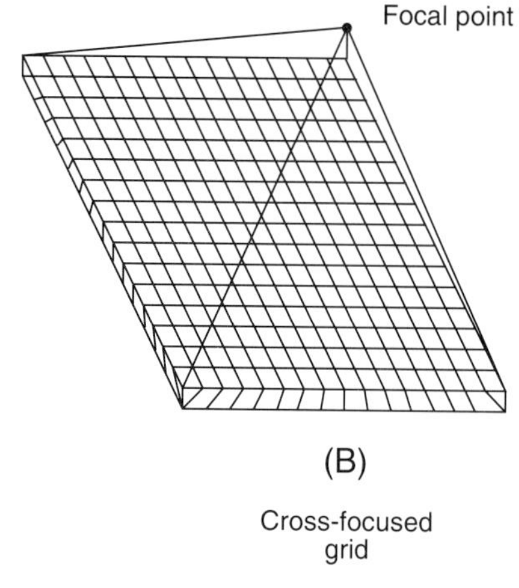


**FIGURE 14–13.** *A,* With a linear-focused grid, the convergence of lines drawn to represent the lead strips produces a focus line. *B,* The convergence of the lines drawn to represent the lead strips in a cross-focused grid produces a focus point. The focal spot can be placed anywhere in the focus line for a linear-focused grid and only at the focus point for a cross-focused grid.

The gK factor depends on the kVp, field size, part thickness, amount of scatter, grid ratio, and grid frequency. The gK factor for most grids ranges from 1.5 to 3.0, with the 16:1 grid producing the highest gK factor. The higher the ratio, the higher the gK factor; the higher the gR factor, the more contrast will increase. In addition, the higher the grid frequency, the higher the gK factor. The contrast improvement factor is most useful when comparing different grids used with the same condition or the same grid used with varying conditions.

### Grid Selectivity (gΣ)

Grid selectivity is used to describe how well a grid will differentiate primary remnant radiation from scatter radiation. Ideally, a grid should absorb all scatter and no remnant rays.

GRID SELECTIVITY DESCRIBES HOW WELL THE GRID WILL DIFFERENTIATE PRIMARY FROM SCATTER RADIATION.

$$\text{Selectivity (g}\Sigma) = \frac{\text{transmitted primary}}{\text{transmitted scatter}}$$

In general, the amount of remnant radiation transmitted by the grid ranges from 60 to 80%. The amount of scatter transmitted by the grid may vary greatly according to the total lead content and the grid ratio to as low as 10% with high-ratio, low-frequency grids. Grid selectivity describes a grid's efficiency.

### Bucky Factor

The Bucky factor (bF) is a practical value that defines the requirement for increasing exposure factors (mAs) to maintain film density. From this point, it is obvious that as lead content in a grid increases, the amount of remnant radiation absorbed increases, resulting in the need to increase exposure factors to maintain adequate density. The Bucky factor is used to determine the increase necessary to achieve this goal.

THE BUCKY FACTOR DEFINES THE REQUIREMENT FOR INCREASING EXPOSURE FACTORS TO MAINTAIN DENSITY WITH THE USE OF A GRID.

$$\text{Bucky factor} = \frac{\text{incident radiation}}{\text{transmitted radiation}}$$

The difference between the bF and grid selectivity is that the bF doesn't differentiate between remnant and scatter rays. Only the total amount of radiation passing through the grid is important to make the evaluation. The bF may range from 2 to 7. If a particular grid has a bF of 2, this means that two times the amount of primary radiation will be needed to maintain density on the film.

The bF increases with an increase in grid ratio. An increase in the cleanup characteristics of the grid will increase with an increase in bF. As the bF increases, so will the need to increase exposure factors, which means an increase in exposure to the patient. Table 14–1 is a guide for changes in exposure factors as required with a change in Bucky factor.

## SELECTION AND USE OF GRIDS

Grids are used to increase contrast and visibility of detail. The general rule is to use a grid for body parts that exceed 10 cm in thickness. To accomplish the goal, grids must be selected for use with specific factors in mind. The thickness of the body part, the kilovoltage selection, FFD, and field size are the major factors used to make the selection. A 16:1 grid would not be appropriate for imaging thicker body parts because of the significant amount of scatter radiation produced. For example, a 16:1 grid would help clean up scatter produced during a kidney, ureters, and bladder (KUB) exposure made with an extremely obese patient as long as high kVp is not used. A 5:1 grid would not be appropriate for fluoroscopic procedures using 100-plus kVp settings.

---

GRIDS ARE SELECTED ACCORDING TO THE PART THICKNESS AND THE EXPOSURE FACTORS.

---

When using a grid, one must take care in placing the focal spot and central ray of the primary beam. This is of particular importance in linear-focused grids. With linear-parallel grids, centering is less of a problem; however, short FFDs are a major concern.

---

GRIDS MUST BE USED WITH CARE IN THE PLACEMENT OF THE CENTRAL RAY.

---

Linear-parallel grids limit radiographic procedures to longer FFD and smaller field sizes (Fig. 14–14).

Linear-focused grids present several problems. The focal spot and central ray must be aligned along the focus line or plane. This will ensure that the remnant rays pass parallel to the lead strips and through the grid without absorption (Fig. 14–15).

The recommended focal range or FFD should be used. For example, an 8:1 focused grid may require a focal range of 38 to 42 inches. The proper FFD must be used to prevent cutoff when using a linear-focused grid (Fig. 14–16).

For a linear-focused grid, the x-ray tube may be angled as long as the angle of the tube is in the direction of the longitudinal lines of the lead strips (Fig. 14–17).

Because the lead strips in the grid correspond to the long axis of the radiographic table, the tube can only be angled with the long axis of the radiographic table (toward the head or toward the feet of the patient).

The focused grid must not be used "off level" with the beam such as may happen with a grid cassette during mobile radiography (Fig. 14–18).

A focused grid must always be used with the proper orientation to the x-ray tube. If the grid is used upside down, the remnant rays will only pass through a very small area at the midline of the grid. There will be almost complete bilateral cutoff (Fig. 14–19). Grids are usually labeled with the tube side identified.

For cross-focused grids, correct centering is absolutely essential. There is only one point for centering the primary beam. Off-centering in either direction will produce grid cutoff. Centering of the primary beam is very important to prevent cutoff on all four sides of the grid. This type of grid provides the best cleanup but at the same time has the greatest limitations in use. Focal-film distance and centering must be exact.

## AIR GAP TECHNIQUE—AN ALTERNATIVE TO GRIDS

An alternative to using grids is a procedure called "air gap." Air gap means leaving a 6 to 10-inch gap between the patient and the recording medium in the place where the grid would normally be located.

---

AIR GAP REQUIRES A GAP BETWEEN THE PATIENT AND THE FILM AND SERVES AS AN ALTERNATIVE TO THE USE OF GRIDS.

---

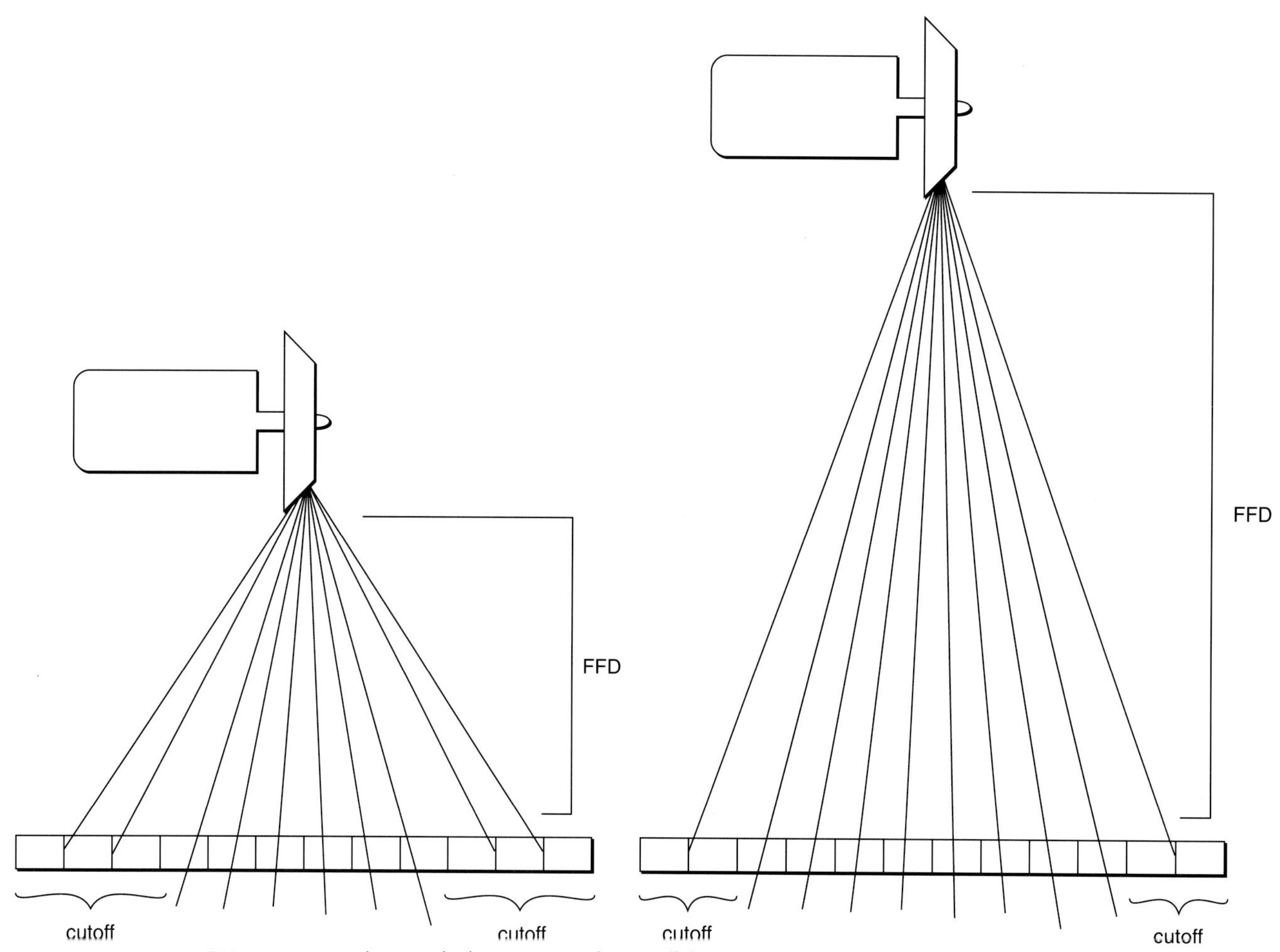



**FIGURE 14–14.** The use of a longer FFD with a parallel grid will reduce cutoff on the lateral edges.

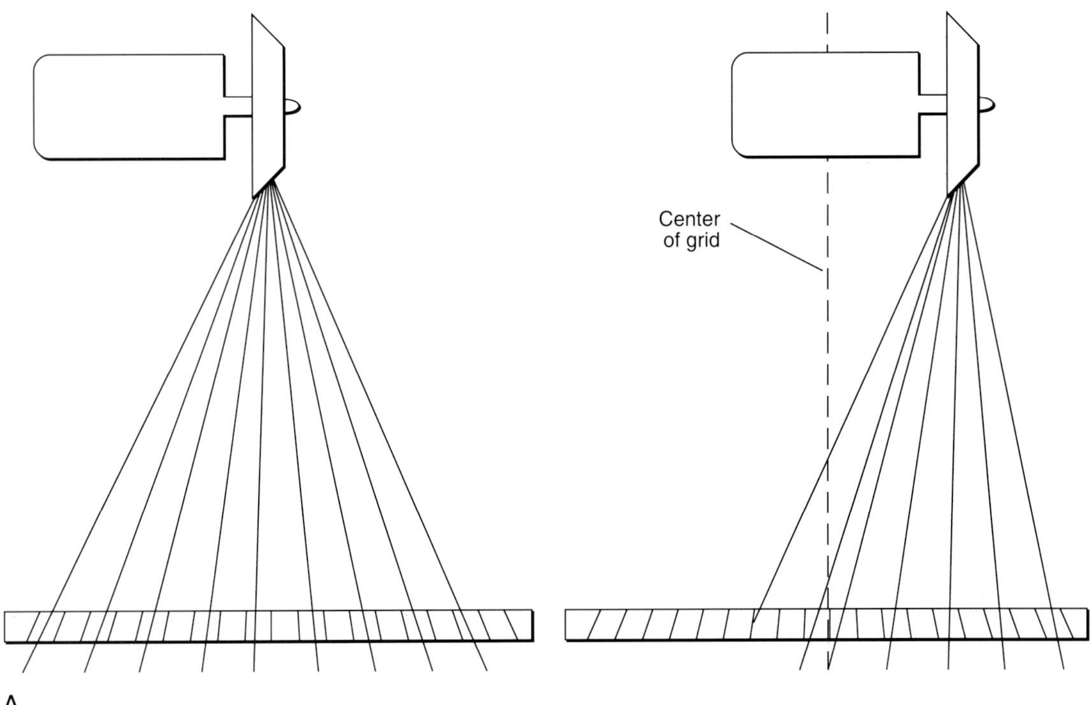


A

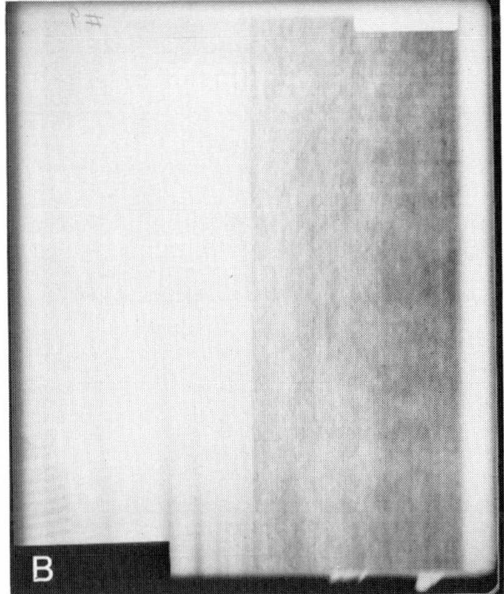

B

**FIGURE 14–15.** *A,* Placement of the focal spot lateral to the focus line will produce cutoff as the x-ray photons are absorbed by the lead strips. *B,* Radiograph demonstrating grid lines produced by improper alignment of the grid.

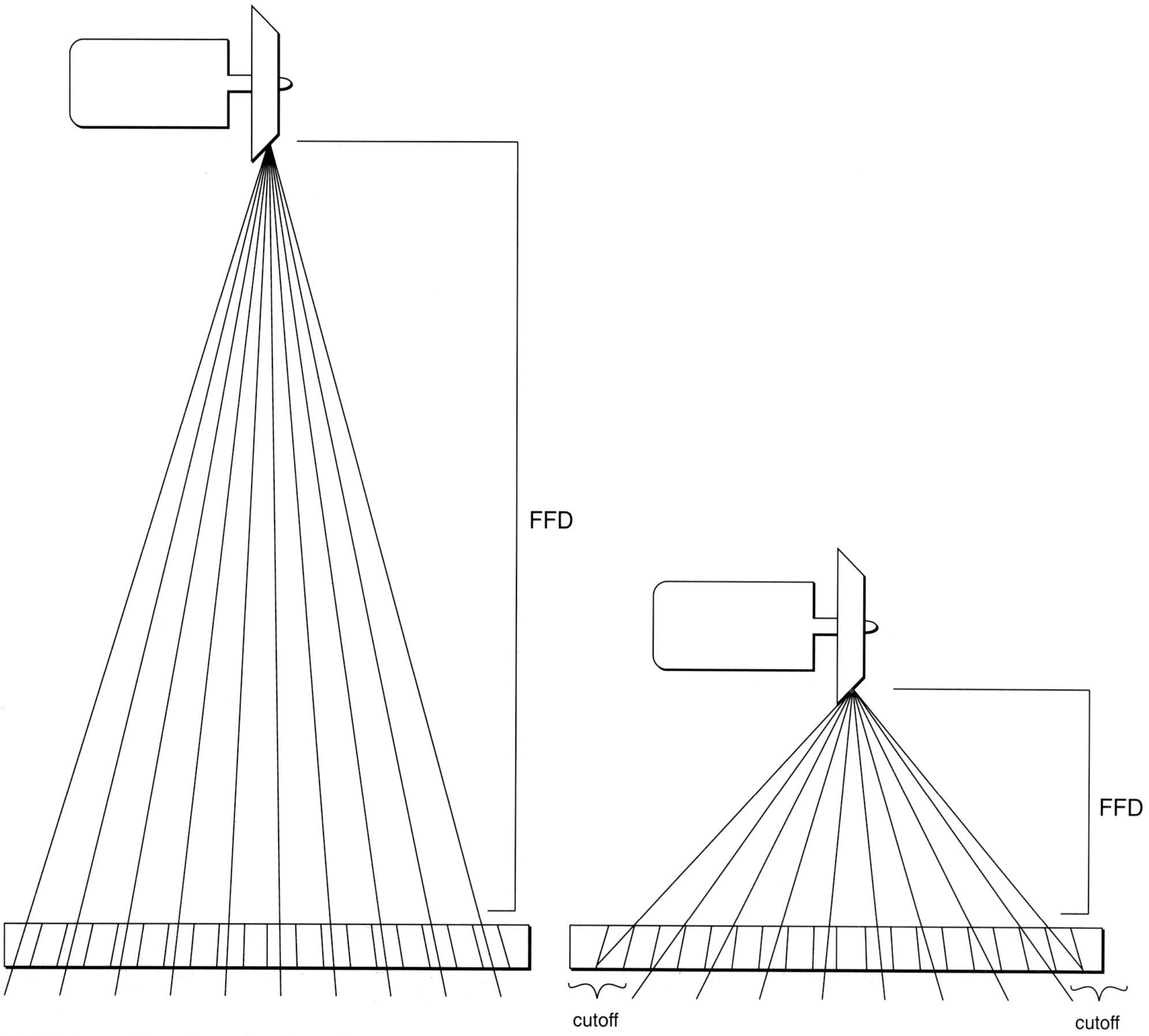

**FIGURE 14–16.** Linear-focused grids are designed for a specific FFD or FFD range. Too short an FFD will produce grid cutoff on the lateral edges of the film.

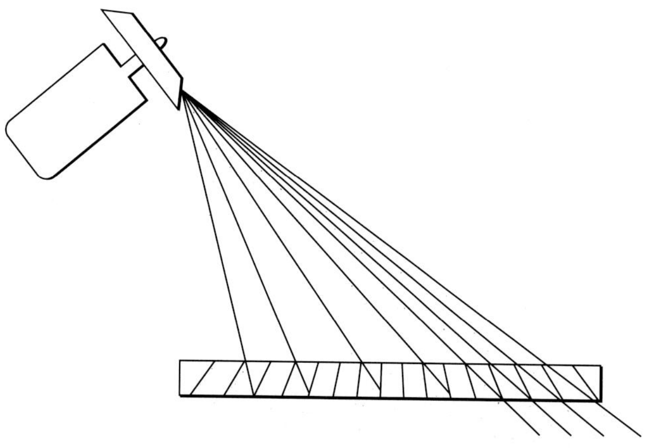


**FIGURE 14–17.** The x-ray tube can be angled as long as the angle is in the direction of the lead strips. An angle directed across the lead strips, as illustrated here, will produce grid cutoff across the film.

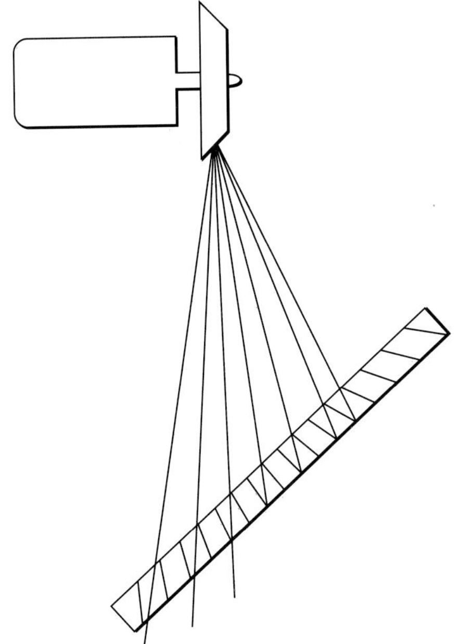

**FIGURE 14–18.** A linear-focused grid performs best when placed perpendicular to the central ray. The use of a tilt or angle of the grid, as illustrated here, will produce grid cutoff across the surface of the film.

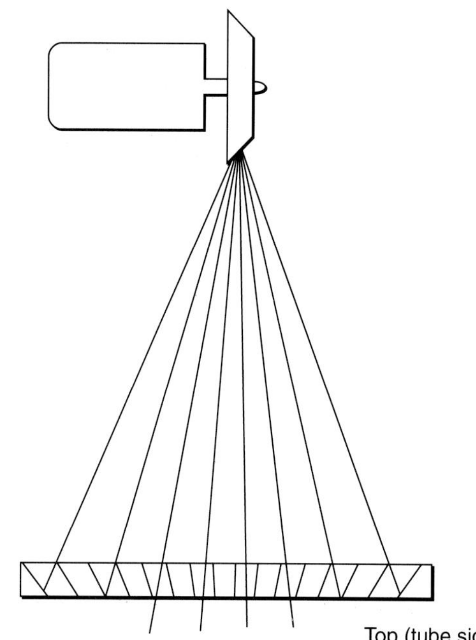



**FIGURE 14–19.** A linear grid mistakenly used upside down will produce almost complete cutoff on both sides. The remnant radiation will pass through the mid portion of the grid.

Scatter radiation is like white light. The closer one gets to the source, the greater the intensity. For scatter, the source is the patient and the first few inches from the object represent the area where scatter is the most intense. As you move further from the source, the scatter travels in multiple directions and would be less likely to strike the recording device (Fig. 14–20). Placement of the film

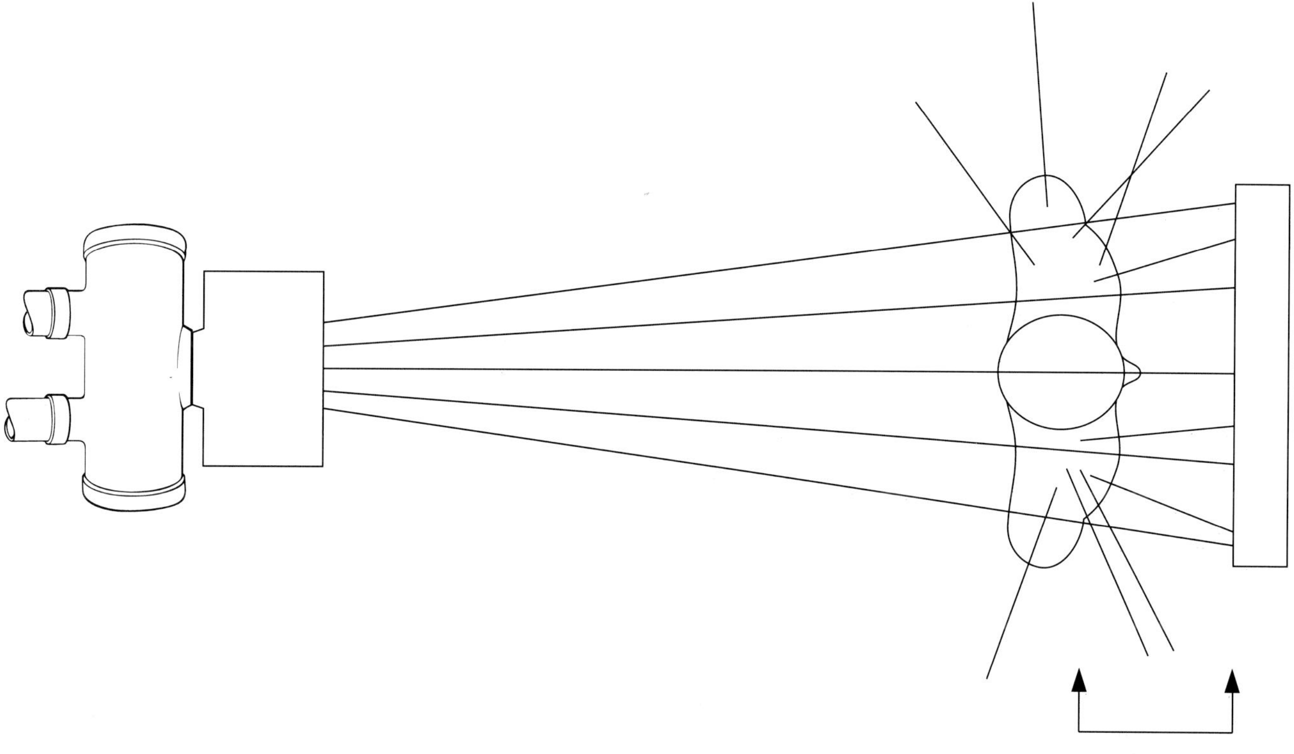



**FIGURE 14–20.** The air gap is approximately 6 to 10″ between the patient and the film. Because the scatter radiation travels in many directions, it is less likely to strike the film. The use of an air gap is an alternative to using a grid.

**TABLE 14–3.** GRID VERSUS NON-GRID EXPOSURE

Changing from non-grid exposure to the use of grids means:
Contrast is increased.
Contrast scale is decreased.
Density is decreased (exposure factors must be increased to compensate).
Visibility of detail is increased.
Magnification is increased as a result of the increase in object-film distance.
Patient exposure is increased because of the requirement to increase exposures to maintain density.

6 inches from the part would be as effective as using an 8:1 grid with a kVp range below 90.

The problem with air gap is that magnification is significant. An increase in the FFD would be necessary to compensate for the increase in object-film distance (OFD). This will require an increase in mAs in accordance with the mAs-distance formula.

Air gap has been used effectively in specialty areas such as angiography. Radiography of the lungs and thorax in diagnostic radiology depart-ments has also been successful using this technique. Air gap would lend itself well for lateral projections of the cervical spine using a 72-inch FFD. Patient exposure is usually lower than with grid techniques. The advantage is that use of an air gap also eliminates all problems related to the use of grids. The disadvantage is the design of most radiographic rooms and equipment does not facilitate the use of air gap exposures.

## GRIDS AND FILM QUALITY

Grids and air gap are major factors associated with the improvement of film quality. In reviewing the details described in this chapter, one realizes that film quality would significantly improve with the application of grids. Table 14–3 summarizes how quality factors are affected by the use of grids.

Grids or air gap are a necessity in radiography and must be used in consideration of the balance between film quality and patient exposure.

# C H A P T E R  15

# Evaluation of Radiographs: Characteristic Curve

## CHAPTER OBJECTIVES

1. Explain the importance of the use of the characteristic curve in radiography.
2. Differentiate between characteristic, sensitometric, and H & D curves.
3. Define sensitometry.
4. Describe the characteristics associated with the toe, shoulder, and straight-line portion of a characteristic curve.
5. Describe the process for plotting density and relative exposure on a graph.
6. Explain the concept of relative exposure.
7. Define $D_{max}$ and $D_{min}$.
8. Define base plus fog.
9. Explain the relationships between film gamma, gradient, and average gradient.
10. Describe the significance for the use of 0.3 increments on a logarithmic scale for relative exposure.
11. Describe the process for producing a radiograph and the graphing of a characteristic curve.
12. Explain how the sensitometer and densitometer are used in the preparation of a characteristic curve.
13. Given a set of exposure density values, plot them on a graph.
14. Calculate the average gradient of a characteristic curve.
15. Explain how density affects light transmission.
16. Describe how each of the following can be evaluated using the characteristic curve:

    contrast          density  
    speed             latitude  
    average gradient

## KEY WORDS AND TERMS

| | |
|---|---|
| Characteristic curve | Straight-line portion |
| Sensitometric curve | Logarithm |
| H & D curve | $D_{max}$ |
| Sensitometry | $D_{min}$ |
| Sensitometer | Film gamma |
| Densitometer | Film gradient |
| Light transmission | Average gradient |
| Base plus fog | Optical density |
| Toe | Relative exposure |
| Shoulder | Step-wedge penetrometer |

## RECOMMENDATIONS FOR GENERAL DISCUSSION QUESTIONS

1. Explain how long and short scale of contrast can be demonstrated by the characteristic curve. Draw examples to represent the explanation.
2. Describe the significance of using the characteristic curve to evaluate changes in exposure factors and image systems.
3. Describe how the characteristic curve can be used to compare and contrast film speed and exposure latitude.

In the preceding chapters, radiographic quality has been described along with the major factors by which it is controlled. To apply quantitative measurement to radiographs, one can use the characteristic or sensitometric curve. The characteristic curve, as shown in Figure 15–1, is an S-shaped curve that represents certain photocharacteristics of x-ray film.

## THE CHARACTERISTIC (SENSITOMETRIC) CURVE REPRESENTS THE PHOTOCHARACTERISTICS AND SENSITIVITY OF X-RAY FILM.

The characteristic curve is also referred to as a sensitometric curve because it represents the sensitivity of the film. The characteristic curve can be used to understand the principles of radiographic exposure and to compare density, contrast, speed, and latitude. It can also be used effectively to evaluate processing methods, especially consistency within automatic processing systems.

The characteristic curve was first used as a tool for measurement by two British photographers in 1890. F. Hurter and V. Driffield used the curve for their work in the analysis of photographs. The curve was originally named the H & D curve in honor of Hurter and Driffield.

The adoption of Hurter and Driffield's work in the evaluation of radiographs has become an extremely valuable tool in understanding how to monitor exposure variables and compare imaging systems. Manufacturers of x-ray film and screens use the characteristic curve to demonstrate how changes in exposure, film type, screen, and processing conditions will affect the final product. In radiography, it can be an important tool used to determine if a selected film-screen combination is being used to its best advantage.

A characteristic curve is obtained by exposing x-ray film to a series of exposures and plotting the density measurements on a graph (Fig. 15–1). The curve becomes a graphic representation of density and exposure to the film. Characteristic curves have also been used to compare and evaluate exposure and identify problems before they become severe.

## SENSITOMETRY

The method used to create a characteristic curve is sensitometry. Sensitometry is the measurement of film sensitivity to exposure and processing.

## SENSITOMETRY IS THE PROCESS USED TO CREATE A CHARACTERISTIC CURVE.

Sensitometry is done by exposing the film to light and/or x-radiation. The film is processed using standardized quality controlled processing methods. Specific areas on the film are identified, and a densitometer is used for measuring the amount of density or blackening in the target areas (Fig. 15–2).

Sensitometry involves the evaluation of light transmission. The amount of light transmitted determines the amount of density on the film. The greater the light transmission, the lower the amount of density (less opaque) on the film. The lower the amount of light transmitted, the greater the density level (more opaque).

## NOMENCLATURE FOR CHARACTERISTIC CURVES

Sensitometry requires the study of certain factors associated with characteristic curves. Before proceeding with the analysis of the curve, one must understand the language (Fig. 15–3).

The *vertical axis* (Y) of the graph represents the density reading obtained by the use of a densitometer. The *horizontal axis* (X) represents the amount of exposure the film received to produce a certain density. Exposure is expressed as a logarithm of relative exposure. It is not so important for the

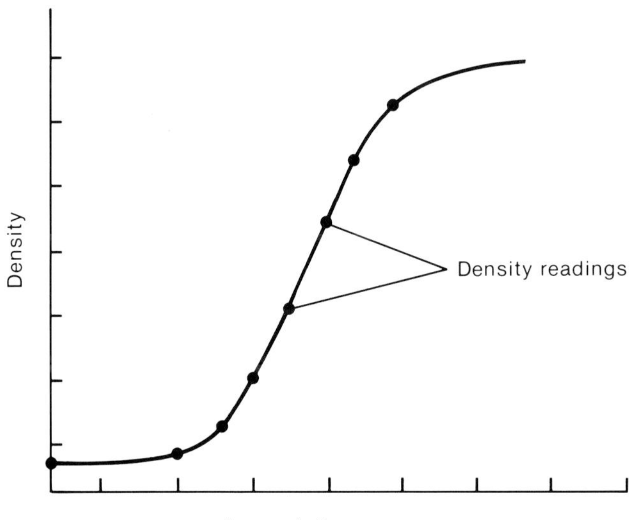

**FIGURE 15–1.** A characteristic curve.

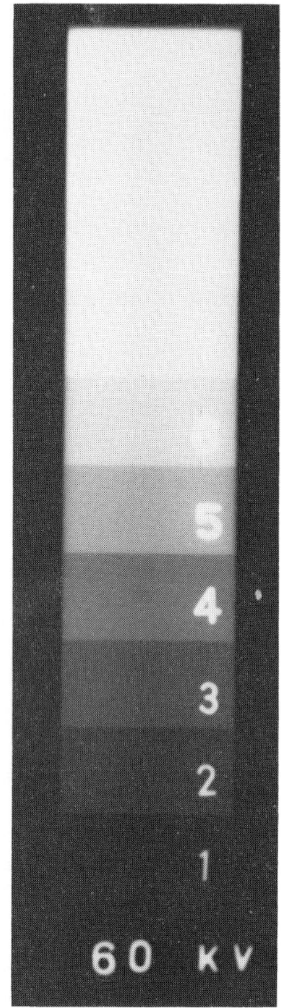

**FIGURE 15–2.** Sample strip to be used for creating a characteristic curve.

radiographer to know the actual amount of exposure. Relative exposure is a more general term used to represent the milliampereseconds (mAs) or amount of photons exposing the film. In day to day work, radiographers use mAs as a relative measurement. To double the density on the film, one can double the mAs. However, the actual amount of exposure or number of photons striking the film is not known. What is important is the relationship between the two exposures. Relative exposure can easily be used in plotting information because the important idea is to know the relationship between the exposures to be plotted on the graph.

The use of logarithms to describe relative exposure and density is very efficient because a broad range of numbers can be represented by a few small numbers.

*Base plus fog* is a key factor in sensitometry. An unexposed processed film will not transmit 100% of light exposing the film. The base of the film will have a small inherent amount of opaqueness or density. In addition, a small amount of fog from the manufacturing process may be present in the emulsion. The total amount of density found to be inher-

ent in the x-ray film before exposure to x-rays or light is called "base plus fog." The amount of base plus fog is obtained by measurement of the so-called "clear" areas on the film. Base plus fog should not exceed a density reading of 0.25. The range for base plus fog is approximately 0.18 to 0.23.

The maximum density present is represented at the highest point on the curve, which is the shoulder region. The maximum density reading is called the $D_{max}$. The minimum density level present is shown in the toe region and is called the $D_{min}$. The $D_{min}$ is recognized as the first measurement made above the base plus fog (Fig. 15–3).

---

$D_{max}$ REPRESENTS THE MAXIMUM DENSITY READING, AND $D_{min}$ REPRESENTS THE MINIMUM DENSITY READING.

---

The *toe* portion of the curve begins in the lower left region and represents an area of underexposure on the film. The toe begins at the vertical axis with the base plus fog measurement, as shown in Figure 15–3. The line moves to the right to a point where density begins to increase. Most of the area identified as the toe region provides little information for the radiographer because the amount of density is too small for information to be evaluated by the human eye.

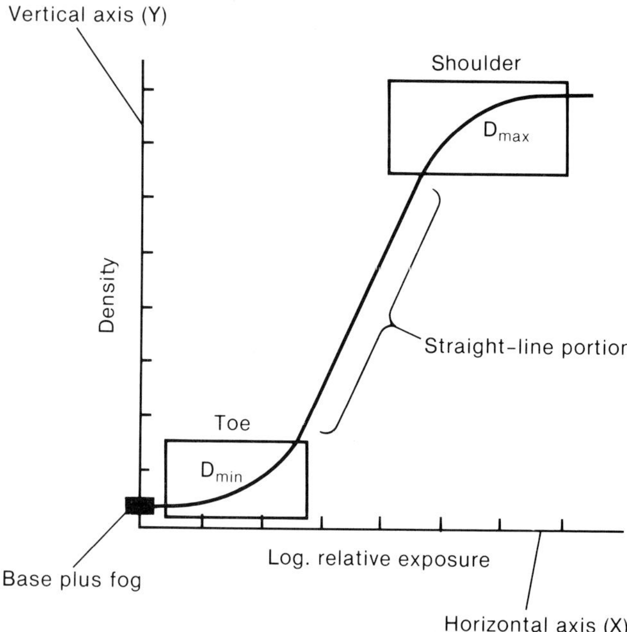


**FIGURE 15–3.** Characteristic curve illustrating the toe, straight-line portion, and shoulder. The $D_{min}$ is represented by the toe region, and the $D_{max}$ is represented by the shoulder region.

The *shoulder* portion is the upper right region of the curve. The shoulder identifies the maximum density levels on the film and represents an area of overexposure. The density levels are so great that the human eye is unable to differentiate between the density readings. Contrast is minimum in the shoulder and toe region, therefore making almost no detail visible.

The shoulder portion of the curve peaks and becomes more parallel with the horizontal axis. This represents the maximum exposure to the film. After all of the silver crystals in the film emulsion have been exposed, no matter how much the exposure increases, the density will not increase.

The *straight-line portion* of the curve is normally to the right and lies between the toe and the shoulder. The straight-line portion of the curve is the most important area for measurement. The slanted straight line represents the increase in density as the relative exposure increases. The slope of the straight-line portion will vary with changes in exposure conditions such as exposure factors, processing, and film-screen systems. As the increase occurs, it forms a straight line; this is known as a linear response. The straight-line portion begins at the level of approximately 0.4 density above base fog and reaches to about 2.5 above base fog.

---

## THE STRAIGHT-LINE PORTION IS THE MOST IMPORTANT AREA FOR EVALUATING THE FILM'S PHOTOCHARACTERISTICS.

---

The maximum slope of the curve is known as the *film gamma*. It is measured at the steepest point on the straight line portion. Gamma is used to measure the *gradient*. Gradient is the slope at any point on the curve and represents the contrast of a film at a specific density level. An x-ray film that has been exposed with the use of intensifying screens has an average film gamma of 2.0 to 3.5. The gamma is seldom used in radiography because the portion of the curve to be included for the calculation is too short and does not reflect the overall sensitivity of the film.

The better method for evaluating the slope of the straight-line portion is to use the portion of the curve between the density levels of 0.25 and 2.0 above the base plus fog. The slope of the straight-line portion between 0.25 and 2.0 is called the *average gradient*. The average gradient is a measure of contrast. In general, as the straight-line portion becomes more vertical, contrast will be enhanced or increased. As the straight-line portion becomes more horizontal, the contrast will decrease.

---

## THE AVERAGE GRADIENT IS EVALUATED BETWEEN THE DENSITY LEVELS OF 0.25 AND 2.0. THE AVERAGE GRADIENT IS A MEASURE OF CONTRAST ON THE FILM.

---

The average gradient is measured from the density levels 0.25 to 2.0 above the base plus fog. Figure 15–4 shows the points of reference for calculating the average gradient.

The average gradient is calculated with consideration given to the amount of base plus fog that is inherent in the film. Once the base plus fog is measured, the amount is always added to the reference points of 0.25 and 2.0.

Base plus fog = 0.18
    Add to 0.25         0.25 + 0.18 = 0.43
    Add to 2.00         2.00 + 0.18 = 2.18

Average gradient is measured with reference points of 0.43 to 2.18

      2.18 is the higher density, or $D_2$
      0.43 is the lower density, or $D_1$

To calculate the average gradient, use the formula:

$$\text{Average gradient} = \frac{D_2 - D_1}{\text{Log exposure}_{E_2} - \text{Log exposure}_{E_1}}$$

$D_2$ represents the upper density reference point, as shown in Figure 15–4, and $D_1$ represents the lower density reference point. $D_2 - D_1$ will always be 1.75. As shown in Figure 15–5, log exposure $E_1$ and log exposure $E_2$ represent the corresponding points on the graph for relative exposure.

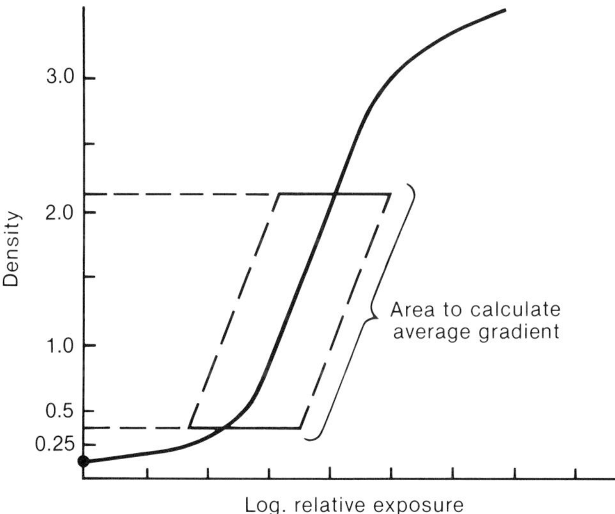


**FIGURE 15–4.** The average gradient is calculated between the density levels of 0.25 and 2.0 above the base plus fog.

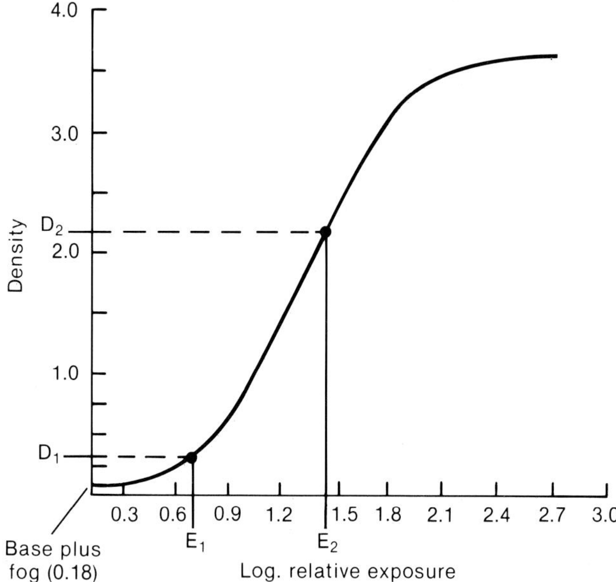

$$\text{Average gradient} = \frac{2.18 - 0.43}{1.40 - 0.70} = \frac{1.75}{0.70} = 2.5$$

**FIGURE 15–5.** The average gradient is calculated between 0.25 and 2.0 above the base plus fog. As illustrated here, the base plus fog is 0.18. The average gradient is measured at 0.43 and 2.18, to equal 2.5.

The average gradient represents contrast. As the average gradient increases, contrast will increase, and as the average gradient decreases, the contrast will also decrease.

---

AS THE AVERAGE GRADIENT INCREASES, THE CONTRAST WILL INCREASE. AS THE AVERAGE GRADIENT DECREASES, THE CONTRAST WILL DECREASE.

---

## LOGARITHMS IN SENSITOMETRY

The use of logarithms has become a very important component in the sensitometric process for the preparation and evaluation of a characteristic curve. The term "logarithm" is derived from the Greek words *logos*, which means proportion, and *arithmos*, which means number. The term *logarithm* means proportional number.

It is not necessary for radiographers to have extensive knowledge of logarithms, but some understanding is required.

On a logarithmic scale, two exposures with a ratio that is always constant can be separated by the same distance on the relative exposure or horizontal axis. For example, if each number in a sequence of

**TABLE 15–1.** THE LOGARITHMIC SCALE

| Number Sequence | 2 | 4 | 8 | 16 | 32 | 64 |
|---|---|---|---|---|---|---|
| Log Scale | 0.3 | 0.6 | 0.9 | 1.2 | 1.5 | 1.8 |

numbers represents twice the amount as the preceding number, this sequence of numbers can be separated by the same distance on the logarithmic scale, as shown in Table 15–1. In sensitometry, density and relative exposure are represented by the use of logarithms.

The logarithm to the base 10 is derived from the number 10 multiplied by itself a number of times or raised to a certain power. Table 15–2 shows that the logarithm of 10 is 1, the logarithm of 100 is 2, and the logarithm of 1000 is 3. The smaller number can be used to represent the big number. Any number between 10 and 100 can be written as 1.xxx to 2.000. For example, 20 would be 1.300. Any real number between 100 and 1000 can be written as 2.xxx to 3.xxx.

Multiplication and division are simplified by using logarithms. For example, Table 15–2 states that the logarithm of 2 is 0.3. If the logarithm 0.3 is added to a number, the sum is the same as multiplying by two. See Table 15–1 to review this principle for using logarithms to represent a sequence of numbers.

---

IF THE LOG 0.3 IS ADDED TO A NUMBER, THE SUM IS THE SAME AS MULTIPLYING BY TWO.

---

EXAMPLE:

From Figure 15–6, the third point on the horizontal axis is log 0.6. The fourth point is 0.9. Adding log 0.3 to 0.6 yields a sum of 0.9; 0.9 represents doubling of the value at 0.6.

Any two numbers on the relative exposure scale where one number is twice the amount of the other can be separated by 0.3 on the scale. Even though the actual value for exposure is not known, the

**TABLE 15–2.** LOGARITHM BASE 10

| | | |
|---|---|---|
| 10 × 1 = 10 | logarithm is 1 | 1 is log of 10 |
| 10 × 10 = 100 | logarithm is 2 | 2 is log of 100 |
| 10 × 100 = 1000 | logarithm is 3 | 3 is log of 1000 |

*Note:* In sensitometry, it is important to know that the logarithm of 2 is 0.3.

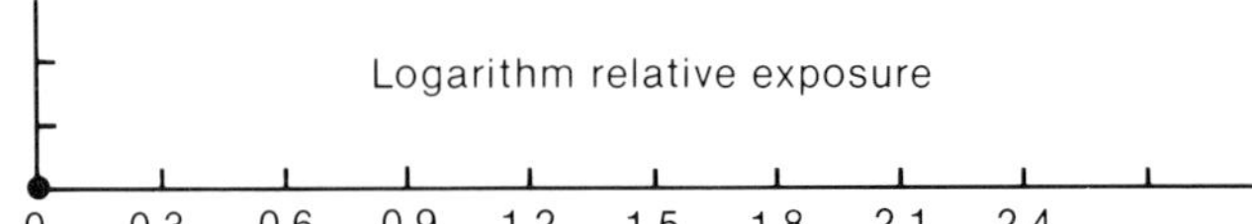



**FIGURE 15–6.** Sequence of logarithms to be marked on the horizontal (X) axis.

logarithmic scale can be used to describe the relationship between each exposure level. To plot log relative exposure for preparing a characteristic curve, one can use Figure 15–6 as an example.

## PREPARATION OF THE CHARACTERISTIC CURVE

Characteristic curves used for evaluating different exposures can be prepared by using a calibrated step-wedge penetrometer (Fig. 15–7). The step-wedge penetrometer is designed in such a way that each step is exactly twice the absorption thickness of the preceding step. In Figure 15–7, for example, step 4 is double the absorption value of step 3. The relative exposure received by the film at step 3 is double the amount received at step 4.

To make the exposure, one uses a standard x-ray film with intensifying screens. The penetrometer is centered over the cassette with the beam restricted to approximately 0.5 inch around the object. The exposure is made using 70 to 75 kilovoltage peak (kVp). After the film is processed, a calibrated densitometer is used to measure base plus fog and each step represented by the image of the penetrometer (Fig. 15–8).

Figure 15–9 demonstrates the corresponding values for plotting on the graph. The step with the least amount of density is marked as corresponding to the level of 0.3 relative exposure. The next step or density level is marked at the point corresponding

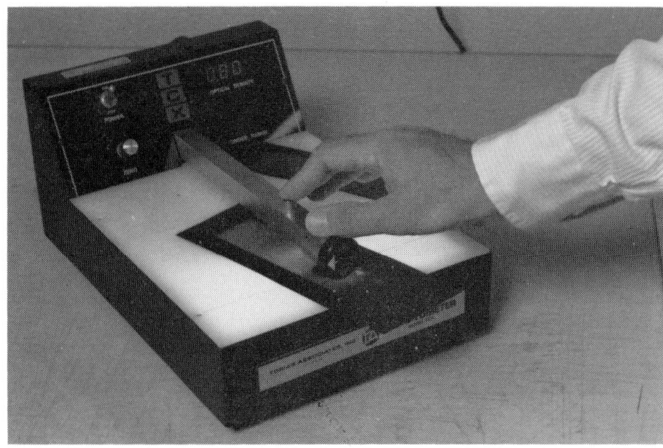

**FIGURE 15–8.** Measuring density levels on the sensitometric strip.

to 0.6, etc. Once the points are marked on the graph, a line is drawn to connect the points. The line should represent a slanted S-shaped curve.

## SENSITOMETER

The sensitometer is a special piece of equipment designed to expose x-ray film with a calibrated amount of light. It can be used as an alternative to the penetrometer. The sensitometer is designed to eliminate any possible variations or fluctuations that may occur with the use of x-ray generators. The finished radiograph resembles the image produced by exposing a penetrometer. Each step or level of density is measured and plotted on a graph in just the same way as described above. The sensitometer is recommended for exposing strips for daily evaluations of the processing system. Figure 15–10 is a photograph of a sensitometer.

## LIGHT TRANSMISSION

To further evaluate the usefulness of the characteristic curve, one must review the relationship of density to the transmission of light through the finished radiograph. It is obvious that greater density levels or blackening will decrease the amount of light that can be transmitted through the radiograph. The higher the density reading, the lower the light transmission. Increased exposure to the film will also reduce the percent of light transmission. Table 15–3 represents this principle.

Ideally, with zero or no exposure to the film, 100% of the light should be transmitted because the film would be clear. However, x-ray film has an inherent base plus fog density level. At a base plus fog reading of 0.2, approximately 80% of the light will be transmitted through the film. Table 15–3 dem-

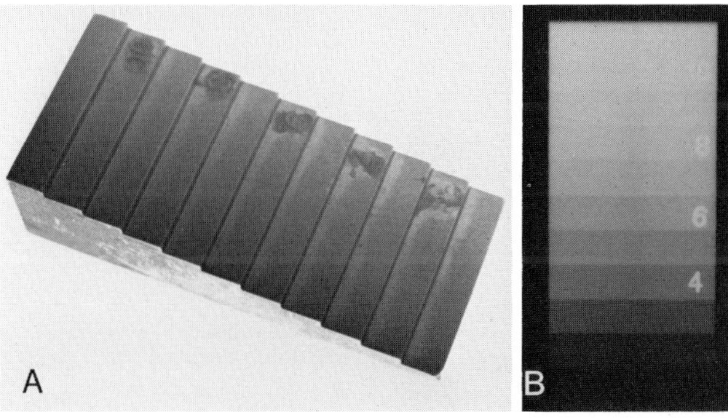



**FIGURE 15–7.** Step-wedge penetrometer can be used to produce sensitometric strips. *A,* Penetrometer. *B,* Radiograph produced using the penetrometer.

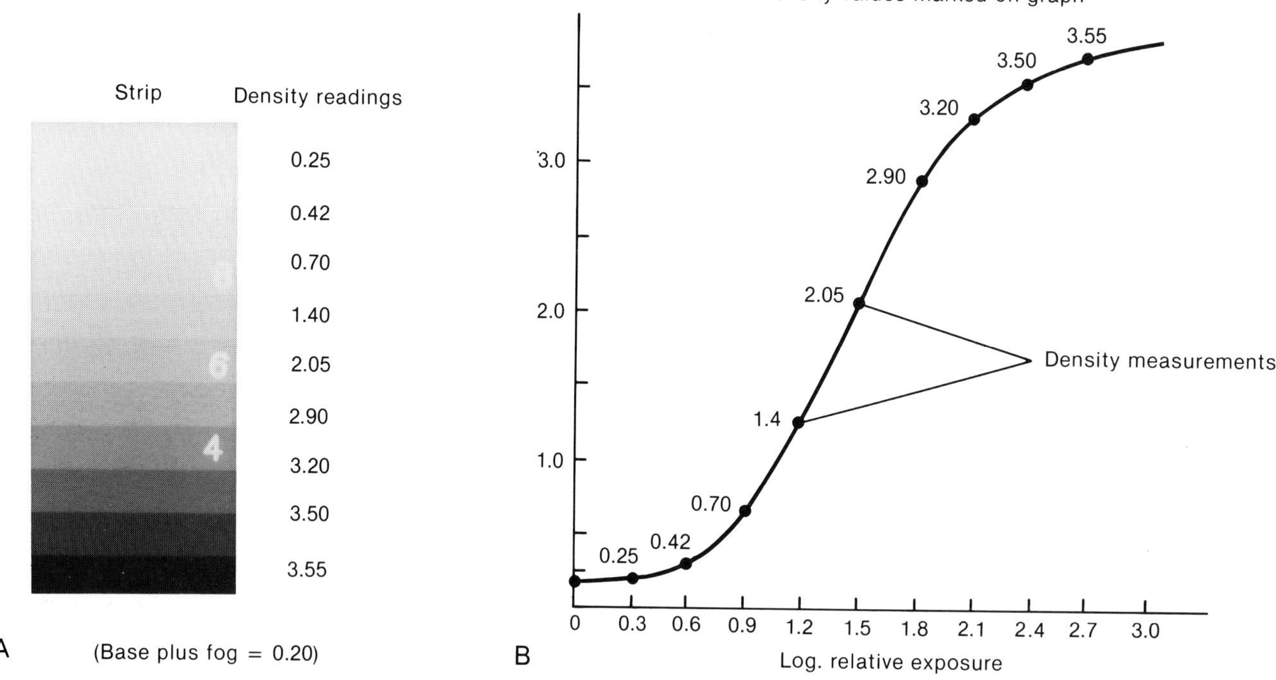



**FIGURE 15–9.** To plot a characteristic curve, one must measure each step of the sensitometric strip using a densitometer. *A,* A strip with the density readings. *B,* Density readings plotted using a graph to produce a characteristic curve.

onstrates how doubling of the amount of exposure to the film will reduce the light transmission by 50%, or one half.

## EVALUATION OF CONTRAST

Radiographic contrast is the difference in density levels of adjacent structures. It is the product of film and subject contrast as well as processing conditions. Sensitometrically, contrast is described by the average gradient or slope of the straight-line portion of the curve.

Film gamma, gradient, and average gradient are measurements used to describe contrast. Average gradient is the term most suitable to the evaluation of radiographic films because contrast is measured within the optical density range of 0.25 to 2.0 above the base plus fog density.

EXAMPLE:

The evaluation of contrast:

Calculate average gradient:

| | |
|---|---|
| Base plus fog | $= 0.20$ |
| $D_2$ — higher density | $= 0.20 + 2.00 = 2.20$ |
| $D_1$ — lower density | $= 0.20 + 0.25 = 0.45$ |
| Log relative exposure at $D_2$ $(E_2)$ | $= 1.50$ |
| Log relative exposure at $D_1$ $(E_1)$ | $= 0.80$ |

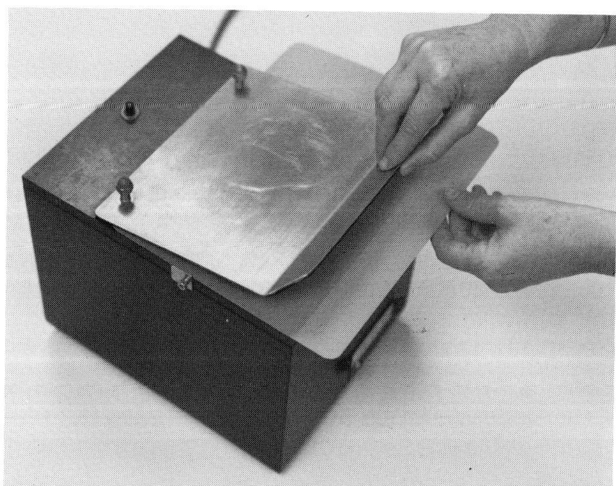

**FIGURE 15–10.** The sensitometer used to produce a sensitometric strip.

**TABLE 15–3.** RELATIONSHIP OF DENSITY TO LIGHT TRANSMISSION

| Density (log) | Light Transmission (percent) |
|---|---|
| 0.0 | 100% |
| 0.2 | 80% |
| 0.3 | 50% |
| 0.6 | 25% |
| 0.9 | 12.5% |
| 1.2 | 6.2% |
| 1.5 | 3.1% |
| 1.8 | 1.5% |

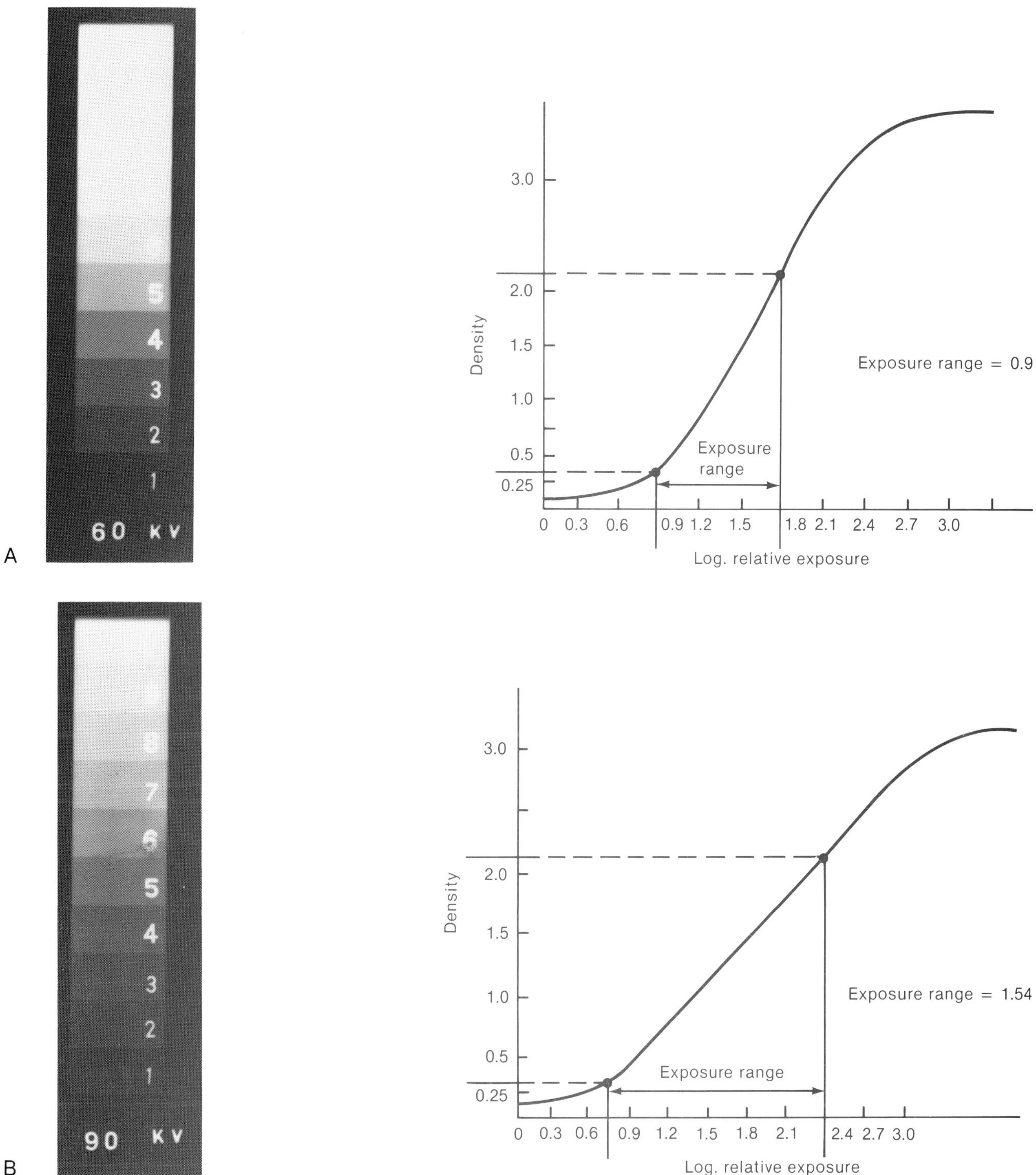



**FIGURE 15–11.** *A,* A sensitometric strip that represents a short scale of contrast. The density measurements have been plotted to produce a characteristic curve. *B,* A radiograph representing a longer scale of contrast. The density measurements have been plotted to produce a characteristic curve. Exposure latitude can be evaluated by comparing the relative exposure range for each curve. The exposure range is 0.9 for film A and 1.54 for film B. Because film B has a broader exposure range, exposure latitude is greater. Radiographs with greater exposure latitude also have a longer scale of contrast.

Formula:

$$\text{Average gradient} = \frac{D_2 - D_1}{\text{Log exp } E_2 - \text{Log exp } E_1}$$

$$\frac{2.20 - 0.45}{1.50 - 0.80} = \frac{1.75}{0.70} = 2.5$$

$$\text{Average gradient} = 2.5$$

If the average gradient is more than 1, contrast will be enhanced or increased. As the average gradient increases, contrast will also increase and the scale of contrast will shorten.

---

AN AVERAGE GRADIENT OF 1 OR ABOVE WILL ENHANCE CONTRAST.

---

Figure 15–11 shows two radiographs with their corresponding characteristic curve. Figure 15–11*A* represents a short scale of contrast, and Figure 15–11*B* represents a long scale of contrast. The average gradient for film A is greater. The straight-line portion of the curve is more vertical than in film B. Film B has a lower average gradient, longer scale, and less contrast.

## LATITUDE

The definition of latitude is the range of exposure that will produce densities between 0.25 and 2.0 above the base plus fog density. Sensitometrically, latitude is determined by the range of a given exposure. For example, in Figure 15–11, film A has a relative exposure range of 0.9 to 1.8. Film B has a relative exposure range of 0.86 to 2.4. Film B has more latitude because the range is greater. The exposure range for film A is 0.9, and the range for film B is 1.54. As latitude increases, the scale of contrast will increase and contrast decreases.

---

AS LATITUDE OR THE RANGE OF RELATIVE EXPOSURE INCREASES, THE SCALE OF CONTRAST WILL LENGTHEN AND THE AMOUNT OF CONTRAST WILL DECREASE.

---

## FILM SPEED

Film speed describes the sensitivity of the film emulsion to exposure. Speed is defined as the rela-

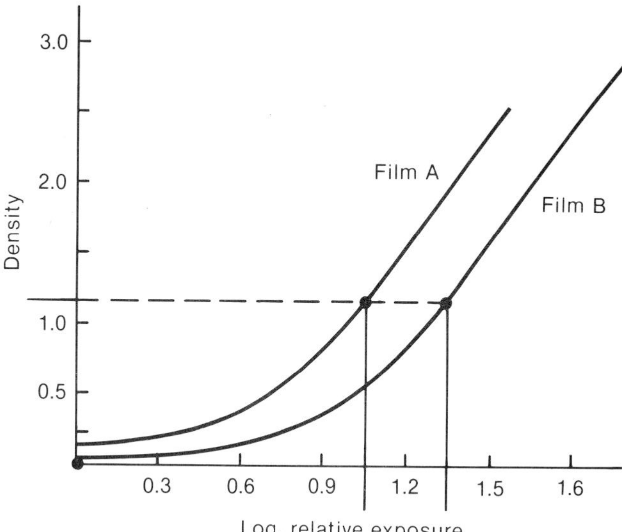


**FIGURE 15–12.** Film speed is evaluated at 1.0 above the base plus fog. Film A has a relative exposure value of 1.1, and film B has a relative exposure value of 1.4. Film A would be considered the faster film because it has the smaller relative exposure value.

tive exposure needed to produce a density of 1.0 plus the base plus fog. Film speed is evaluated on the characteristic curve at the density level of 1.0.

In Figure 15–12, film A has a log relative exposure of 1.1, and film B has a log relative exposure of 1.4. Film A has a relative exposure of 0.3 less than film B; therefore, film A is the faster film because less exposure is required to produce the same density as film B. When one compares two or more film curves, the curve nearest the vertical axis or to the left (at density level of 1.0) will be the fastest film.

---

WHEN ONE COMPARES TWO OR MORE CURVES, THE CURVE NEAREST THE VERTICAL AXIS AT THE DENSITY LEVEL OF 1.0 WILL BE THE FASTEST EXPOSURE.

---

## PROCESSING SYSTEM

The sensitometric characteristics used to evaluate the characteristic curve can be very useful in daily assessment of the processing system in the department. The sensitometer is the best instrument to use for preparing curves for automatic processing monitoring. The slope of the curve may be influenced by aging chemicals, poor replenishment rates, etc., resulting in a decrease in contrast and speed.

# Critique of the Radiographic Image

## CHAPTER OBJECTIVES

1. Describe the radiographer's role in assessment of the image.
2. Explain the process for evaluating radiographs for adequate density, contrast, and scale of contrast.
3. Describe what is meant by the phrase "moderate scale of contrast."
4. Explain how the radiographer determines if adequate penetration is present along with subject contrast.
5. List the parameters for evaluating visibility of detail on radiographs.
6. Describe how the degree of image distortion may be evaluated.
7. Explain possible causes for image distortion.
8. Describe the method for assessment of beam restriction.
9. Describe the purpose of making radiographs.
10. Identify common radiographic artifacts and give their cause.

## KEY WORDS AND TERMS

Critique

Criteria for assessment

Moderate contrast scale

Evidence of beam restriction

Marker

Radiographic artifacts

Handling artifacts

Artifacts from the patient

## RECOMMENDATIONS FOR GENERAL DISCUSSION QUESTIONS

1. Prepare a document for new students entering the radiology department that describes how a radiograph should be assessed for its technical quality.
2. Describe how a radiographer can assure patients that high-quality radiographs with good radiation protection have been accomplished.
3. Prepare a procedure guide for the darkroom personnel to eliminate handling artifacts.

To this point, this text has presented basic concepts for producing high-quality radiographs. One of the most important aspects for the radiographer is to be able to visually inspect the image and make an assessment of quality. This skill permits the image to be inspected and judged for its merits or weaknesses. The goal is to produce high-quality radiographs. However, conditions do not always present themselves with an environment that results in the "perfect" image. Radiographers must be skilled in using judgment for the evaluation of radiographs.

To critique the image, radiographers should be able to assess density, contrast, and the overall image definition to include recorded detail and visibility of detail (Table 16–1). The position of the tube, film, and part of interest must be assessed along with the selection of appropriate accessories. Evidence of beam restriction must also be evaluated. Artifacts must be identified and the cause eliminated. Finally, film identification markers must be visible.

**TABLE 16–1.** MEDICAL IMAGING DEPARTMENT

**Image Critique Checklist**

| Image Characteristics | Excellent | Accept | Needs to Improve |
|---|---|---|---|
| 1.  Density | | | |
| 2.  Contrast | | | |
| 3.  Recorded detail | | | |
| 4.  Visibility of detail | | | |
| 5.  Position of tube | | | |
| 6.  Position of part | | | |
| 7.  Position of cassette | | | |
| 8.  Beam restriction | | | |
| **Other Factors** | | | |
| 9.  Grid selection | | | |
| 10.  Film-screen system | | | |

Artifacts: If present, give origin and corrective action to be taken.

_______________________________________________

Comments: ______________________________________

_______________________________________________

Radiographer: ___________________________ Date: _______

## DENSITY

In Figure 16–1, three radiographs with different density levels are shown. Film A has the proper density levels to make contrast visible. Film B has too much density, which is the result of overexposure. Film C has too little density, or underexposure. Adequate density is present when the object of interest is visible. It should not be obscured by too much or too little blackening on the film. Density is the result of exposure to the silver halide crystals in the film emulsion, and it is controlled by the milliampereseconds (mAs) selection.

## CONTRAST

Radiographic contrast results from the combination of film contrast and subject contrast. Careful

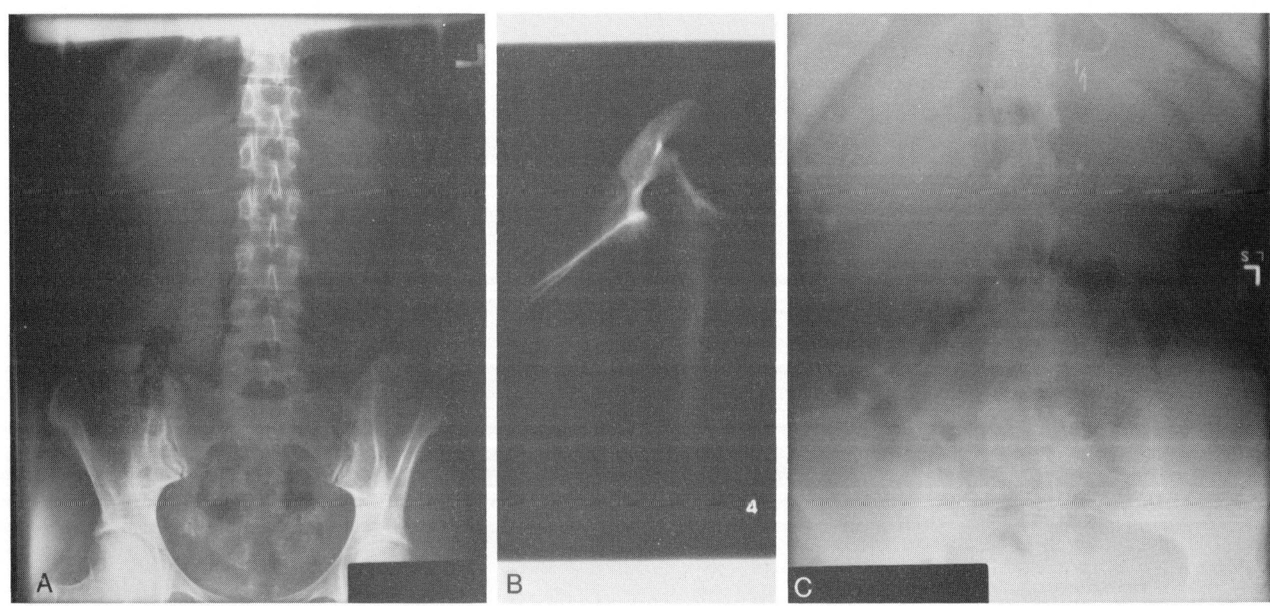

**FIGURE 16–1.** Radiographs demonstrating different amounts of density. *A,* A radiograph with good density. *B* demonstrates too much density, and *C* represents too little density.

examination of the radiograph and the part of interest should reveal tissue or skeletal markings. The density differences of the adjacent structures should be sufficient to reveal borders. Contrast makes detail visible. Contrast may be exhibited as a long range of gray tones (long scale of contrast) or a short range of mostly black and white areas (short scale of contrast). Ideally, a moderate scale of contrast, as shown in Figure 16–2, would be achieved.

A scale of contrast that is extremely short or long may exhibit areas of underexposure or overexposure, as shown in Figure 16–3. Tissue or subject contrast would not be adequate, and the detail of the image will not be visible. A scale of contrast that is too long, as shown in Figure 16–3, will exhibit numerous gray tones and decrease the subject contrast. The skilled eye of the radiographer must be able to assess the image and determine that contrast is adequate to make detail visible.

## DEFINITION AND VISIBILITY OF DETAIL

The process of judging a radiograph will include an inspection of the edges of the object(s). For example, radiographs of the skeleton must exhibit images of bones that are well defined. Contrast must be adequate to demonstrate the tiny markings that make up the cancellous bone tissue, compact bone, etc. As described in Chapter 11, the geometric factors (focal spot, focal-film distance [FFD], and object-film distance [OFD]) play a primary role in producing a well-defined image.

Producing an image with good definition may be very straightforward. However, allowing for maximum visibility of the image detail provides the radiographer with a greater challenge.

To examine a radiograph for visibility of detail, one must use the following questions as a guide:

1. Is the amount of blackening on the film at the proper level? too much? or too little? Was the appropriate mAs selected?
2. Is sufficient contrast present? Can tissue markings be seen? Was the appropriate kilovoltage peak (kVp) selection made to adequately penetrate the part?
3. Is the amount of scatter acceptable? Is there too much scatter present? Was the grid that was used adequate for cleanup of the scatter? Is a border for the beam restrictor visible? Was it adequate for reducing scatter?
4. Was the best possible selection of a film-screen combination used?

The ability to answer "yes" to each question should be the measure for assuring that excellent visibility of detail has been achieved.

## TUBE, FILM, AND PART ALIGNMENT

The radiographer must now examine the image to assess distortion. How much magnification and shape distortion is present that may interfere with the evaluation of the image?

If the correct FFD and tube alignment were achieved, minimum distortion would be present. The normal anatomic shape and size should be compared with the image present on the radiograph. Poor alignment or placement of the cassette and/or the part of interest will result in shape distortion. Evaluate the image for magnification, elongation, and foreshortening (Fig. 16–4).

## EVIDENCE OF BEAM RESTRICTION

Careful examination of the image should show a border indicating the field size of the x-ray beam. Good radiation safety practices will be evident when the outline of the primary x-ray beam can be identified. For extremities, the primary x-ray beam should be limited to the actual size of the part to be

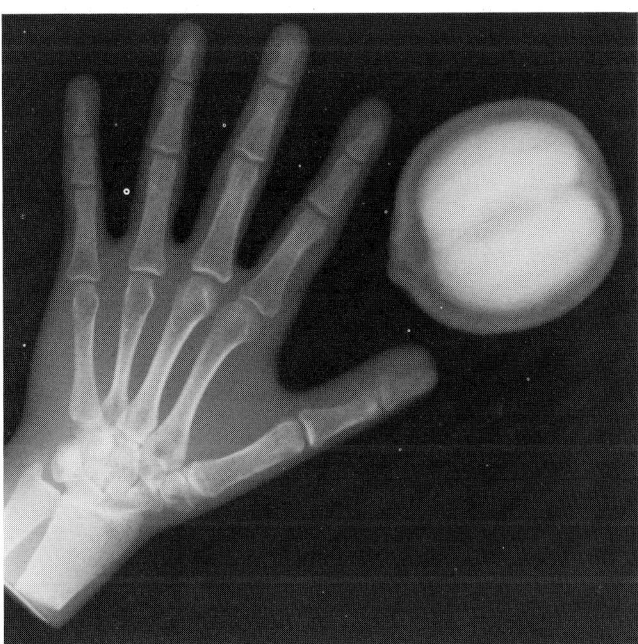

**FIGURE 16–2.** Radiograph with a moderate scale of contrast. The exposure was made using a hand phantom and an orange. The differences in subject contrast between the two objects are visible. The skeleton and soft tissue shadows are present in the hand. The peel and segments of the orange are also visible.

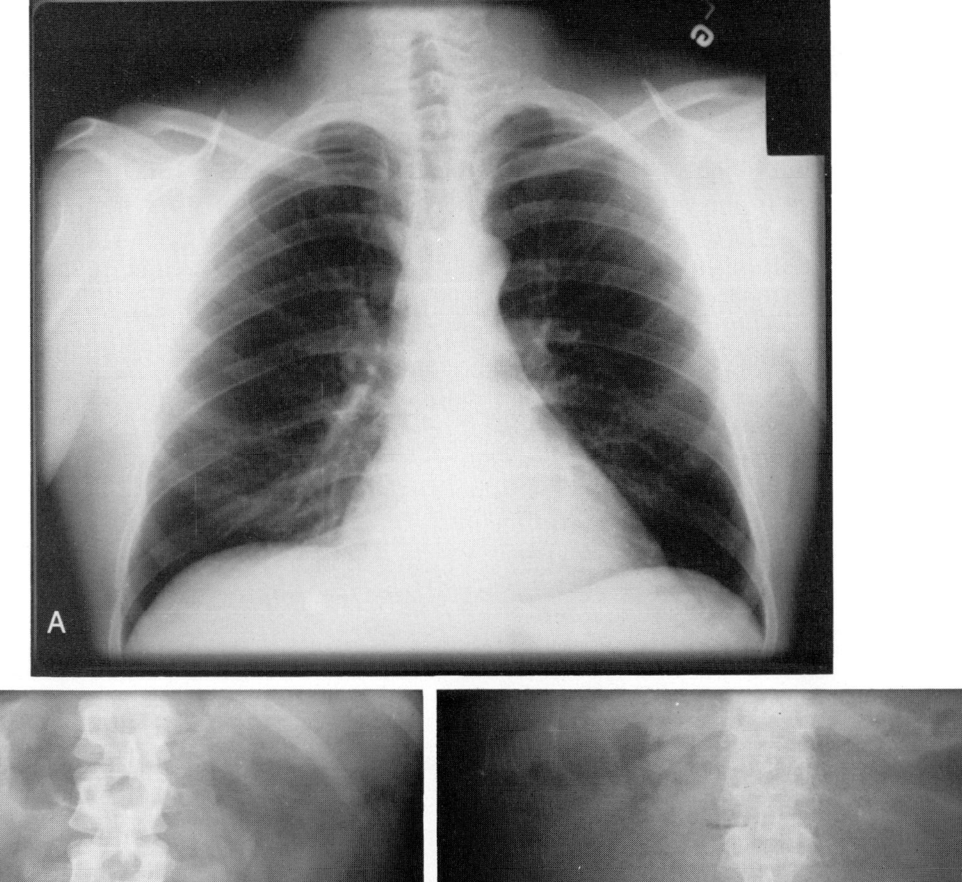

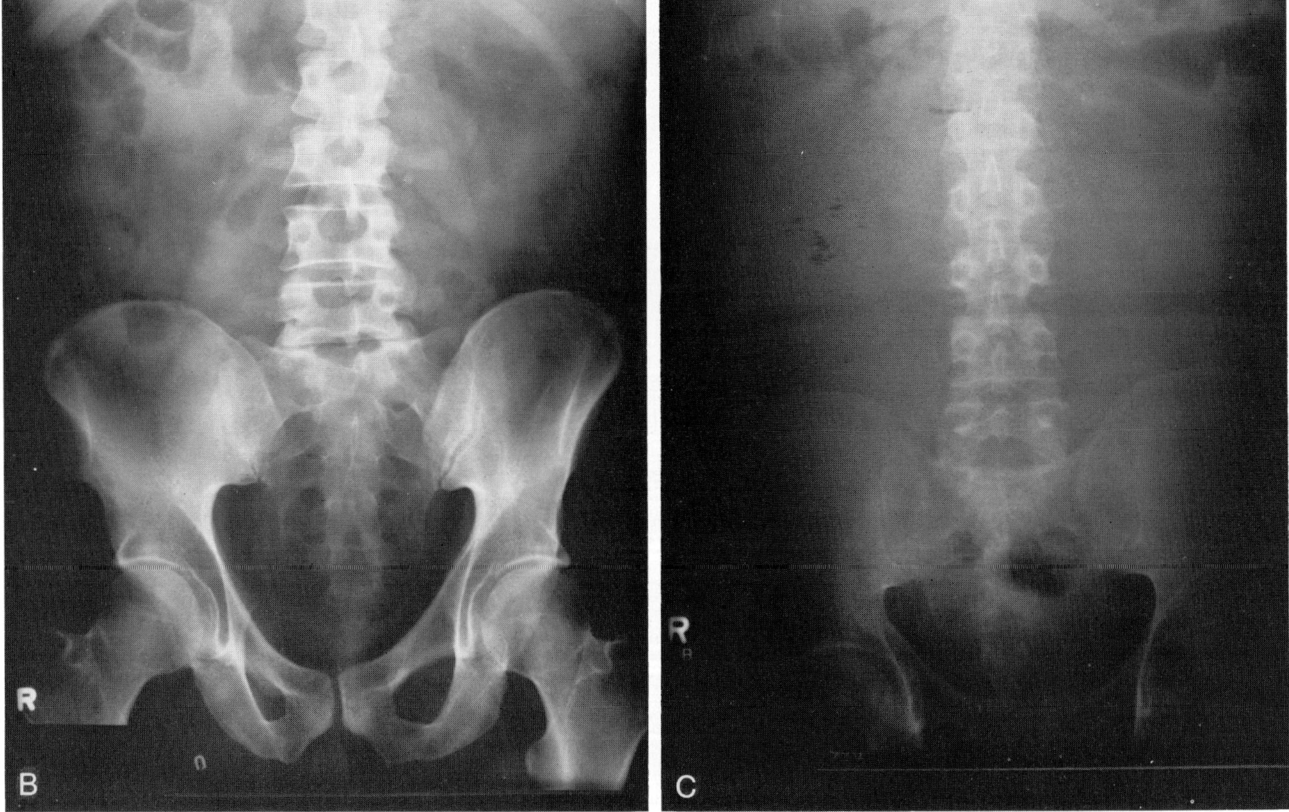

**FIGURE 16–3.** A good radiograph must have sufficient contrast to make detail visible. *A,* A radiograph of the chest with a shorter scale of contrast. *B,* A radiograph of the abdomen with a moderate scale of contrast. *C,* A radiograph with a longer scale of contrast.

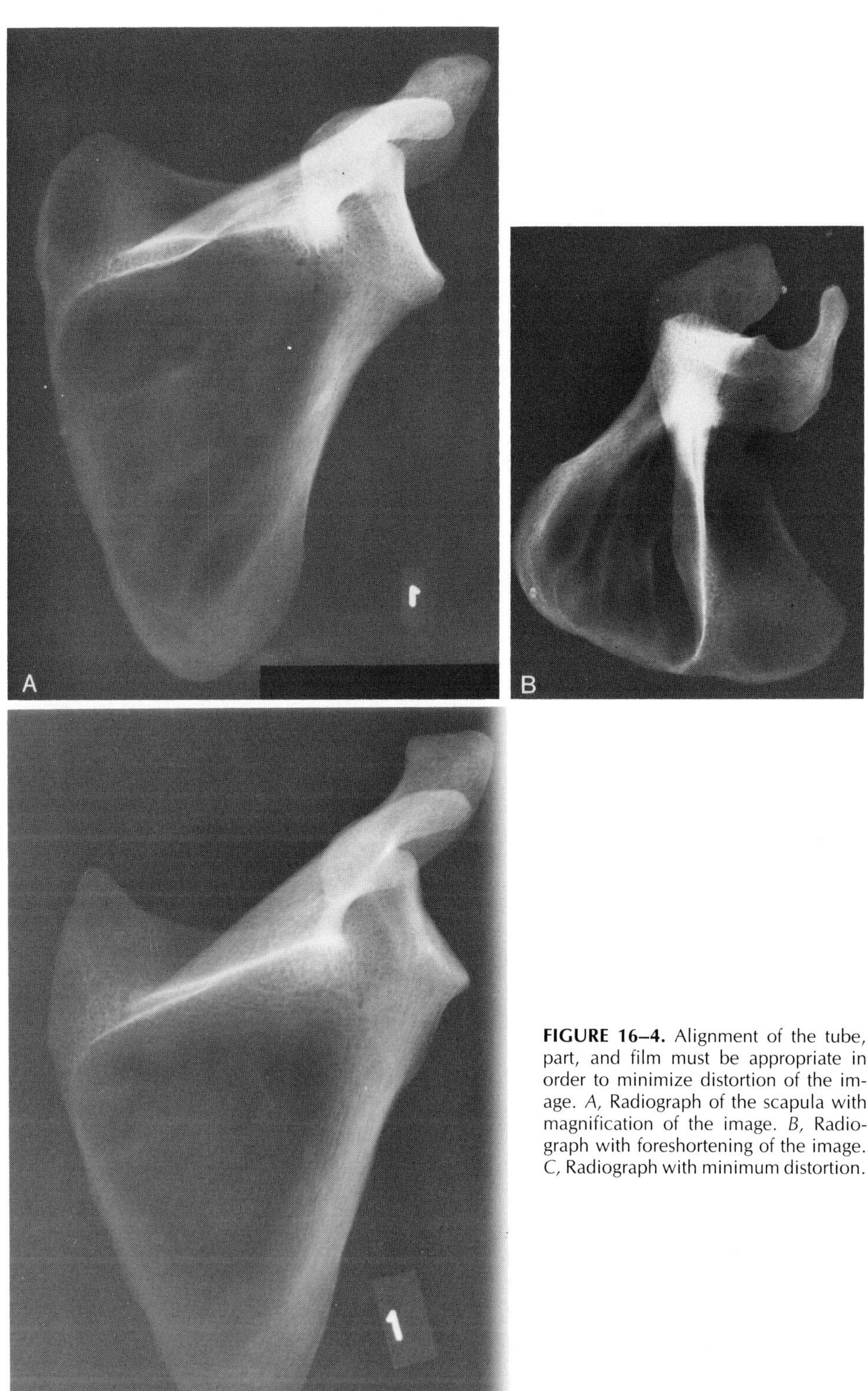

**FIGURE 16–4.** Alignment of the tube, part, and film must be appropriate in order to minimize distortion of the image. *A,* Radiograph of the scapula with magnification of the image. *B,* Radiograph with foreshortening of the image. *C,* Radiograph with minimum distortion.

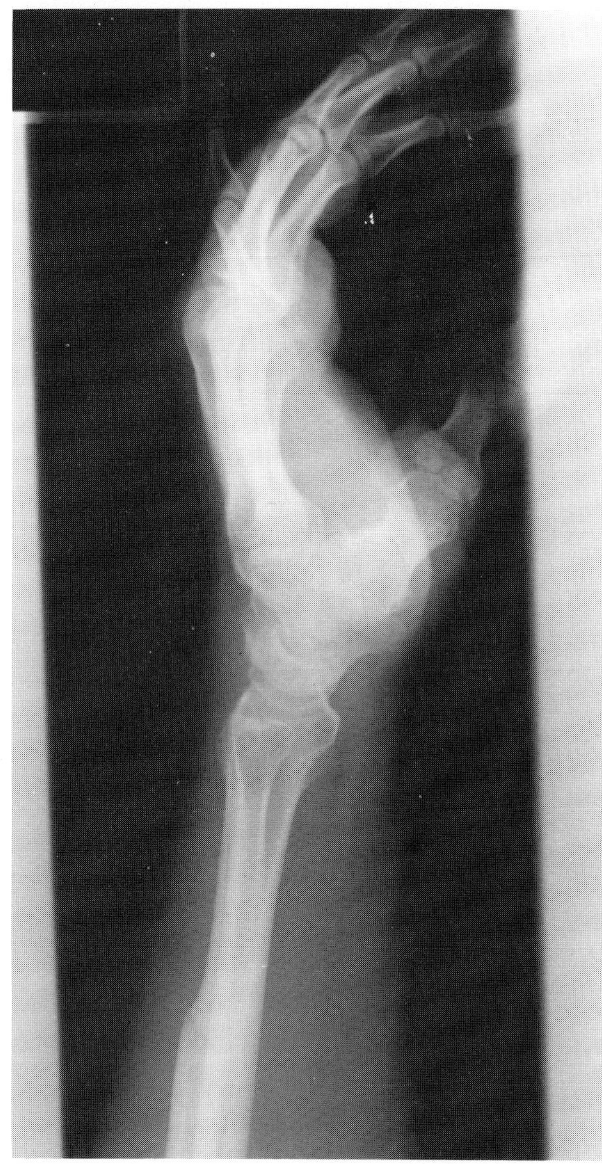

FIGURE 16–5. Evidence of beam restriction is shown here in an examination of the hand.

imaged as opposed to the film size, as demonstrated in Figure 16–5.

## MARKERS

It is not within the scope of this text to present the rules for the use of radiographic lead markers. Radiographers learn the guidelines along with positioning skills. In the critique of the radiographic image, it is important for the radiographer to acknowledge the presence and verify the placement of markers. Markers for right, left, upright, prone, etc., are important for assessing the quality of the image. The markers must be visible and must ad-

here to standards required by the department (Fig. 16–6).

## RADIOGRAPHIC ARTIFACTS

Radiography is not a perfect art and science. Artifacts may frequently interfere by obscuring parts of the image. An artifact is any extraneous agent that changes the character of an object. Radiographically, an artifact is unwanted or undesirable information that limits the interpretation of the image. Artifacts may have multiple or unlimited origins. Artifacts caused by processing conditions, patient preparation, and technical errors are more common.

### Film Handling Artifacts

It is extremely important for radiographers and darkroom personnel to be given clear instructions for handling x-ray film. The methods used for handling the film properly must be understood to prevent artifacts that obstruct the viewing of the image.

Static electricity artifacts, as shown in Figure 16–7, may be caused by moving or sliding the film and/or cassette across the surface of the darkroom cabinet work area or dropping the cassette on the floor. Static build-up is released, causing a spark that exposes the emulsion. Static electricity artifacts are more common in areas of dry climate.

Dirt and smudge marks, as shown in Figure 16–8, are a result of the film being dropped on a wet and dirty floor.

As described in Chapter 5, x-ray film must be handled carefully to prevent damage to the emulsion. Figure 16–9 demonstrates tiny "half-moon" marks caused by bending the film.

From time to time, cassettes and intensifying screens are the cause of artifacts. Figure 16–10 is an example of the result of dirty screens. Tiny white specks are present, caused by tiny dirt particles inside the cassette.

Figure 16–11 shows an artifact caused by a small piece of paper left inside the cassette during the exposure.

Figure 16–12 demonstrates light fog, resulting from improper placement of the film in the cassette. A small strip along the side remained outside to be exposed to light.

Figure 16–13 shows a radiographic artifact caused by the film being folded over when it was loaded in the cassette.

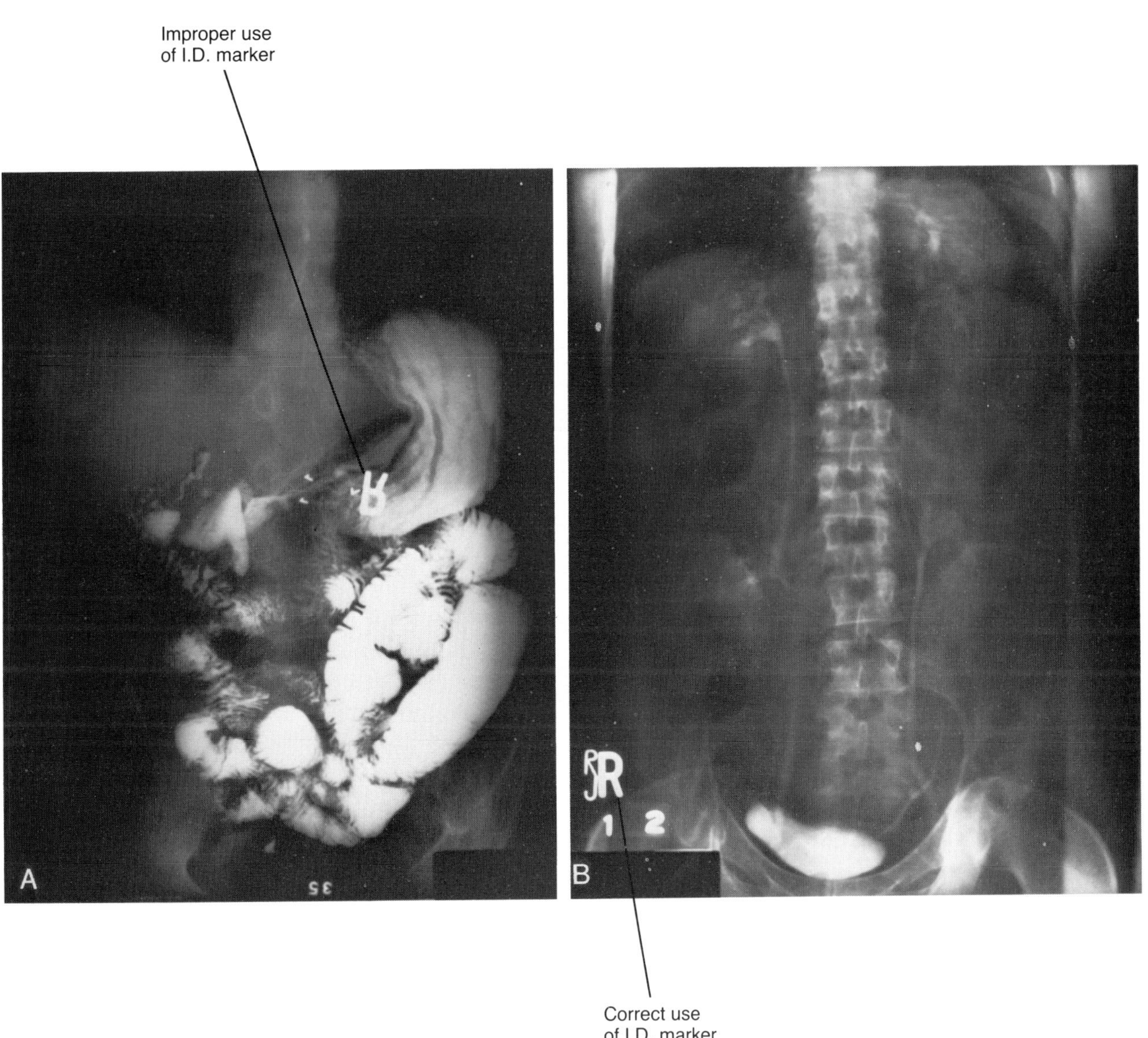


**FIGURE 16–6.** *A* demonstrates improper marker identification. *B* shows proper marker identification with an ''R'' marker, radiographer I.D., and minute marker. Markers must be placed to prevent superimposition over the anatomic parts of interest.

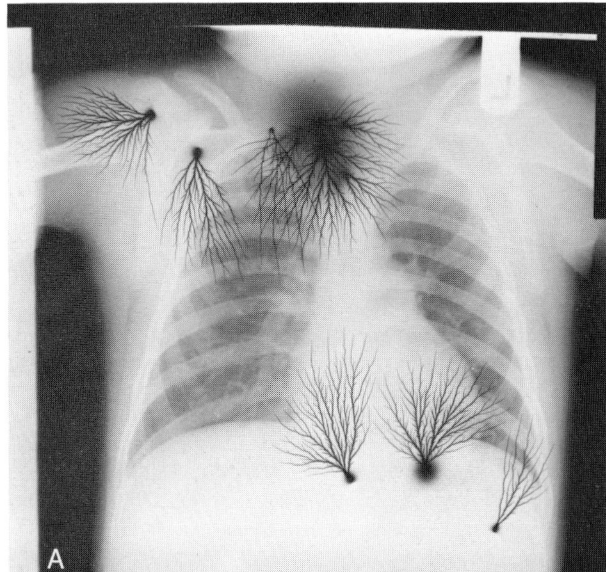

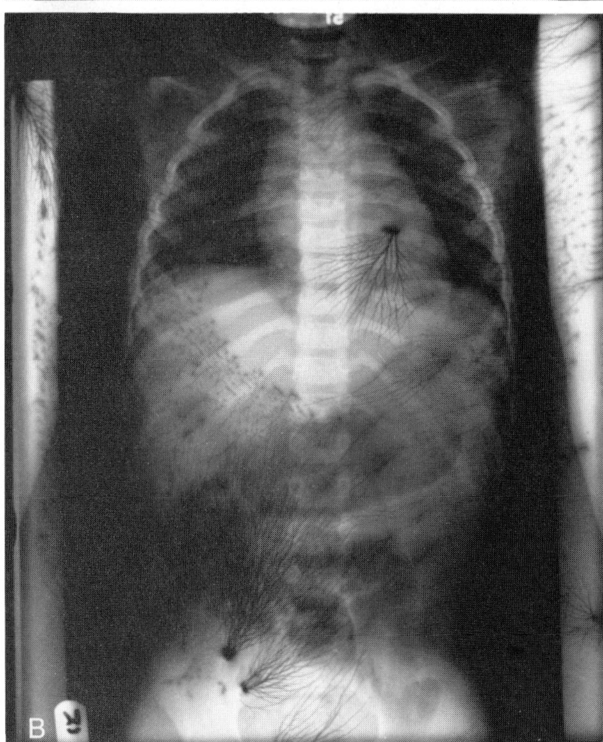

FIGURE 16–8. Artifacts produced by being dropped on an unclean surface before processing.

FIGURE 16–7. Static artifacts produced by improper handling of the film.

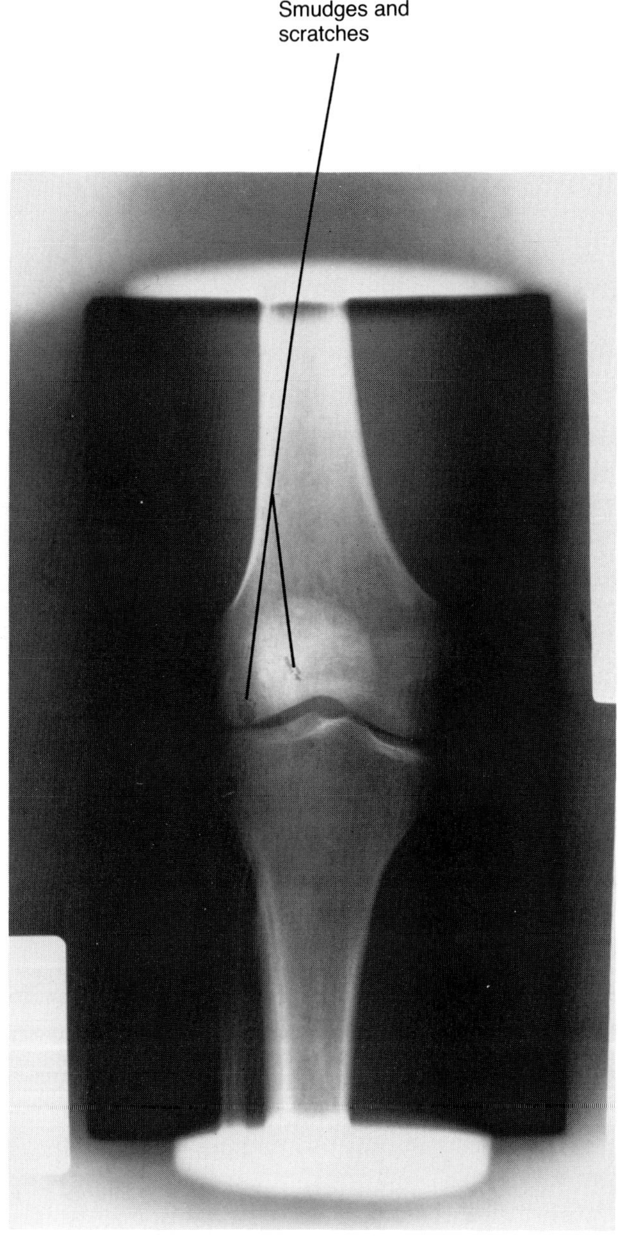

**FIGURE 16–9.** Artifacts that resemble ''half moons'' are present as a result of bending the film before processing.

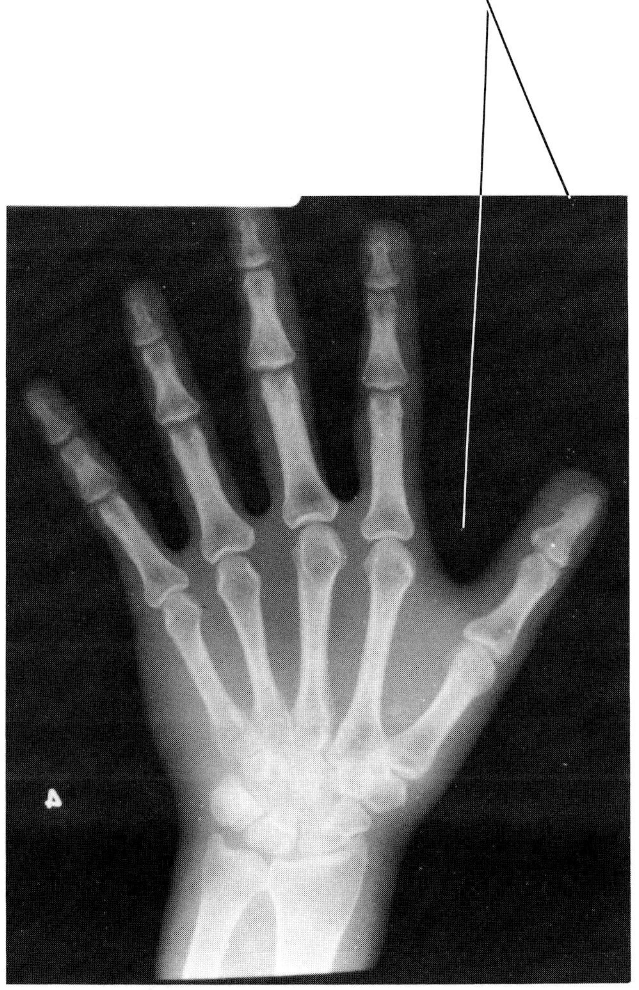



**FIGURE 16–10.** Dirty intensifying screens produce tiny white specks on the film.

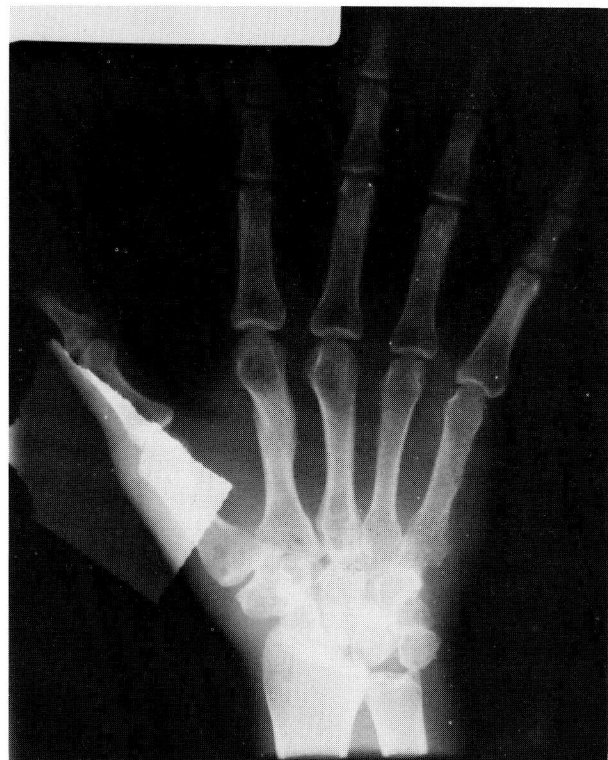

FIGURE 16–11. The radiograph shows an artifact resulting from a small piece of paper that was mistakenly placed in the cassette in the darkroom.

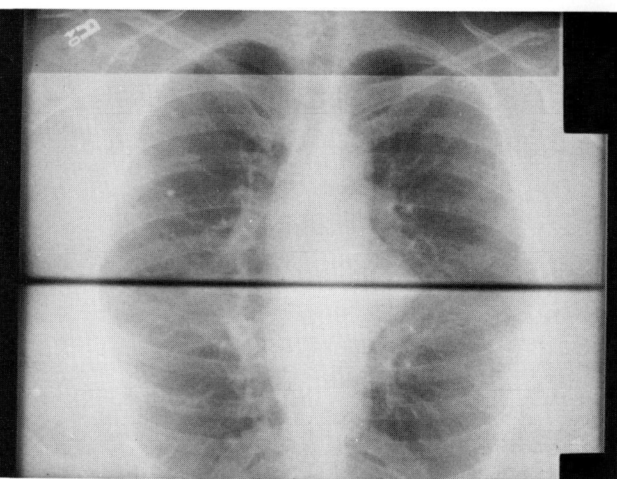

FIGURE 16–13. Carelessness in the darkroom produced this artifact. The film was folded in the cassette for the exposure.

Figure 16–14 is another example of light fog; in this instance, it resulted from opening the cassette in a lighted room.

## DARKROOM AND PROCESSING ARTIFACTS

The processor system may also be a common source for artifacts, especially when all components are not operating in unison. "Pi" lines and hesitation marks are artifacts caused by the transport system.

Pi lines are thin lines of increased density that occur at right angles to the film travel. These lines may occur just after a thorough cleaning of the rollers and the addition of fresh chemicals. Hesitation marks are also lines of increased density that may be present in a uniform pattern of lines that occur at right angles to the film travel. The hesita-

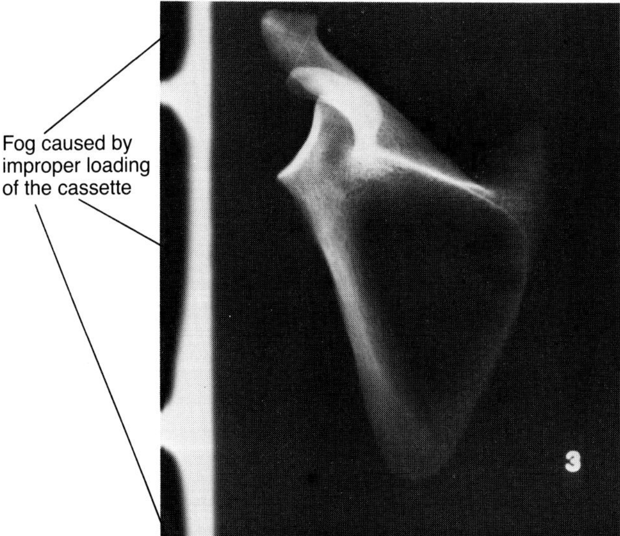


FIGURE 16–12. Fog on the edge of the film resulted from improper placement of the film in the cassette. The edge of the film was exposed to light even though the cassette was properly closed.

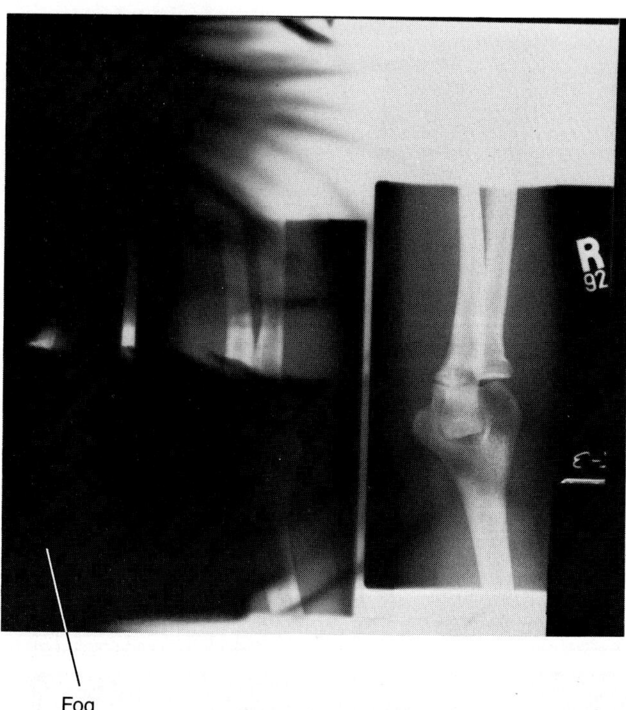


FIGURE 16–14. The cassette was opened in the darkroom before the overhead illumination was turned off.

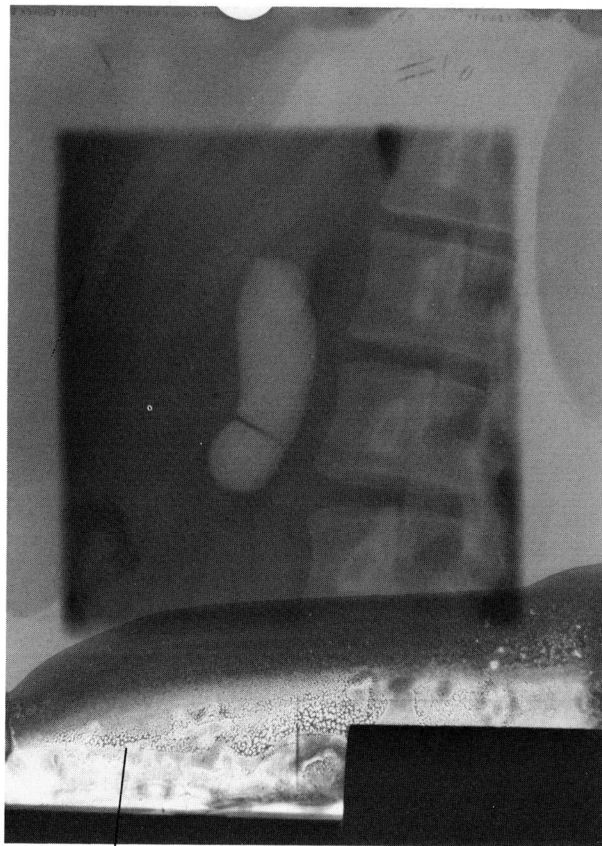

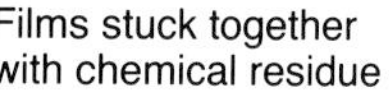


**FIGURE 16–15.** This artifact was created by two radiographs that were stuck together while passing through the processor.

**FIGURE 16–16.** Artifact produced by dirty rollers in the processor.

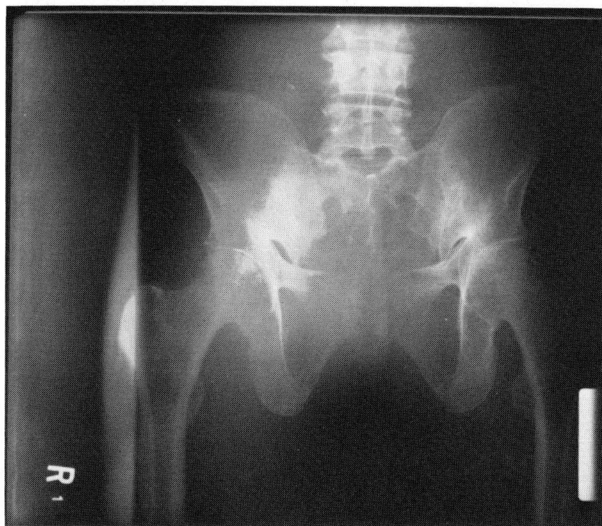

FIGURE 16–17. This radiograph is deteriorating as a result of improper washing. Part of the image detail has disappeared owing to the presence of chemicals that were not washed away.

tion marks result from improper operation or uneven travel speed of the processor transport system.

Figure 16–15 is an example of two films superimposed on top of each other in the processor. They became stuck together in the transport system and were not processed adequately.

Figure 16–16 demonstrates the result of a dirty roller. Debris was collected on the rollers because of the absence of water in the wash tank.

Chemical deterioration, as shown in Figure 16–17, is a result of poor washing of the film.

Figure 16–18 shows light fog from the darkroom. The door was opened before the film had completely traveled into the processing unit.

## ARTIFACTS FROM THE PATIENT

Pacemakers, nasogastric tubes, intravenous tubes, metal implants, safety pins, etc., are opaque devices

FIGURE 16–18. Light fogged the film as it was moving into the processor. The outside door to the darkroom was accidentally opened.

that become artifacts in radiography. Any foreign object that is radiopaque becomes an artifact and may obscure anatomic parts of interest. Figure 16–19 demonstrates examples of metal objects remaining on the patient at the time the exposure was made.

The number of artifacts in radiographic imaging is endless. Each day a new artifact may appear. Figure 16–20 demonstrates four conditions that cause artifacts.

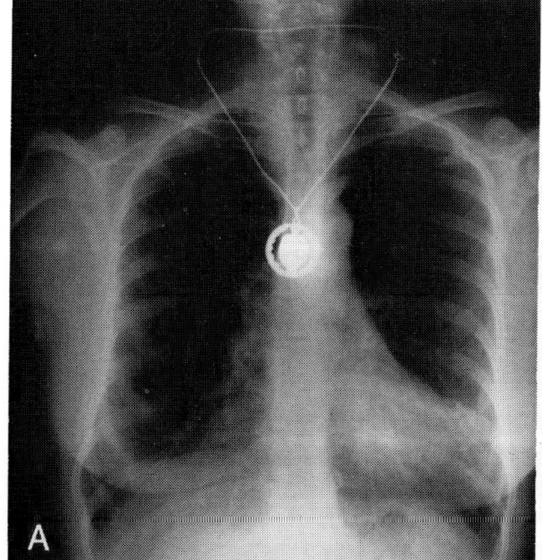
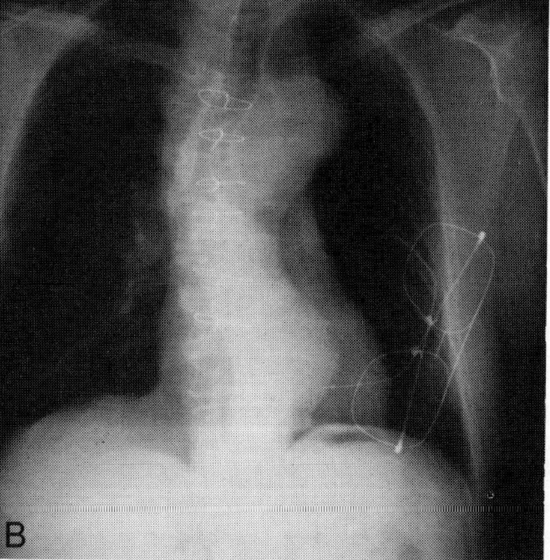
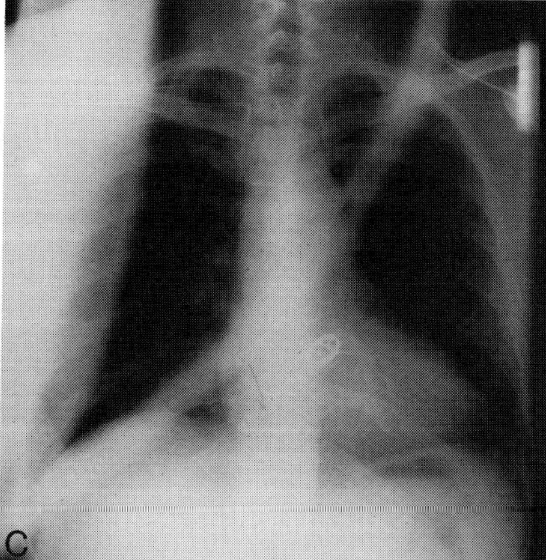

FIGURE 16–19. Preparation of the patient requires that all jewelry and other metal objects be removed from the clothing. *A* and *B* show artifacts produced by objects on the patient in a pajama pocket. *C* is an artifact produced by cables from the x-ray tube that were accidentally placed in the path of the primary x-ray beam.

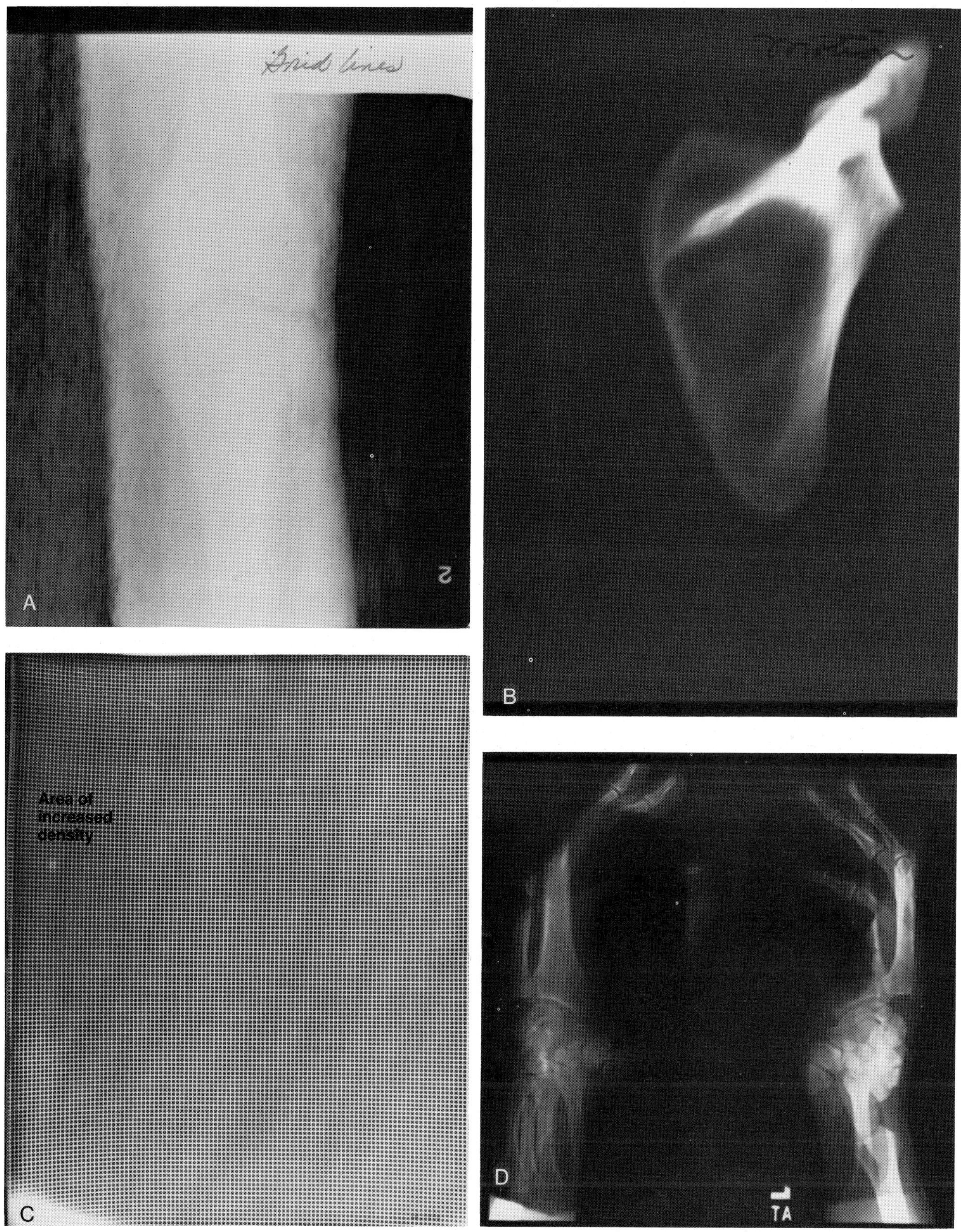


**FIGURE 16–20.** Examples of radiographic artifacts. *A* shows grid lines that were produced as a result of improper alignment of the grid. *B* is blurred as a result of motion. *C* demonstrates inadequate film-screen contact. The image shows increased density on the left, which is a result of poor screen contact. *D* shows two images superimposed.

# Preparation of Radiographic Exposure Guides

## CHAPTER OBJECTIVES

1. Explain the importance for the use of radiographic exposure guides.
2. Describe the basic characteristics of exposure guides.
3. Describe how the use of exposure guides is considered a form of radiation protection.
4. List the characteristics of the four basic exposure guides.
5. Describe the eight steps recommended for the preparation of exposure guides.
6. Describe the necessary procedures used to prepare variable and optimal kilovoltage guides.
7. Compare and contrast radiographs made with each of the four guides for the degree of contrast, contrast scale, visibility of detail, and exposure to the patient.

## KEY WORDS AND TERMS

Exposure guide                  Automated exposure guide
Technique chart                 Variable kilovoltage guide
Standardized exposures          Optimal kilovoltage guide
Optimal performance             "Fixed" kilovoltage guide
High kilovoltage guide          Caliper

## RECOMMENDATIONS FOR GENERAL DISCUSSION QUESTIONS

1. Describe what should be included in a department procedure manual section for the use of exposure guides.
2. Select the "best" guide and describe its strengths and weaknesses.
3. If the department is site surveyed by the Bureau of Radiological Health Department, how should the preparation of exposure guides be explained to the site visitors? Describe the content that should be included in the explanation.
4. Explain the differences that should be present in a guide for a fluoroscopic room compared with a guide for a general radiographic room.

Radiology departments continue to become more and more complex or "high tech," using sophisticated computerized equipment and extremely sensitive imaging systems. However, radiographers still face the basic problem of preparing and assessing basic exposure guides or technique charts. Technique chart is another name for an exposure guide, usually referring to a guide posted on the wall or in a notebook located in the radiographic room. The chart lists recommended exposure factors for a variety of thicknesses of anatomic parts for specific positions and procedures. The term "exposure guide" is more appropriate because it implies guidance and usually contains more comprehensive information.

With all the new and modern trends, high-quality radiographs can only be obtained by proper exposure techniques. It is no longer acceptable to use guessing games to select factors and hope that the first exposure hits the mark. Skilled radiographers must be able to create exposure guides that provide flexibility in consideration of the characteristics of the room design, equipment, and type of procedure to be done. The steps presented in this chapter are intended to serve as a guide based on a systematic process using a standard single-phase generator with a 400-speed imaging system. The principles presented in this chapter can easily be adapted for slower or faster systems.

## DESCRIPTION OF THE EXPOSURE GUIDE

The exposure guide is a group of recommended exposure factors and accessories to be used for specific radiographic procedures. It is based on average thickness of tissue and bone without pathology or disease present. An exposure guide should never be considered the absolute; it is only one consideration in the selection of exposure factors. The patient must be considered for body type, tissue composition, water content, and pathology.

---

THE EXPOSURE GUIDE IS A GROUP OF RECOMMENDED EXPOSURE FACTORS AND ACCESSORIES TO BE USED FOR SPECIFIC PROCEDURES.

---

The radiographic exposure guide is considered the standardization of exposure factor selection and serves as a useful aid for the orientation of new personnel to a radiographic room.

## FUNCTION OF THE EXPOSURE GUIDE

When properly prepared and tested, the exposure guide becomes the primary tool for consistently producing excellent quality radiographs. Quality is established by determining the type of contrast scale desired. The use of a standard guide allows the radiographer to attain his or her best work. If the radiographer is not informed of the patient's condition, in regard to air, fluid content, or pathology, there will be errors in exposure to the patient and to the film.

The type of guide selected will also determine the amount of exposure to the patient and the amount of latitude in exposure settings.

The standardization of exposure with the use of a guide permits the radiographer to give optimal performance. The radiographer will be more confident in the selection of factors and able to provide better patient care.

The old phrase "button pusher" has historically been used as an argument against the use of traditional exposure guides, implying that the radiographer needs less skill and knowledge when using

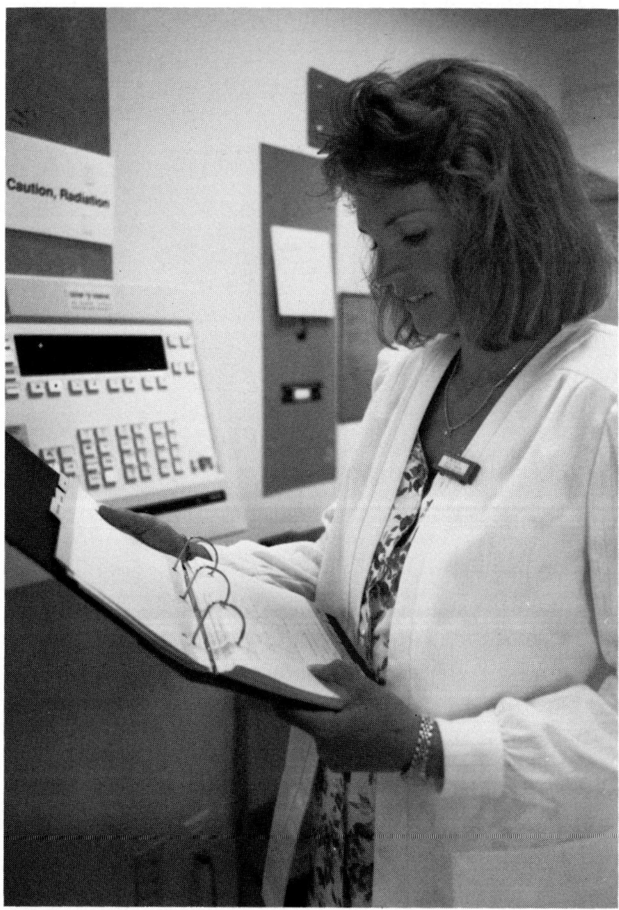


**FIGURE 17–1.** Radiographer using an exposure guide to select exposure factors.

exposure guides. The radiographer would magically produce factors each time an exposure was made. A more realistic analysis of the radiographer's duties shows that the selection of factors requires skill, judgment, and knowledge even with the use of exposure guides (Fig. 17–1).

Interpretation of the guide must be made by the radiographer. This can be accomplished only if the radiographer has a strong background in the principles of radiographic exposure techniques.

Radiation protection for the patient is an important reason for the use of a standardized exposure guide. Standardization of exposures will decrease the number of repeat exposures, therefore increasing the accuracy of the radiographer.

## TYPES OF EXPOSURE GUIDES

There are four basic types of exposure guides. They are high kilovoltage, automated exposure, variable kilovoltage, and optimal or fixed kilovoltage (Table 17–1). In most radiology departments, a selection is made from the four guides. The guide becomes the basis for the selection of exposure factors for most examinations. The same type of guide may be used for all general radiographic rooms and another type of guide may be used for all barium procedures or specialty rooms.

## High-Kilovoltage Guide

The high-kilovoltage exposure guide offers settings of 100 to 130 kilovolts. The increase in energy and penetrating ability of the primary x-ray beam can be advantageous. Contrast is reduced, producing radiographs with longer scale. The use of this type of guide allows shorter exposure times, therefore reducing the possibility of motion.

Exposure techniques that require a high degree of contrast, such as intravenous urography, contrast studies, and angiography, do not lend themselves very well to this type of exposure guide. High-speed imaging systems would not be ideal with a high-kilovoltage exposure guide because of increased quantum mottle. The use of high-kilovoltage exposure guides has been very successful with chest radiography and barium studies. High-kilovoltage exposures are recommended with barium studies because of the increased penetrating ability of the x-ray photons.

## Automated Exposure Guide

As described in Chapter 3, the automated exposure system contains a timer that is designed to terminate the exposure automatically when the desired amount of exposure reaches the film. The choice of exposure setting is determined by the size of the patient to be imaged, the kilovoltage needed for adequate penetration, and the milliampereseconds (mAs) that will give sufficient density. On most automated exposure systems, the procedure control is selected first. This will activate the sensors designated for the procedure and the desired density level. The kilovoltage selection is made as indicated by the exposure guide. Together these factors allow the automated timer device to control the actual length of the exposure.

Anatomic exposure controls would be considered in this category. The anatomic control system is like an automatic technique chart. The control panel has anatomic parts to select from when the exposure factors are established. For example, if the shoulder is to be imaged, the radiographer selects the shoulder button. The exposure is preset to provide adequate density for an average shoulder.

The automated exposure guide must include the recommended kilovoltage level, density selection, and back-up timer selection.

**TABLE 17–1.** EXPOSURE GUIDES

| Type | Kilovoltage | Milliampereseconds | Characteristics |
|---|---|---|---|
| 1. High kilovoltage (kVp) | 100–130 | Low (adjust to patient) | ↑ latitude<br>↓ patient exposure<br>Longer scale of contrast<br>Less contrast |
| 2. Automated exposure | 70–90 | Set by density control | Moderate scale of contrast |
| 3. Variable kVp | 45–75 | Higher | ↓ latitude<br>↑ patient exposure<br>Shorter scale of contrast<br>Higher contrast |
| 4. Optimal kVp | 75–90 | Varies for patient size | ↑ latitude<br>↓ patient exposure<br>Longer scale of contrast<br>Less contrast |

## Variable Kilovoltage Exposure Guide

The variable kilovoltage exposure guide is used more frequently than either of the two guides listed above. The principle driving this type of guide is the variety of kilovoltage settings used to produce proper density. The size of the part is an important factor. As the size of the part changes, so will the kilovoltage. The size of the part becomes the basis for changing the penetration of the beam.

The quantity of radiation, or mAs, remains the same from the smallest to the largest part.

Except for the very thick body parts that require higher kilovoltage settings, short scale of contrast is prevalent on most radiographs. Radiographs made using this type of exposure guide generally have a higher degree of contrast with very little gradation or shades of gray.

In some areas on the radiograph, density readings of less than 0.25 are present as a result of underexposure of the area. The radiation did not have sufficient energy to penetrate the part. On the same radiograph, there may be areas with density readings of 3.0 or higher, which are overexposed. These will be areas of no real optical value inasmuch as the human eye cannot differentiate between density levels that are overexposed or underexposed. If the kilovoltage used is extremely low (below 50), fewer density readings may be present when compared with radiographs having a more moderate scale.

Variable kilovoltage exposure guides require increased mAs settings and therefore a higher dose of radiation exposure to the patient. This can be compensated for with the use of 800- or 1200-speed imaging systems.

Exposures made with the variable kilovoltage exposure guides have less exposure latitude and require that each part be measured correctly using the caliper.

## Optimal Kilovoltage Exposure Guide

The fourth type of exposure guide is the optimal or fixed kilovoltage. The term "fixed" stems from the principle that kilovoltage is selected to penetrate an average body thickness or part and then remains fixed or unchanged no matter what variations may occur from patient to patient.

The mAs is selected as needed to produce the proper density level. Milliampereseconds is used as a variable when there is too little or too much density present. Kilovoltage is not changed to control density on the radiograph, as described in the variable exposure guide. This type of exposure guide generally produces radiographs with a longer scale of contrast than those produced by using a variable kilovoltage exposure guide.

To some radiographers, radiographs made with the optimal kilovoltage guide are considered to be less attractive owing to their lower degree of contrast and gray appearance (Fig. 17–2). Closer examination reveals increased diagnostic value because all areas of the anatomic part of interest have been penetrated and contrast is present.

## REQUIREMENTS FOR THE PREPARATION OF EXPOSURE GUIDES

The goal of every radiology department is to consistently produce high-quality radiographs. In order to attain such a goal, the department must prepare, test, and post exposure guides for all radiographic rooms. These should be used by the radiographers when selecting exposure factors.

Before the exposure guide can be prepared, eight steps must be completed. First, the radiologists and radiographers must come to common agreement on what are acceptable characteristics of a radiograph. Selection of exposure guides will determine the degree of contrast and patient exposure. It is important to have complete agreement on the quality of radiographs to be produced in all areas of the radiology department.

---

### STEP 1. AGREE ON CHARACTERISTICS OF FILM QUALITY.

---

Second, the radiographic equipment should be tested and calibrated to assure proper function. Milliampere (mA), timer, and kilovoltage stations must be tested to determine that each station is functioning properly. Collimators and grids should also be checked to confirm accuracy. Any malfunctioning equipment should be tested and adjusted to provide accurate results.

---

### STEP 2. TEST AND CALIBRATE EQUIPMENT.

---

Third, obtain exposure rating charts from the department service engineer or manufacturer to assure that exposures to be used for the guide do not exceed the recommended operational limits of the equipment. Heat capacity and anode-thermal cooling charts should also be reviewed.

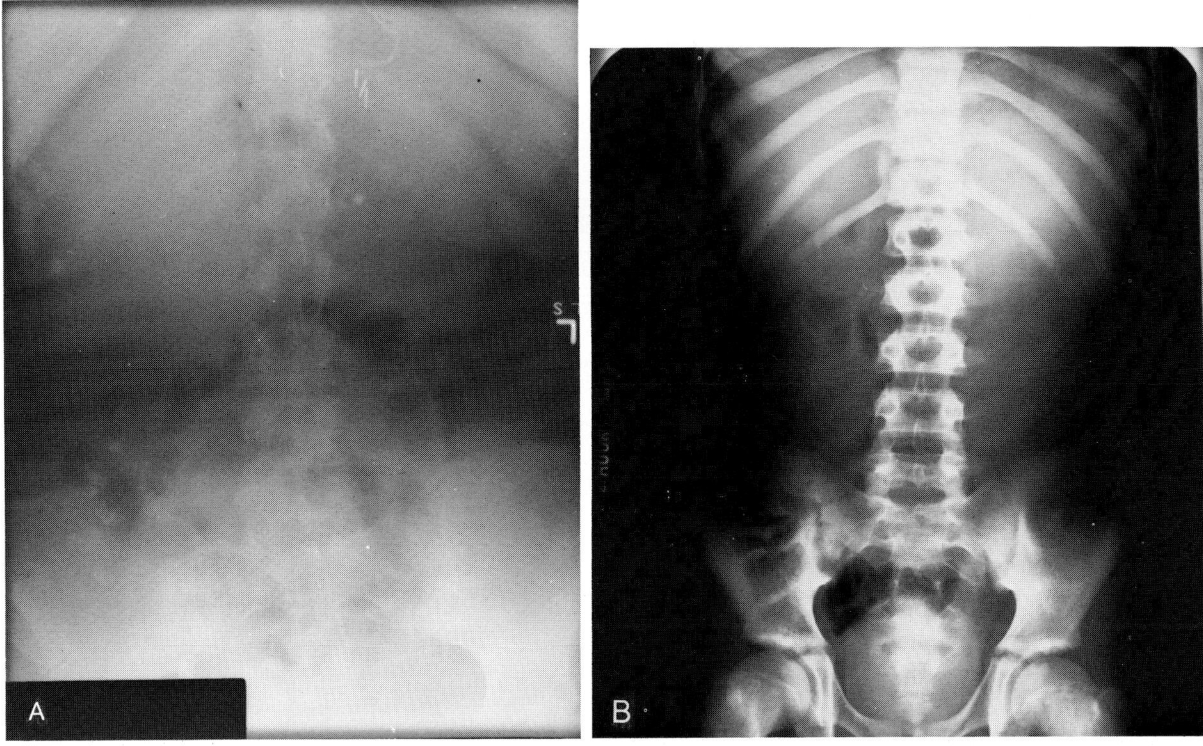

FIGURE 17–2. *A*, Radiograph with long scale of contrast. *B*, Radiograph with shorter scale of contrast.

## STEP 3. REVIEW TUBE RATING AND HEATING CHARTS

Fourth, the processing system must be standardized. A program for frequent and regular testing of the processing system must be established.

## STEP 4. STANDARDIZE THE PROCESSING SYSTEM.

Fifth, calipers for measuring the thickness of the body parts must be made available in each radiographic room. The use of exposure guides eliminates the guessing game. The best results are obtained by accurate measurement of the body part to be imaged (Fig. 17–3).

## STEP 5. PLACE CALIPERS IN EVERY RADIOGRAPHIC ROOM.

Sixth, the appropriate grid selection must be made to accommodate the procedures to be per-formed in a specific radiographic room. High-frequency stationary grids with ratios of 8:1 to 10:1 are selected for general radiographic rooms using a kilovoltage range from 70 to 90. Radiographic rooms selected for high-kilovoltage exposures may require grids with a ratio of 12:1 or higher.

## STEP 6. MAKE GRID SELECTION.

Seventh, the imaging system or film-screen com-bination must be selected. The choice may be a 200-,

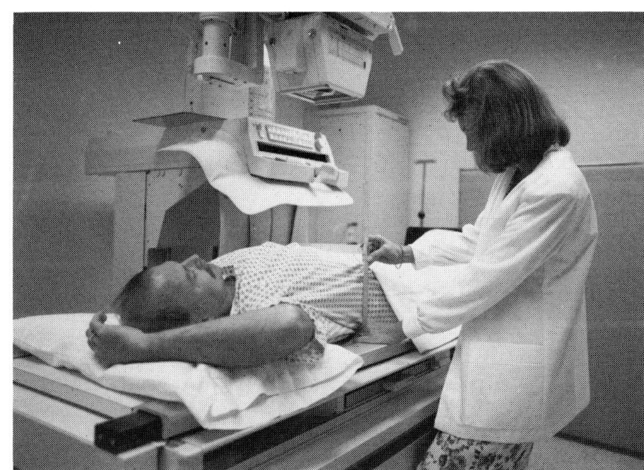

FIGURE 17–3. Calipers used to measure the thickness of the part to be radiographed.

400-, or faster speed system. Rare earth screens are rapidly becoming the screens of choice because of their efficiency and reliability of performance. The exposure guide must reflect the type of imaging system that has been selected.

## STEP 7. SELECT FILM-SCREEN SYSTEM.

Eighth, phantoms for testing the exposure settings must be obtained. It is ideal to have many parts of the body represented by phantoms, such as skull, chest, knee, foot, hand, and pelvis. At frequent intervals, exposures are made to test the exposure guide and its reliability (Fig. 17–4).

## STEP 8. USE BODY PHANTOMS TO TEST RELIABILITY OF GUIDE.

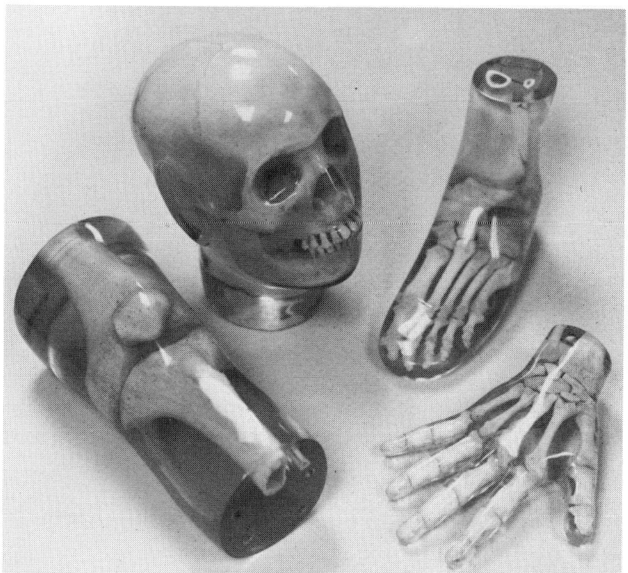

**FIGURE 17–4.** Radiographic phantoms used to test exposure guides.

## PREPARATION OF THE EXPOSURE GUIDE

When the preliminary steps have been completed, the exposure guide can be prepared. The two most common guides are the variable and optimal kilovoltage guides.

### Variable Kilovoltage Exposure Guide

The fundamental factor for making a variable kilovoltage exposure guide is that an increase of 1 cm in tissue thickness is equal to an increase of 2 kV. The test for establishing the basic factors is performed with an average size patient without pathology present that could affect the exposure factors. To test these factors, one uses a phantom. Beginning with a skull phantom, measure the part accurately in centimeters. Multiply the centimeter measurement by 2 and add 30.

EXAMPLE:

Measurement of a lateral skull is 15 cm.

$$15 \times 2 = 30 + 30 = 60 \text{ kV}$$

The kilovoltage to be used for the exposure is 60.

For a lateral skull measuring 15 cm, the kilovoltage will be 60.

The next step is to select the mAs. Three radio-graphs are made, each with the same kilovoltage but with a different mAs selection. The first exposure is made using the estimated amount of mAs needed for producing adequate density. The second exposure is made with two times the amount used for the first exposure. The third exposure is made with one half the mAs for the first exposure. For a 200-speed system, the estimated mAs selection could be 20, 40, and 80, using 60 kV. For a 400-speed system, the mAs setting for the three exposures could be 10, 20, and 40.

After processing the three exposed films, review and evaluate the density. If none of the three radiographs shows adequate density levels, select the midway point of the two mAs selections that are nearest the ideal density. Process and review all of the radiographs. Continue this process until the ideal mAs selection has been attained. After the mAs has been selected, the fundamental factors have been identified to begin the exposure guide (Table 17–2).

If the centimeter measurement is more or less than 15, the kilovoltage is changed by 2 kV for each centimeter to maintain proper density (Table 17–3). Table 17–3 shows that for each measurement, the kilovoltage varies and the mAs remains

**TABLE 17–2.** BEGINNING THE EXPOSURE GUIDE

| Lateral Skull | | | | | | |
|---|---|---|---|---|---|---|
| Centimeters | 12 | 13 | 14 | 15 | 16 | 17 |
| Kilovoltage | | | | 60 | | |
| Milliampereseconds | | | | 15 | | |

**TABLE 17–3.** COMPLETING THE EXPOSURE GUIDE

| Lateral Skull | | | | | | |
|---|---|---|---|---|---|---|
| Centimeters | 12 | 13 | 14 | 15 | 16 | 17 |
| Kilovoltage | 54 | 56 | 58 | 60 | 62 | 64 |
| Milliampereseconds | 15 | 15 | 15 | 15 | 15 | 15 |

**TABLE 17–4.** OPTIMAL KILOVOLTAGE SELECTIONS FOR BODY PARTS

| Body Part | Kilovoltage |
|---|---|
| Upper extremity (nongrid) | 60 |
| Leg and foot | 60 |
| Shoulder (grid) | 80 |
| Knee (grid) | 80 |
| Femur | 80 |
| Hip | 80 |
| Vertebrae (AP/PA)* | 75 |
| Vertebrae (Obl/Lat)† | 85 |
| Skull (Lat) | 80 |
| Skull (AP/PA) | 85 |
| Sinuses | 80 |
| Abdomen | 75 |
| Chest | 85 |

*AP/PA, anterior-posterior/posterior-anterior.
†Obl/Lat, oblique/lateral.

constant. The exposure guide for a lateral skull has been prepared. The focal-film distance (FFD), grid type, and film-screen system should also be identified on the guide. Notations should be made to allow for increase or decrease in mAs when pathologic processes are present that have changed the tissue density.

For patients who measure the same as the average patient but whose body tissue appears to be more dense than normal, an increase in the mAs of 30 to 40% may be required. This is especially true for athletes. Those patients who measure the same as an average patient, but whose body tissue density is less than normal as a result of age or pathology, may require a reduction of the mAs by 30 to 60%. These changes in tissue density should not require changes in the kilovoltage selection.

Accurate measurement of the part is necessary for the variable kilovoltage guide. This is accomplished by correct use of calipers. A 2-cm error in the measurement may result in a 4-kV error, and the density would be affected.

The steps outlined above are used to continue the preparation of exposure guides for other parts of the body. Remember, periodic exposures should be made using phantoms to assure the staff radiographers that the guide maintains its accuracy.

## Optimal Kilovoltage Exposure Guide

The optimal or fixed kilovoltage guide was first described by Arthur Fuchs. The term "optimal" refers to a kilovoltage level that assures that all parts of the tissue are adequately penetrated and latitude is such that consistent, high-quality radiographs are produced.

Kilovoltage is selected for penetration of a particular body part and remains unchanged. Milliampereseconds is used to increase or decrease density. For example, a kilovoltage selection of 80 is made for the lateral skull. For each patient to be imaged, the kilovoltage setting will be 80 and the mAs will vary according to the size of the patient.

The mAs selection is made for groups. For example, one mAs setting is established for the average patient thickness. Another setting of lesser amount is established for the small patient, and one

of higher amount is established for the large patient. This type of guide permits the exposure factors to have greater latitude with fewer variables, resulting in fewer errors.

The first step is to classify body measurements into small, medium, and large groups. The lateral skull groups could be small (12 to 13 cm); medium (14 to 16 cm); and large (17 to 18 cm). For all three classifications, the recommended kilovoltage would be 80. Table 17–4 provides recommended kilovoltage settings for the optimal kilovoltage exposure guide.

The kilovoltage selection is identified for each body part/position and remains unchanged.

The mAs is selected for each size group. To begin preparation of the exposure guide, use the skull phantom in the lateral position. Employing a 400-speed imaging system, select 80 kV and make four exposures, using 5 mAs, 10 mAs, 20 mAs, and 40 mAs. Process and evaluate each radiograph for adequate density levels. If none of the exposures provides the ideal density, select the midpoint between the two exposures nearest the ideal density level. Make exposures and evaluate the radiographs. The process continues until the ideal density is achieved. The radiographs produced by this method will have a longer scale of contrast than radiographs produced by the variable kilovoltage method.

When the ideal mAs selection is made, the guide is prepared (Table 17–5).

**TABLE 17–5.** PREPARING THE GUIDE

| Part Size | Lateral Skull Kilovoltage | Milliampereseconds |
|---|---|---|
| Small | 80 | 6 |
| Medium | 80 | 12 |
| Large | 80 | 24 |

For a small patient, the lateral skull would be exposed with one half the mAs as for the medium-sized patient. The large patient would be exposed with the mAs double that for the medium-sized patient. All groups will require the same kilovoltage selection.

For some body parts such as the abdomen and chest, it may be necessary to classify body measurement into more than three groups.

The same principle for increasing and decreasing mAs for pathology, age, and tissue thickness, used for the variable kilovoltage guide is used to make adjustments on the optimal kilovoltage guide.

## Automated Exposure Guide

Automated exposure guides are very similar to the optimal kilovoltage guide. Most exposures use a standard kilovoltage selection along with a density selection. The back-up timer must be set. The exposure guide will include the kilovoltage, density control (determines the mAs), and a standard exposure time. The back-up timer will not be activated unless the automated exposure device fails. The exposure is terminated when maximum density level is reached. To make the ideal kilovoltage and density selections, one uses phantoms in the same manner as they are used for the preparation of the optimal kilovoltage guide. Specific guidelines will depend on the type of automated exposure system (Table 17–6).

The positioning of the patient must be accurate when the automated exposure system is used. The body part to be examined must be perfectly centered over the sensing device. Measurement of the part is highly recommended to determine the density selection. The density selection controls should be checked periodically by the department service engineer for accuracy.

## High-Kilovoltage Exposure Guide

As the name implies, high-kilovoltage exposure guides use high kilovoltage selections for all exposures. Most exposures are made with 100 to 130 kV. For example, chest radiography can be very effectively done using 100 to 110 kV. The method for

**TABLE 17–6.** AUTOMATED EXPOSURE SYSTEM GUIDE

| Body Part | Kilovoltage | Milliamperes | Time |
|---|---|---|---|
| Skull (Average) | 75 | Density II | 1 sec (back-up) |

**TABLE 17–7.** HIGH-KILOVOLTAGE EXPOSURE GUIDE

| Posterior-Anterior Chest (72″ with grid) | | |
|---|---|---|
| *Patient Size* | *Kilovolts* | *Milliampereseconds* |
| Small | | |
| Below average | | |
| Average | 110 | 5 |
| Above average | | |
| Large | | |

preparing the guide is the same as for the optimal kilovoltage exposure guide (Table 17–7).

Because the kilovoltage selection is high, a grid is recommended, and the focal-film distance (FFD) is 72 inches.

Employing a chest phantom, one makes exposures using 3, 5, 10, 15, 20, and 30 mAs. The radiographs are evaluated for the ideal density. The mAs producing the ideal density is identified. The mAs is adjusted with a below-average setting that is 30% less than average, and less another 30% for the small patient. The above-average patient requires an increase of 30% mAs, and the large patient requires another increase of 30%.

The high-kilovoltage guide is also very effective for use with barium studies.

## COMPARISON OF EXPOSURE GUIDES

Distinct differences may be visible with the variable, optimal, and high-kilovoltage guides. To determine if the film quality objective has been achieved, the radiographer must have the ability to determine how and why the type of guide has achieved its purpose.

## Variable Exposure Guide

The variable kilovoltage guide produces radiographs with a short scale of contrast and a higher degree of contrast. For some of the exposures made with lower kilovoltage selection (below 55), areas with thick anatomic parts (especially skeletal tissue) may not be adequately penetrated. Inadequate penetration eliminates the presence of contrast and visibility of detail. Exposure latitude is decreased, requiring extreme accuracy on the part of the radiographer.

Because the use of lower kilovoltage requires higher mAs selections than for the other types of exposure guides, the exposure to the patient increases.

## Optimal Kilovoltage Exposure Guide

Radiographs produced using the higher kilovoltage selection from the optimal kilovoltage guide will have a longer scale and lower contrast. The kilovoltage selection assures that all anatomic parts are penetrated. Tissue contrast and visibility of detail are present. Latitude increases with higher kilovoltage selections. The lower mAs selection reduces exposure to the patient.

## Automated Exposure Guide

The greatest disadvantage of the automated exposure guide is the requirement for positioning accuracy. Inaccurate position of the part may result in too much or too little density. The patient may receive more exposure when accurate positioning of the part over the sensing device is not achieved or when the proper density control is not selected.

The scale of contrast is usually moderate for automated exposure guides.

## High-Kilovoltage Exposure Guide

Maximum exposure latitude is achieved with this guide. The scale of contrast is long as a result of the high kilovoltage selection. The great advantage is the low patient dose. Penetration is always adequate and the mAs is very low, resulting in a reduction of the amount of exposure to the patient.

## CHAPTER 18

# Basics of a Radiologic Quality Assurance Process

•　•　•　•　•　•　•

## CHAPTER OBJECTIVES

1. Describe the need for implementing a quality assurance process in radiology departments.
2. Describe the quality assurance process.
3. Differentiate between quality assurance and quality control.
4. List the six phases of a quality assurance process.
5. Name and describe the elements for each phase of the quality assurance process.
6. Describe a quality control program.
7. List five quality control tests and explain their relationship to film quality.
8. Explain how the staff radiographer can become directly involved in the quality assurance process.

## KEY WORDS AND TERMS

Accountability
Responsibility
Quality care
Quality assurance (QA)
Quality control (QC)
Quality patient care services (QPCS)
Consumer
Competency
Department culture
Reject film analysis
Preventive maintenance

Record log
W. Edwards Deming
Joseph Juran
Philip B. Crosby, Sr.
Tom Peters
Management leadership
Inservice education
Quality control training
Quality control tests
Analysis

## RECOMMENDATIONS FOR GENERAL DISCUSSION QUESTIONS

1. Describe the procedure for organizing and implementing a QA process, to include the personnel involved, duties, training, and evaluation of the process.
2. Explain how a radiology department can determine the effectiveness of a QA process.
3. Name the most common QC tests used in radiology. In order of priority, list the factors necessary to maintain film quality. Be able to defend each item on the priority list.

Radiology department professionals are members of the team that provides health care to consumers and are part of the growing service industry in the United States. It is imperative that each employee in the radiology department provide the best possible service to patients at the lowest possible cost.

In the early 1990s, accountability has become a key word. *Accountability* implies that radiographers must be responsible for providing high-quality service and must answer to consumer demands for high-quality care.

The professional staff in the radiology department includes the radiologists and radiographers. They must be able to provide evidence that quality of care and technical expertise are present for all members of the staff. This is called the quality assurance (QA) process. QA is a comprehensive process that includes a description of the activities to be carried out by radiology personnel that will assure patients that services received will be of the highest quality. The services include patient care, responsiveness, radiation protection, equipment operation, and competency of the staff operating the equipment.

In 1968, the Radiation Health and Safety Act was passed. It required that the United States Department of Health, Education and Welfare (now the Health and Human Services Department) set up and administer standards for a radiation control program. The operation of the program became the responsibility of the Bureau of Radiological Health. In 1974, quality control guidelines for the manufacture and installation of x-ray equipment were first made available. In 1981, Congress passed the Consumer Patient Radiation Health and Safety Act, which required the implementation of programs to reduce repeat exposures and unnecessary radiation exposure to patients along with minimum standards for radiography training programs. The Act also required certification for the operators of x-ray equipment. Congress responded to consumer concerns about excessive exposure to radiation resulting from the lack of accountability for radiology personnel and inconsistency in the procedures used to produce radiographs.

The QA process has been expanded by the Joint Commission for Accreditation of Healthcare Organizations (JCAHO) to include quality of overall care of the patient while he or she is receiving services in a radiology department (Fig. 18–1).

## PURPOSE

Quality assurance is a systematic process to reduce variables in providing radiologic services to

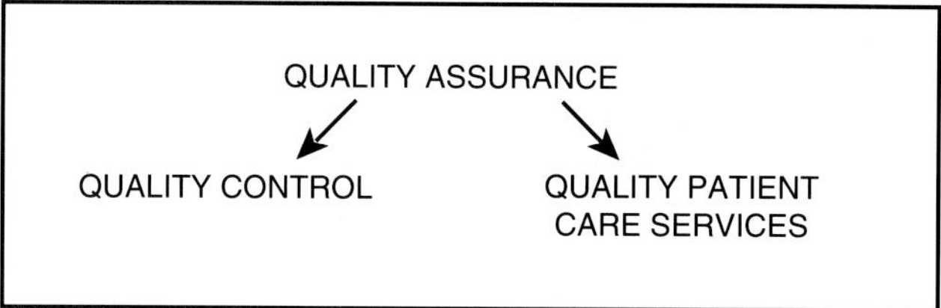



**FIGURE 18–1.**

consumers. The central theme is to reduce exposure to the patient and operator while providing high-quality radiographs to help diagnose and evaluate diseases and disorders. Quality assurance is designed to encompass all aspects of patient care from the time the patient enters the department until the time the patient leaves. It also includes communication and interaction with consumers and other health care specialists and team members.

## QUALITY ASSURANCE IS A SYSTEMATIC PROCESS TO PROVIDE QUALITY SERVICES TO CONSUMERS.

The personal aspect of QA includes measuring the culture and morale of the department. Employees must feel important and that their opinion counts. Everyone must be committed to efficiency in providing services to their patients. A good QA process must include assessment of employee morale. Unhappy employees will not be able to give high-quality services at all times.

Radiologists must depend on the commitment and competency of the radiographers. Radiographers depend on the competency and commitment of the department support staff. The QA process begins with a comprehensive review of the department activities and attitudes. A reject-film analysis is also included in the original assessment.

The QA process will also include a preventive maintenance program that reduces the downtime for radiographic rooms. Each room has its own record log. The record log provides a history of maintenance procedures, dates, and other such data to identify the performance record of the particular piece of equipment. Small or subtle changes can be detected before they become a big problem.

To begin talking about a comprehensive QA process, one must ask several questions. Do patients expect to get the same quality of care and competency from every radiology department? Do patients actually receive the same quality of care from every radiology department? Consumers are continually shopping around for the best care and service. Corporations are also looking for the best care and services for their employees, with cost a major factor. Competition is rapidly becoming an important element in services provided by radiology departments. The "moment of truth" comes when patients come to the radiology department and something less than the best is delivered.

## QUALITY EXPERTS

The "quality" factor is not a new concept in the American workplace. High-quality service is expected by every patient who enters a radiology department. To provide this service, everyone becomes involved—the receptionist who greets the patient, the radiographer who produces the best possible radiograph, the support staff in the darkroom and records room, and file clerks. Managers must be directly involved by keeping all the groups working together to serve the patient well.

HIGH-QUALITY SERVICE IS EXPECTED BY EVERY PATIENT WHO ENTERS THE RADIOLOGY DEPARTMENT.

The best-known quality experts in American business organizations are Dr. W. Edwards Deming, Joseph M. Juran, Philip B. Crosby, and Tom Peters. All of their philosophies include the belief that all employees must participate in the development and implementation of a QA process.

Dr. Deming is best known for his work in developing high quality within Japanese organizations. His philosophy is that productivity must be uniform to ensure high quality.

Mr. Juran emphasized the need for management within the organization to be involved in many aspects of quality because he believes that approximately 80% of the problems in the organization are caused by management. He advocates the use of specialists in quality control to coordinate activities for the QA process.

Philip Crosby, Sr., created the concepts of "zero defects" and "do it right the first time." He also points to management, not workers, for poor performance of an organization. In radiology departments, this means that management is responsible for providing the environment and equipment for radiographers to be able to produce the best possible radiograph with the first exposure.

The focus on management is again emphasized

by Tom Peters. He stresses the need for innovation and leadership by managers in order to have a healthy organization.

A good radiologic QA process must include visible managers who are publicly committed to providing high-quality services to every patient who walks through the doorway.

RADIOLOGY DEPARTMENT MANAGERS MUST BE PUBLICLY COMMITTED TO PROVIDING HIGH-QUALITY SERVICES TO EVERY PATIENT WHO ENTERS THE DEPARTMENT.

## OPERATING A QUALITY ASSURANCE PROCESS

Quality assurance is a process, not a program. The word "program" implies that it has a beginning and end, whereas "process" implies ongoing.

QUALITY IS A PROCESS, NOT A PROGRAM.

Figure 18–2 and Table 18–1 represent the QA process. The QA process is composed of six phases: planning, assignment of duties and responsibilities, reject-film analysis and patient care survey, education and training, program implementation of quality control tests and high-quality patient care ser-

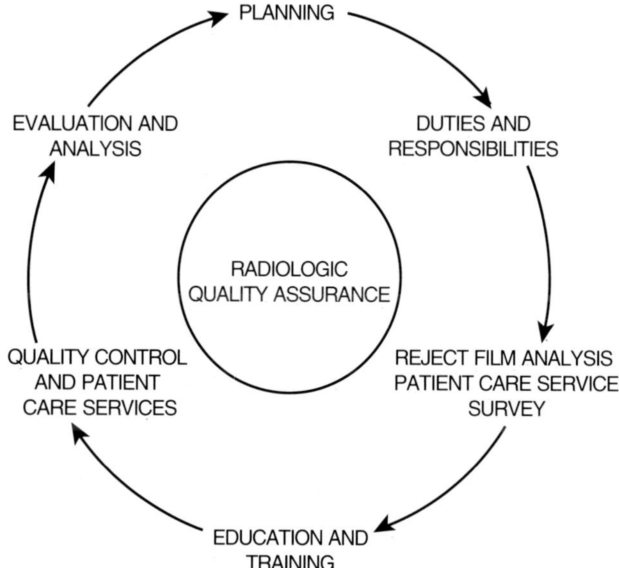


**FIGURE 18–2.** Quality assurance is a continuous process—a process that is ongoing.

**TABLE 18–1.** QUALITY ASSURANCE PROCESS

**Characteristics of Each Quality Assurance Phase**

***Phase I—Planning***
- Appoint advisory committee
- Goals and objectives
- Evaluation of objectives
- Develop plan for education and training
- Complete morale survey
- Management commitment

***Phase III—Reject-Film Analysis and Patient Care Survey***
- Record all repeat films
- Identify reason for repeat
- Analyze results and report
- Prepare questionnaire for patient care survey
- Complete survey
- Compile results of survey

***Phase V—Quality Control and Quality Patient Care Services***
- Perform QC tests
- Keep record logs for each room
- Preventive maintenance program
- Use department "report card" for patient survey
- Complete ongoing repeat film analysis

***Phase II—Assignment of Duties and Responsibilities***
- Appoint QA supervisor
- Appoint QC coordinator
- Appoint QPCS coordinator
- Job duties for coordinators
- Job duties for service engineer

***Phase IV—Education/Training***
- Information QA process
- Present goals and objectives
- Results of patient care survey
- Results of repeat film analysis
- Overview of QC tests
- Train coordinators
- Train staff in patient care services

***Phase VI—Evaluation and Analysis***
- Periodic review of repeat film analysis and patient care surveys
- Complete periodic morale survey
- Periodic review of QC tests
- Recognition ceremonies
- Review and revise goals and objectives

vices, and evaluation and analysis. The diagram in Figure 18–2 shows the continuous process, and Table 18–1 lists the elements of each step.

## Phase I—Planning

Radiology management must take the initiative to develop the QA process. The first step in the process would be to establish an in-house or intradepartment advisory committee. The advisory committee would oversee the planning of the QA process. The committee should be composed of radiologists, managers, supervisors, staff radiographers, and support personnel from the darkroom, reception area, file room, and records area. Input should be sought from the hospital or clinic medical staff, and other departments within the organization that directly communicate with radiology.

It is also recommended that a survey to measure morale and attitudes of every department employee be completed. This would be of great importance in a large radiology department with many employees. Pockets of disgruntled employees can spell danger to a QA process. The advisory committee should review the results of the survey and recommend action by the management based on the results.

Goals and operational objectives should be established by the committee. The goals and objectives should spell out what is expected in such areas as patient care, film quality control, preventive maintenance, and overall efficiency. Inservice education programs and training activities should be established to assure that everyone is expecting the same results.

Finally, management must demonstrate commitment to making the QA process successful. This is vital for each phase of the process.

## Phase II—Assignment of Duties and Responsibilities

Accountability and responsibility are extremely important components of a QA process. A QA supervisor must be appointed. Duties and responsibilities must be identified. Coordinators for the quality control (QC) program and quality patient care services (QPCS) must also be identified. The job duties for each coordinator must be identified and made public for all department employees. The network for information flow or QA organization chart must be defined so that each employee can understand his or her role in the process.

## Phase III—Reject-Film Analysis and Patient Care Survey

In order to determine the initial direction for the QA process, one must evaluate the present status of the department. Two activities need to be completed. First, a reject-film analysis must occur. A 3- to 4-week period is identified. The radiographer appointed to lead the QC program should oversee the process of analyzing and documenting the reason for every repeat or rejected radiograph done in the department. The room number and radiographer must be identified. This must be done in a non-threatening environment with the assistance of every department employee.

The documentation for the reject-film analysis must include identification of repeats according to errors with positioning, exposure factors, processing, motion, fog, static, or other artifacts. At the end of the designated time period, the report must be analyzed to determine the immediate problems that need to be addressed.

Second, a patient care services survey should be conducted. For hospitals, inpatients and outpatients should be surveyed. For clinics and offices, all patients should be included. It is important to determine how the patient consumers define high-quality services, expectations, and perceptions of the radiology department personnel. Elements of the survey should include respect, responsiveness, access, courtesy, appearance of facility, professional demeanor of the staff, competency, communication skills, and credibility. It would also be advisable to survey other departments that radiology personnel interact with on a regular basis.

The results of the reject analysis and patient care services survey should be reported to all department employees. The best forum could be an inservice education program.

## Phase IV—Inservice Education and Quality Assurance Training

The philosophy and purpose of the QA process could serve as the introduction for the education of the department employees. As the QA process is introduced, threats and open criticism of individual performance must be eliminated.

Contents of the inservice education program must include the goals and operational objectives, QA organizational chart, job duties and responsibilities, and technical training if needed.

The QC program should be fully explained, and limited training for the employees should be outlined to ease the concerns or insecurities of the staff. Each radiographer should have a basic understanding of the QC tests to be carried out in the radiographic rooms and darkroom.

Staff development with advanced skills training in patient care services and new innovations in radiology are also suitable topics for inservice programs.

## Phase V—Implementation of Quality Control Program and Quality Patient Care Services

### Quality Control

The radiographer in charge of the QC program works closely with the QA supervisor and advisory committee to establish the QC tests for the radiographic equipment. The department service engineer must also be involved in this process.

The QC program will include a series of tests to be performed routinely in each radiographic room. A series of tests, including sensitometry, must be established for the automatic processor. Accessories used in radiology such as grids, screens, and collimator must also be tested. Quality control procedures must be completed, with the results recorded in a log book and tracked to assure that each radiographic room, as well as the darkroom, provides consistent performance.

---

## QUALITY CONTROL IS A SERIES OF TESTS FOR MONITORING AND EVALUATING RADIOGRAPHIC EQUIPMENT AND ACCESSORIES.

---

The repeat analysis procedures as described earlier in this chapter must become a routine part of QC. The film-screen contact and beam alignment tests, described in earlier chapters of this text, should be done as the QA process is implemented. In addition, grid evaluation should be performed. This can be done by placing the grid over a loaded $14 \times 17$ cassette. Expose at 40-inch focal-film distance (FFD) with a minimal exposure. Examine the radiograph for uneven density level in the grid lines that may be caused by warping of the grid.

Timer accuracy, kilovoltage peak (kVp), and linearity test for consistency in milliamperes (mA) output are more complex tests completed by the QC coordinator and service engineer. Special equipment and instruments are required. It will also be important to evaluate the consistency of similar radiographic rooms.

The focal spot size can be evaluated by using either a star-test pattern or pinhole camera. The purchase of these and other QC instruments will include instructional guides with a step-by-step process to complete the tests.

The radiographic darkroom and processor unit are frequent sources for repeat radiographs. Periodic tests for light leaks and safelight protection must also be conducted, as described in Chapter 6.

Sensitometry is the method recommended for routine testing of the processor. Strips produced by a sensitometer or pre-exposed strips are recommended for producing the strip for density measurements. Caution must be exercised with the use of pre-exposed strips. Transportation and storage conditions could affect the quality of the strip. A mid-density level on the strip is used daily as the density measurement recorded for processor performance. The processor should be performing with a plus or minus limit of 0.1 of the mid-density level. The processor must be tested daily and the results placed in the processor record log. Trends can be observed before major problems occur.

Most radiology departments utilize routine QC tests for the processor; however, too often this procedure is described as the QA process without other procedures taking place. Processor testing is an extremely important element of QA but only one of the many activities that must occur to ensure the consistency of high-quality radiographs.

## Preventive Maintenance Program

The QC coordinator and service engineer design a schedule for each radiographic room to be evaluated. Frequent evaluation and maintenance procedures are scheduled to prevent major equipment failures, especially during peak work loads.

A record log for each radiographic room and processor unit must be compiled. Review of the record logs by the QC coordinator and service engineer becomes a valuable aspect in detecting problems and also in determining if equipment should be replaced.

At the completion of each repeat film analysis cycle, the results should be reviewed with each radiographer.

Update reports of the QC tests could become a regular information item during inservice sessions. Good work by the staff members should be recognized and rewarded.

## Quality Patient Care Services

Optimal patient care practices and interactions must be part of the QA process. A coordinator for QPCS should be appointed to oversee the objectives for the improvement of patient care services. Areas of weakness can be improved by inservice training. Role-playing of the do's and don't's provides an excellent format for presenting the ideals of patient care. Surveys or "report cards" should be made available for patients when they arrive in the radiology department. By receiving the evaluation at the beginning of the visit, patients are alerted to their importance to the department personnel. Patients know that their opinion of the care received is important. Follow-up reports should be compiled

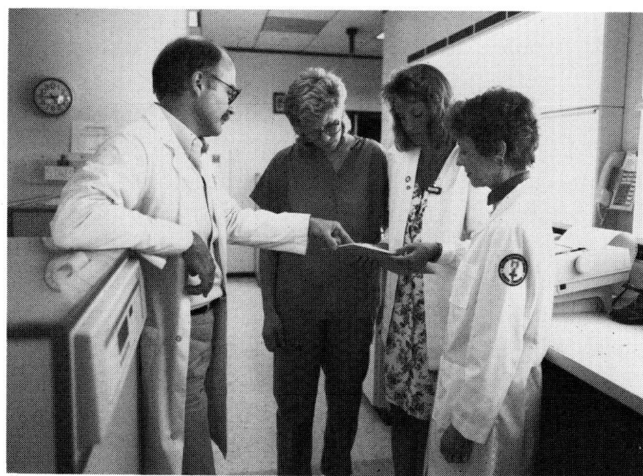

**FIGURE 18–3.** Quality assurance team working together.

and presented to the department personnel. Again, outstanding performance should be rewarded.

## Phase VI—Evaluation and Analysis

The final phase becomes the beginning of the QA cycle. Evaluation methods for the QA process must be implemented to include input from all employees, patients, radiologist, and appropriate outside groups that work directly with radiology personnel (Fig. 18–3).

Evaluation should include a cost analysis to determine the costs and savings of the QA process. The QC coordinator and service engineer need to provide data relating to the performance of radiographic equipment, including accuracy and reliability and the competency of the staff. The QPCS coordinator should compile periodic reports from patient care surveys used to monitor the services provided by the department.

Periodic review of the QA process is done by the advisory committee. Recommendations are made to the department manager to assist in the planning and goal setting of the continuous process.

The QA process is management in action. Management makes it happen. Quality assurance makes the difference between mediocre and excellent radiology departments.

---

QUALITY ASSURANCE IS THE DIFFERENCE BETWEEN A MEDIOCRE RADIOLOGY DEPARTMENT AND AN EXCELLENT DEPARTMENT.

# Bibliography


Albrecht, Karl, and Zemke, Ron: Service America. Homewood, Ill: Dow Jones-Irwin, 1985.

Burns, Evelyn F: Concepts of Image Quality. Chicago: PEP Packet, American Society of Radiologic Technologists, 1979.

Bushong, Stewart C: Radiologic Science for Technologists: Physics, Biology, and Protection, 4th ed. St Louis: CV Mosby, 1988.

Carroll, Quinn: Fuchs' Principles of Radiographic Exposure, Processing and Quality Control, 3rd ed. Springfield, Ill: Charles C Thomas, 1985.

Cullinan, Angeline: Producing Quality Radiographs. Philadelphia: JB Lippincott Co, 1987.

Curry, Thomas, et al: Christensen's Physics of Diagnostic Radiology, 4th ed. Philadelphia: Lea & Febiger, 1990.

Eastman, Terry: Radiographic Fundamentals and Technique Guide. St Louis: CV Mosby, 1979.

Fodor, Joseph, III, and Malott, Jack: The Art and Science of Medical Radiography, 6th ed. St Louis: The Catholic Health Association of the United States, 1987.

Fundamentals of Radiography. Eastman Kodak Publication, Number M1-18.

Gray, Joel, et al: Quality Control in Diagnostic Imaging. Baltimore: University Park Press, 1983.

McKinney, William E: Radiographic Processing and Quality Control. Philadelphia: JB Lippincott Co, 1988.

Morgan, James: The Art and Science of Medical Radiography, 5th ed. St Louis: The Catholic Hospital Association, 1977.

Morris, William (ed): The American Heritage Dictionary of the English Language. Boston: Houghton Mifflin Co, 1976.

Myers, Patricia: An Introduction to Radiographic Technique. New York: Praeger Publishers, 1980.

Selman, Joseph: The Fundamentals of X-ray and Radium Physics, 6th ed. Springfield, Ill: Charles C Thomas, 1977.

Spanbauer, Stanley J: Quality First in Education . . . Why Not? Appleton, Wis: Fox Valley Technical College Foundation, 1987.

Sweeney, Richard J: Radiographic Artifacts: Their Cause and Control. Philadelphia: JB Lippincott Co, 1983.

# Index